Saving Mothers' Lives: Reviewing maternal deaths to make motherhood safer – 2003-2005

The Seventh Report of the Confidential Enquiries into Maternal Deaths in

Director and Editor

Gwyneth Lewis
MSc MRCGP FFPH FRCOG

Central Assessors and Authors

Thomas Clutton-Brock
MRCP FRCA

Griselda Cooper
OBE FRCA FRCOG

James Drife
MD FRCOG FRCPEd FRCSEd FCOG(SA)

Grace Edwards
RN RM ADM Cert Ed Med PhD

Ann Harper
OBE MD FRCPI FRCOG

Diana Hulbert
FRCS FFAEM

William Liston
FRCOG

Alison Macfarlane
BA Dip Stat C Stat FFPH

James Neilson
MD FRCOG

Catherine Nelson-Piercy
FRCP FRCOG

John McClure
FRCA

Margaret Oates
DPM FRCPsych

Gillian Penney
MD FRCOG MFFP

Judy Shakespeare
MRCP FRCGP

Michael de Swiet
MD FRCP FRCOG

Harry Millward-Sadler
FRCPath MHSH

Robin Vlies
FRCSEd FRCOG

Other authors and contributors

Naufil Alam
BSc (Hons) MSc

Valerie Beale
RN RM Dip Man MSc

David Bogod
FRCA LLM

Victoria Brace
MRCOG

Nirupa Dattani
BSc MPhil

Dawn Kernaghan
MRCOG

Alison Miller
RN RM RDM

Jo Modder
MRCOG

Judy Myles
BAO FRCPsych

Jane Rogers
BA PhD DPSM SRN RM

Kate Sallah
MBE RN RM ADM MPH

Contents

Contents

Maternal deaths *Indirectly* related to pregnancy

Deaths *unrelated* to pregnancy

Key issues and lessons for specific health services and/or health professionals

Appendices

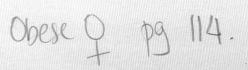

Obese ♀ pg 114.

Acknowledgements

Thanks are due to all the health care professionals and staff who assisted with the individual cases and who have contributed their time and expertise and without whom this Report would not have been possible. With their help this Enquiry remains an outstanding example of professional self-audit, and will continue to improve the care provided to pregnant and recently delivered women and their families.

In particular, thanks are due to:

- All Central Authors and Assessors, and other authors and contributors

- All Regional Assessors

- The Office of National Statistics

- All CEMACH Regional Managers and Assistants for liaising with local clinicians and managing the data collection process (listed in Appendix 2)

- The National Perinatal Epidemiology Unit (NPEU) for providing external review to this Report, and in particular, Jenny Kurinczuk

- Rosie Houston, Projects Manager, for managing the publication of this Report

- Shona Golightly, Director of Research and Development; Richard Congdon, CEMACH Chief Executive; Dharmishta Parmar, Data Manager and all other staff at CEMACH Central Office for their support and advice during the development of this Report.

Foreword

Having a baby is a joyous and fulfilling experience and, nowadays, a safe one for the great majority of women in the United Kingdom. This safety has been hard won. It is the result of many years of painstaking work to identify and reduce risks, and to define the best treatment when complications do occur. Nevertheless some mothers still die, and these deaths are all the more shocking because they are now so uncommon.

It is our duty to learn all we can from such tragedies. Confidential enquiries into maternal deaths began in England and Wales more than fifty years ago and have covered the United Kingdom since 1985. The triennial reports have become essential reading for health professionals, and a model for similar enquiries in many other countries. The Enquiry, however, is continually evolving and the present report has a new title, Saving Mothers' Lives. The previous name, Why Mothers Die, failed to emphasise that these reports not only describe the reasons for maternal mortality but also make important recommendations to reduce the risk of death in the future.

We are concerned that the UK maternal mortality rate has not fallen in recent years. This is partly due to the changing nature of our mothers' overall health. In general, the women who died appeared to be in poorer general health and smoked more, and over half were overweight or obese. Many also had chaotic lifestyles and found it hard to engage with maternity services. The rate is almost certainly influenced by the increasing number of deaths amongst migrant women, whose numbers have also risen.

For this triennium the Report not only identifies areas of substandard care but also, even though the overall percentage of such cases has not increased, includes for the first time a list of ten overall recommendations highlighting the key issues to be addressed as a matter of priority by commissioners, providers and policymakers. We expect these, and the other recommendations in the Report, to lead to action.

Other innovations include contributions from a general practitioner and a consultant in emergency medicine. These new chapters emphasise the need for wider awareness of risk factors and early signs and symptoms of problems which may be crucial in pregnancy. The broad range of specialties represented in the writing panel reflects the teamwork required in modern maternity care. The team also includes the woman herself. Women who are socially excluded, such as asylum seekers or homeless people, have a disturbingly high risk of death.

Publication of this report has been achieved on schedule despite pressures from health service reorganisation. This is due to the hard work and enthusiasm of many people but we are particularly grateful to Dr Gwyneth Lewis, the National Clinical Lead for Maternal Health and Maternity Services in England. As well as directing the UK Enquiry and making insightful innovations she has personally collated the data and prepared the report. We thank her for her continuing commitment and dedication.

Saving Mothers' Lives has important messages for everyone involved in maternity care. It is essential that we do not become complacent. Although some maternal deaths are unavoidable, other women are still dying needlessly in the UK. This can be prevented in future only if lessons are learned and acted upon, and the process begins here.

Sir Liam Donaldson
Chief Medical Officer – England

Dr Tony Jewell
Chief Medical Officer – Wales

Dr Michael McBride
Chief Medical Officer – Northern Ireland

Harry Burns
Chief Medical Officer – Scotland

Top ten recommendations

The overwhelming strength of successive Enquiry Reports has been the impact their findings have had on maternal and newborn health in the United Kingdom and further afield. Over the years there have been many impressive examples of how the implementation of their recommendations and guidelines have improved policies, procedures and practice and saved more mothers' and babies' lives.

The 'top ten'

Over time, as new specialties have come on board and with the expansion of the Enquiry into the wider social and public health determinants of maternal health, the number of recommendations has inevitably grown. Whilst this is as it should be, the increasing numbers make it difficult for commissioners and service providers to identify those that require action as a top priority. Therefore, in order to ensure the key overarching or most crucial issues are not lost, this Report contains a list of the new 'top ten' recommendations which every commissioner, provider, policy maker and other stakeholder involved in providing maternity services should plan to introduce, and audit, as soon as possible.

This new list adds to, but does not replace, recommendations made in earlier Reports.

Baseline data and audit of progress

The data needed to audit these 'top ten' recommendations are not currently collected routinely in all units. This Report proposes that baseline data in the form of numbers and percentages are collected continuously from April 2008 onwards. These data can then form the baseline by which progress can be measured.

The more specific individual Chapter recommendations

Whilst these 'top ten' recommendations are of general importance, the individual Chapters in this Report contain more targeted recommendations for the identification and management of particular conditions for specific services or professional groups. These are no less important and should be addressed by any relevant national bodies as well as by local service commissioners, providers and individual health care staff.

The Confidential Enquiry into Maternal and Child Health (CEMACH) will be working with key stakeholders, including the Health Care Commission for England, to consider how the implementation and auditing of the 'top ten', as well as the more specific recommendations, might best be achieved.

The 'top ten' key recommendations

Pre-conception care

1. **Pre-conception counselling and support, both opportunistic and planned, should be provided for women of child-bearing age with pre-existing serious medical or mental health conditions which may be aggravated by pregnancy. This includes obesity. This recommendation especially applies to women prior to having assisted reproduction and other fertility treatments.**

Rationale

This Report has identified that many of the women who died from pre-existing diseases or conditions which may seriously affect the outcome of their pregnancies, or which may require different management or specialised services during pregnancy, did not receive any pre-pregnancy counselling. In particular, this was the case for several women with major risk factors for maternal death who received treatment for infertility. This Report has also demonstrated that obese pregnant women with a body mass index (BMI) > 30 are far more likely to die. Where possible, obese women should be helped to lose weight prior to conception or receiving any form of assisted reproductive technologies (ART).

The commoner conditions that should require pre-pregnancy counselling and advice include:

- Epilepsy

- Diabetes

- Congenital or known acquired cardiac disease

- Auto-immune disorders

- Obesity BMI of 30 or more

- Severe pre existing or past mental illness.

Baselines and auditable standards

- *Maternity service commissioners, maternity trusts and any centre, NHS or private, which provides maternity services and/or assisted reproduction:*

    - *Number and percentage of pregnant women with pre-existing medical conditions for whom specialist pre-conception counselling is offered at April 2008 and then by the end of 2009.*

    - *Number and percentage of pregnant women at booking, or women attending for ART or pre-pregnancy counselling, who have their Body Mass Index (BMI) calculated and noted. Target 100% by April 2008.*

Access to care

2. **Maternity service providers should ensure that antenatal services are accessible and welcoming so that all women, including those who currently find it difficult to access maternity care, can reach them easily and earlier in their pregnancy. Women should also have had their first full booking visit and hand held maternity record completed by 12 completed weeks of pregnancy.**

3. **Pregnant women who, on referral to maternity services, are already 12 or more weeks pregnant should be seen within two weeks of the referral.**

Rationale

Around 20% of the women who died from *Direct* or *Indirect* causes either first booked for maternity care after 20 weeks' gestation, missed over four routine antenatal visits, did not seek care at all or actively concealed their pregnancies. This contrasts starkly with the 98% of women overall who reported having "booked" with NHS maternity services by 18 weeks of gestation in a recent study undertaken by the National Perinatal Epidemiology Unit (NPEU)[1]. Identifying and overcoming the barriers to care women face in reaching and staying in touch with maternity services will help improve both the accessibility and continuity of local care for all women and outcomes for maternal and newborn health.

Some of the women who died were let down because, although the GP referral was timely, they did not receive a first maternity service appointment until they were around twenty weeks gestation. This delay denied them the opportunities that early maternity care provides for mother, baby and family.

Baseline and auditable standards

-   *Number and percentage of women who have had an antenatal care "booking visit" and hand held maternity record completed by 12 completed weeks of gestation.*

-   *Number and percentage of women referred who were sent a date for their first booking appointment by 12 weeks of their pregnancy, or within two weeks of referral for women with gestations greater than 12 weeks.*

Baseline measurement by April 2008, review December 2009, by when 80% coverage should be attained.

Migrant women

4. **All pregnant mothers from countries where women may experience poorer overall general health, and who have not previously had a full medical examination in the United Kingdom, should have a medical history taken and clinical assessment made of their overall health, including a cardio-vascular examination at booking, or as soon as possible thereafter. This should be performed by an appropriately trained doctor, who could be their usual GP. Women from counties where genital mutilation, or cutting, is prevalent should be sensitively asked about this during their pregnancy and management plans for delivery agreed during the antenatal period.**

Rationale

An increasing number of migrant women are seeking maternity care in the UK. Women who have recently arrived from countries around the world, particularly those from Africa and the Indian sub-continent, but also increasingly from central Europe and the Middle East, may have relatively poor overall general health and are at risk from illnesses that have largely disappeared from the UK, such as TB and rheumatic heart disease. Some are also more likely to be at risk of HIV infection. All of these conditions, alone or in combination, contributed to a number of the maternal deaths identified in this Report. None of the women who died of these causes had a routine medical examination during their pregnancy and the opportunity for remedial treatment was lost.

Further, the prevalence of female genital mutilation, or cutting, amongst the pregnant population is increasing due to inward migration of women from countries or cultures where it is still routine practice, despite almost universal international condemnation at government level. It can affect women's pregnancies in a number of ways and the deaths of at least four women were directly or indirectly associated with the consequences of such procedures in this triennium. Specialist services and reversal procedures are available for these women in their antenatal period, which make childbirth and postnatal recovery easier.

Baseline and auditable standard

- *Number and percentage of pregnant women new to the UK, and who have not previously had a full medical examination in the UK, who have had a complete medical history taken and physical examination performed during their pregnancy and which is recorded in their notes.*

Baseline measurement by April 2008, review December 2009 by when 100% coverage should be attained.

Systolic hypertension requires treatment

5. **All pregnant women with a systolic blood pressure of 160mm/Hg^2 or more require anti-hypertensive treatment. Consideration should also be given to initiating treatment at lower pressures if the overall clinical picture suggests rapid deterioration and/or where the development of severe hypertension can be anticipated.**

Rationale

In the current triennium the single most serious failing in the clinical care provided for mothers with pre-eclampsia was the inadequate treatment of their systolic hypertension. In several cases this resulted in a fatal intracranial haemorrhage. Systolic hypertension was also a key factor in most of the deaths from aortic dissection. The last Report suggested that clinical guidelines should identify a systolic pressure above which urgent and effective anti-hypertensive treatment is required. Since then a publication from the US has made a convincing case that that threshold should be 160 mm/Hg^2. Clinically, it is also important to recognise increases in, as well as the absolute values of, systolic blood pressure. In severe and rapidly worsening pre-eclampsia, early treatment at less than 160 mm/Hg is advisable if the trend suggests that severe hypertension is likely.

Auditable standard

- *The number and proportion of women with pre-eclampsia and a systolic blood pressure of 160 mm/Hg or more on two or more occasions who were given anti-hypertensive treatment.*

Caesarean section

6.1 **Whilst recognising that for some mothers and/or their babies caesarean section (CS) may be the safest mode of delivery, mothers must be advised that caesarean section is not a risk-free procedure and can cause problems in current and future pregnancies.**

6.2 **Women who have had a previous caesarean section must have placental localisation in their current pregnancy to exclude placenta praevia, and if present, to enable further investigation to try to identify praevia accreta and the development of safe management strategies.**

Baseline and auditable standards

- *Number and % of women having a CS, its type and underlying indication, as classified in the National Institute for Clinical Excellence guideline on Caesarean Section[3].*

- *Number and % of women who have had a previous CS and who have had a placental localisation scan. Baseline measurement by April 2008 and the % increase by December 2009; target 100%.*

Clinical skills

7. Maternity service providers and clinical directors must ensure that all clinical staff caring for pregnant women actually learn from any critical events and serious untoward incidents (SUIs) occurring in their Trust or practice. How this is planned to be achieved should be documented at the end of each incident report form.

Rationale

In some cases in this Report, where lessons could have been learnt, a critical incident report or serious untoward incident (SUI) review was not undertaken. Without such reviews lessons cannot be learnt and practice cannot improve. Even when reviews were carried out their quality was extremely variable. Although there were many examples of very good internal reviews, this was not always the case. It was also not always evident who was involved in such reviews. In some cases the hospital enquiries were improperly conducted: investigatory panels did not include clinicians from relevant disciplines (including anaesthesia) and therefore lacked clinical insight and relevance, or included clinicians who were directly involved in the death and were therefore potentially biased in their assessments. In other cases, it was clear the review only involved those directly associated with the woman's care and lessons may not have been widely disseminated to others in the maternity service. Hospital managers should consider whether unbiased external input would assist real learning from individual deaths: it is often only after this has been received that the benefit is realised.

If lessons are to be learnt, it is important that all clinical staff are made aware of the findings of such reviews, particularly those who may not have ready access to internal meetings e.g. GPs and community midwives.

Auditable standards

- *Every maternal death, and serious untoward incident, should be critically reviewed and the lessons learnt actively disseminated to all clinical staff, risk managers and administrators. The precise educational actions taken as a result must be recorded, audited and regularly reported to the Trust board by the clinical governance lead.*

- *The percentage of staff who have participated or contributed to an SUI review and who confirm having received feedback from the clinical governance lead about the actions taken as a result.*

8. **All clinical staff must undertake regular, written, documented and audited training for:**

   - **The identification, initial management and referral for serious medical and mental health conditions which, although unrelated to pregnancy, may affect pregnant women or recently delivered mothers**

   - **The early recognition and management of severely ill pregnant women and impending maternal collapse**

   - **The improvement of basic, immediate and advanced life support skills. A number of courses provide additional training for staff caring for pregnant women and newborn babies.**

   There is also a need for staff to recognise their limitations and to know when, how and whom to call for assistance.

Rationale

A lack of clinical knowledge and skills amongst some doctors, midwives and other health professionals, senior or junior, was one of the leading causes of potentially avoidable mortality. This triennium the assessors were particularly struck by the number of health care professionals who failed to identify and manage common medical conditions or potential emergencies outside their immediate area of expertise. Resuscitation skills were also considered poor in an unacceptably high number of cases.

Auditable standards

   - *The provision of courses and a record of attendees should be regularly audited to reinforce, familiarise, and update all staff with local procedures, equipment and drugs.*

   - *Number and percentage of staff who have their training requirements in relation to safety and clinical skills identified and addressed in their annual appraisal report. Target 100%.*

   - *Number and percentage members of all cardiac arrest teams who know where the maternity unit is and how to gain immediate access to it. Target 100%.*

Early warning scoring system

9. There is an urgent need for the routine use of a national obstetric early warning chart, similar to those in use in other areas of clinical practice, which can be used for all obstetric women which will help in the more timely recognition, treatment and referral of women who have, or are developing, a critical illness. In the meantime all trusts should adopt one of the existing modified early obstetric warning scoring systems of the type described in the Chapter on Critical Care, which will help in the more timely recognition of woman who have, or are developing, a critical illness. It is important these charts are also used for pregnant women being cared for outside the obstetric setting for example in gynaecology, Emergency Departments and in Critical Care.

Rationale

In many cases in this Report, the early warning signs of impending maternal collapse went unrecognised. The early detection of severe illness in mothers remains a challenge to all involved in their care. The relative rarity of such events combined with the normal changes in physiology associated with pregnancy and childbirth compounds the problem. Modified early warning scoring systems have been successfully introduced into other areas of clinical practice and a system which has been modified for obstetric mothers is discussed in Chapter 19, together with an example of such a chart. These should be introduced for all obstetric admissions in all clinical settings.

In developing this recommendation, a consultant from a hospital where staff are trying to get such a scheme introduced said *"we have had three near misses related to unrecognised sepsis in the last two months, all of which would have been picked up by this chart. All three women came close to featuring in the next edition of your Report".*

Auditable standards

*   *A National Modified Obstetric Early Warning System (MEOWS) chart developed and piloting started by December 2008.*

*   *In the interim, the number of trusts who have adopted a version of any existing MEOWS charts and trained all staff in its use by the end of 2008.*

National guidelines

10. Guidelines are urgently required for the management of:

- The obese pregnant woman

- Sepsis in pregnancy

- Pain and bleeding in early pregnancy

Rationale

National clinical guidelines are especially useful where there are unexplained variations in practice, emerging problems, and the recognition of persisting sub-standard care. The increasing prevalence of obesity in the UK has been widely publicised, and the risks of maternal death among pregnant obese women have been highlighted in this Report. There are many aspects of the care of overweight women in pregnancy, beyond maternal risks, that require guidance including the difficulties of prenatal diagnosis, the enhanced risk of gestational diabetes, the increased chance of caesarean section and the challenges of analgesia and anaesthesia. With deaths from sepsis and ectopic pregnancies the issues are different and there are persisting failures to recognise these conditions promptly. These have been highlighted in several Reports and guidelines would help by addressing diagnostic issues in a more extensive, evidence-based format, than is possible in this Report.

Additionally

International definitions

The next revision of the International Classification of Diseases, ICD 11, should recognise that, in more developed countries at least:

- The current arbitrary cut off point for the definition of a maternal death, 42 days postpartum, is unhelpful and Enquiries limited by this definition will miss learning lessons from some important *Direct* and *Indirect* deaths which occur later than this.

- Deaths from peripartum cardiomyopathy, ovarian hyper-stimulation syndrome (OHSS) and suicide from puerperal psychoses, at any time after pregnancy, should be recognised as *Direct* maternal deaths. These deaths would not have occurred if the woman had not been, or sought to become pregnant.

References

1   Redshaw M, Rowe R, Hockley C, Brocklehurst, P. *Recorded delivery: a national survey of women's experience of maternity care 2006*. National Perinatal Epidemiology Unit. Oxford; NPEU; 2007. ISBN 978 0 9735860 8 0. www.npeu.ac.uk

2   Martin Jr JN, Thigpen BD, Moore RC, Rose CH, Cushman J, May W. *Stroke and pre-eclampsia and eclampsia: a paradigm shift focusing on systolic blood pressure*. Obstet Gynecol 2005;105:246-54.

3   National Institute for Clinical Excellence. National Collaborating Centre for Women's and Children's Health. *Caesarean section: clinical guideline*. Royal College of Obstetricians and Gynaecologist Press. April 2004. www.nice.org.uk or www.rcog.org.uk

Introduction and aims, objectives and definitions used in this Report
Gwyneth Lewis

Introduction

A new title; a renewed purpose

The change of title of this, the seventh Report of the United Kingdom (UK) Enquiries into Maternal Deaths, from "Why Mothers Die" to "Saving Mothers' Lives" more aptly reflects the purpose of this continuing, crucial, component of maternity service provision in the UK. To underline the proactive nature of this Enquiry, this Report, for the triennium 2003-2005, differs in other ways as well. It sets out ten overarching recommendations, which, where possible, are accompanied by suggested benchmarks and/or auditable standards to ensure more consistent implementation, monitoring and feedback. Whilst this does not take away the importance of the more specific recommendations and learning points made in each chapter, it will enable a more focused and strategic approach to implementing, and monitoring the key overarching recommendations which aim to provide every mother and her baby with high quality, safe and accessible maternity services.

Each Report's recommendations are acted on by different people at many different levels. Examples include individual health practitioners, the Royal Colleges and other professional organisations, health authorities, commissioners, Trust risk and general managers, the Clinical Negligence Scheme for Trusts (CNST), the Welsh Risk Pool (WRP), the Health Care Commission (HCC) as well as central Government and its affiliated agencies. For example, in England, the National Service Framework for Maternity Services[1] and its implementation strategy "Maternity Matters"[2], both acknowledge the key part the findings of previous Reports have played in policy development. The Welsh National Service Framework for Maternity Services is similar[3]. Their recommendations help in protocol development, clinical audit and maternity service design and delivery.

In recent years, the Enquiry has expanded its remit to cover wider public health issues, and its findings and recommendations in this area have played a major part in helping in the development of other, broader, policies to help reduce health inequalities for the poorest families and for socially excluded women. Without this current Report for example, it would not be known that, even in the UK in the twenty-first century, the most deprived pregnant women have a risk of dying which is seven times higher than that of the broad majority of other pregnant women. And, by acting on similar findings in past Reports, this Enquiry has played a major part in re-defining the philosophy that now expects each individual women and her family to be at the heart of maternity services designed to meet their own particular needs, rather than vice versa.

Telling the story

The methodology used by the Enquiry goes beyond the scientific. Its philosophy, and that of those who participate in its process, also recognise and respect every maternal death as a young woman who died before her time, a mother, a member of a family and of her community. It does not demote women to numbers in statistical tables; it goes beyond counting numbers to listen and tell the stories of the women who died in order to learn lessons that may save the lives of other mothers and babies, as well as aiming to improve the standard of maternal health overall. Consequently, its methodology and philosophy now form part of a key strand in the World Health Organisations (WHO) overall global strategy to make pregnancy safer. A maternal mortality review tool kit, and programme, "Beyond the Numbers"[4], has been introduced which includes advice and practical steps in choosing and implementing one or more of five possible approaches to maternal death reviews adaptable at any level and in any country. These are facility and community death reviews, Confidential Enquiries into Maternal Deaths, near miss reviews and clinical audit[5].

Working together to save mothers' lives and improve maternity care

It is because of the sustained commitment of all health professionals who provide maternity and other services for pregnant women in the United Kingdom that this Enquiry is able to continue as the highly respected and powerful force for change and improvement as it is today. Reading the Report or preparing a statement for an individual enquiry also forms part of individual, professional, self-reflective learning. As long ago as 1954 it was recognised that participating in a confidential enquiry had a "powerful secondary effect" in that "each participant in these enquiries, however experienced he or she may be, and whether his or her work is undertaken in a teaching hospital, a local hospital, in the community or the patient's home must have benefited from their educative effect"[6]. Personal experience is therefore a valuable tool for harnessing beneficial changes in individual practice.

Learning lessons for continual improvement

This Enquiry is the first, and possibly best, example of use of the maternal mortality and morbidity surveillance cycle, now internationally adopted by the World Health Organisation's programme "Beyond the Numbers" which promotes the use of maternal deaths or morbidity reviews to make pregnancy safer[4]. The cycle, shown in Figure 1, is an ongoing process of deciding which deaths to review and identifying the cases, collecting and assessing the information, using it for recommendations, implementing these, evaluating their impact before refining and improving the next cycle. The ultimate purpose of the surveillance process is **action**, not to simply count cases and calculate rates. All these steps: identification, data collection, analysis, action and evaluation are crucial and need to be continued in order to justify the effort and to make a difference. The impact of previous findings of this Report continually demonstrate the contribution of such an observational study to both maternal and child health and the overall public health, and emphasise the need for it to continue in the future.

Figure 1.1 The maternal mortality or morbidity surveillance cycle

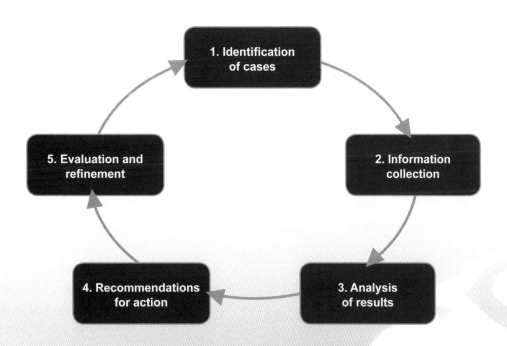

The Enquiry process is best described as an observational and self-reflective study which identifies patterns of practice, service provision, and public health issues that may be causally related to maternal deaths. This method of reviewing individual deaths has been described as "sentinel event reporting". As Rutstein et al[7], stated:

> "Just as the investigation of an aeroplane accident goes beyond the immediate reasons for the crash to the implications of the design, method of manufacture, maintenance and operation of the plane, so should the study of unnecessary undesirable health events yield crucial information on the scientific, medical, social and personal factors that could lead to better health. Moreover, the evidence collected will not be limited to the factors that yield only to measures of medical control. If there is clear cut documented evidence that identifiable social, environmental, "life-style", economic or genetic factors are responsible for special varieties of unnecessary disease, disability, or untimely death, these factors should be identified and eliminated whenever possible".

It is this "Saving Mothers' Lives" aims to achieve.

The evidence base

In the past some have questioned whether the Reports are 'evidence based'. The highest level of evidence of clinical effectiveness comes from systematic reviews of randomised controlled trials. The most comprehensive and up-to-date systematic reviews of relevance to these Enquiries are produced by the Cochrane Pregnancy & Childbirth Group, whose editorial structure is funded by the NHS Central Programme for Research & Development. The Co-ordinating Editor of the Group is a member of the editorial board of this Enquiry.

Some Cochrane reviews are of direct relevance to topics highlighted by deaths described in recent Reports, and have been cited to support recommendations. These include treatments for eclampsia and pre-eclampsia, and antibiotic prophylaxis before caesarean section. However, many problems tackled in successive Reports have not been addressed by randomised trials, including prevention of thrombo-embolic disease and treatment of amniotic fluid embolism or massive obstetric haemorrhage.

An important limitation of randomised trials is that, unless they are very large, they may provide little information about rare, but important, complications of treatments. Safety issues are, therefore, sometimes better illuminated by observational studies than by controlled trials.

Many causes of maternal death are very rare and treatment options for these may never be subjected to formal scientific study. Inevitably, recommendations for care to avoid such deaths in the future rely on lesser levels of evidence, and frequently on 'expert opinion'. This does not mean that the Report is not evidence based, merely that, necessarily, the evidence cannot be in the form of a randomised control trial or case control study due to the relative rarity of the condition.

Severe maternal morbidity, "near misses"

The Enquiry has long wanted to extend its work to also review the cases of mothers who suffered severe obstetric morbidity and complications; so called "near misses", but for lack of resources this has not yet been possible. However, this Report contains a chapter on the latest results of the Scottish Confidential Audit of Severe Maternal Morbidity[8], and a summary of the first report of the United Kingdom Obstetric Surveillance System (UKOSS) for rare obstetric events, run by the National Perinatal Epidemiology Unit (NPEU) is contained in the relevant chapters of this Report[7,9].

The United Kingdom Obstetric Surveillance System (UKOSS)

This new national system to study rare disorders of pregnancy was launched in February 2005. It enables the surveillance of a range of uncommon obstetric disorders, including conditions which may be classified as "near miss" events for maternal mortality. Descriptive, case-control and cohort studies are conducted.

Each month a reporting card including a simple tick box list of conditions under surveillance is sent to the nominated reporting clinicians (anaesthetists, midwives, obstetricians and perinatal risk managers) in each consultant-led maternity unit in the UK. The nominated clinicians are asked to return the card indicating whether there have been any women with any of the conditions seen in their hospital over the past month. The card also includes a box to indicate 'nothing to report'. A data collection form is then sent back to any clinicians reporting cases to obtain details confirming the case definition, risk factors, management and outcomes. For some conditions, similar information is also collected about control or comparison women. All hospitals in the UK with consultant-led maternity units are participating in UKOSS, and hence these studies effectively survey the entire cohort of women giving birth in the UK. Several studies conducted through UKOSS provide incidence information which reveals some of the morbidity underlying the deaths detailed in this Report; this information is included in the relevant chapters.

The aims and objectives of the Enquiry

The **aim** of the Enquiry is to save mothers and newborns lives by reviewing maternal deaths in order to learn lessons and formulate and disseminate recommendations which will lead to improvements in clinical care and beneficial health system changes for all women in the UK. Its **objectives** are:

- Through the use of the maternal morbidity and mortality surveillance cycle, to assess the main causes of, and trends in maternal deaths; to identify any avoidable or sub-standard factors; to promulgate these findings and recommendations to all relevant health care professionals and, in future, to ensure the update of these are audited and monitored.

- To improve the care that pregnant and recently delivered women receive and to reduce maternal mortality and morbidity rates still further as well as the proportion of deaths due to substandard care.

- To make recommendations concerning the improvement of clinical care and service provision, including local audit, to commissioners of obstetric services and to providers and professionals involved in caring for pregnant women.

- To suggest directions for future areas for research and audit at a local and national level.

- To produce a triennial Report for the funding bodies in all four countries.

The Enquiry's role in setting clinical standards and contributing to clinical governance

The Enquiry is the longest running example of national professional self-evaluation in the world. Whilst much has changed since its inception in 1952, the lessons to be learnt remain as valid now as in the past. Whilst the Enquiry has always had the support of professionals involved in caring for pregnant or recently delivered women, it is also a requirement that all maternal deaths should be subject to this confidential enquiry and all health professionals have a duty to provide the information required.

In participating in this Enquiry, all **health professionals** are asked for two things:

- If they have been caring for a woman who died, to provide the Enquiry with a full, accurate and unbiased account of the circumstances leading up to her death, with supporting records, and

- Irrespective of whether they have been caring for a woman who died, or not, to reflect on and take any actions that may be required, either personally, or as part of their wider institution, as a result of the recommendations and lessons contained within this Report.

At a **local commissioning level** maternity health care commissioners, such as Primary Care Trust (PCTs,) and Local Health Boards (LHBs) should commission services which meet the recommendations set out in this, and previous, Reports and ensure that all staff participate in the Enquiry if required, as part of their contract.

At **service provider level** the findings of the Enquiry should be used to:

- Ensure all staff are regularly updated and trained on the signs and symptoms of critical illness, such as infection, and the early identification, management and resuscitation of seriously ill women

- Develop and regularly update multidisciplinary guidelines for the management of complications during or after pregnancy

- Review and modify, where necessary, the existing arrangements for the provision of maternity or obstetric care

- Ensure all *Direct* and unexpected *Indirect* maternal deaths are subject to a local review and critical incident report, which is made available to the Enquiry as part of its own process of review, as well as disseminating its key findings and recommendations to all local maternity staff

- Introduce an obstetric early warning system chart as recommended in this Report

- Promote local audit and clinical governance.

At a **national** level

In every country, the findings of successive Reports have been used to develop national maternal and public health policies. For example, in England and Wales the findings of the Enquiry are used:

- To help develop government policy. For example, in England, the National Service Framework for Maternity Services[1] and its implementation strategy "Maternity Matters"[2], both acknowledge the key part the findings of previous Reports have played in policy development. In Wales, the National Service Framework for Young People and Maternity Services addresses similar issues[3]

- To inform NICE or other guideline or audit development

- To inform guideline and audit development by the relevant Royal Colleges

- To set minimum standards of care, for example as set out in the criteria for the management of maternity services by the Clinical Negligence Scheme for Trusts (CNST) for England and the Welsh Risk Pool (WRP)

- To contribute to the Health Care Commission's review on maternity services

- As part of post graduate training and continuous professional self-development syllabus for all relevant health professionals

- To identify and promulgate areas for further research.

In Scotland, the findings of the Enquiry inform the work of equivalent bodies responsible for national quality initiatives. These include NHS Quality Improvement Scotland (NHS QIS), the Scottish Intercollegiate Guidelines Network (SIGN) and the Clinical Negligence and Other Risks Indemnity Scheme (CNORIS).

In Northern Ireland the findings of the Enquiry similarly inform policy development through the Department of Health, Social Services, and Public Safety for Northern Ireland (DHSSPS), inform quality and standards through the DHSSPS and other bodies including the Clinical Resource Efficiency Support Team (CREST) and the Regulation and Quality Improvement Authority (RQIA) and are included in postgraduate education.

Definitions of, and methods for, calculating maternal mortality

The ninth and tenth revisions of the International Classification of Diseases, Injuries and Causes of Death, (ICD9/10) define a maternal death as "the death of a woman while pregnant or within 42 days of termination of pregnancy, from any cause related to or aggravated by the pregnancy or its management, but not from accidental or incidental causes". This means that there was both a temporal and a causal link between pregnancy and the death. When the woman died she could have been pregnant at the time, that is, she died before delivery, or within the previous six weeks have had a pregnancy that ended in a live or stillbirth, a spontaneous or induced abortion or an ectopic pregnancy. The pregnancy could have been of any gestational duration. In addition, this definition means the death was caused by the fact that the women was or had been pregnant. Either a complication of pregnancy or a condition aggravated by pregnancy or something that happened during the course of caring for the pregnant woman caused her death. In other words, if the woman had not been pregnant, she would not have died at that time.

Maternal deaths are subdivided into further groups as shown in Table 1. **Direct** maternal deaths are those resulting from conditions or complications or their management which are unique to pregnancy, occurring during the antenatal, intrapartum or postpartum period. **Indirect** maternal deaths are those resulting from previously existing disease or disease that develops during pregnancy, not due to direct obstetric causes, but which were aggravated by physiologic effects of pregnancy. Examples of causes of *Indirect* deaths include epilepsy, diabetes, cardiac disease and, in the UK only, hormone dependent malignancies. The Enquiry also classifies most deaths from suicide as *Indirect* deaths as they were usually due to puerperal mental illness although this is not recognised in the ICD coding of such deaths. The UK Enquiry assessors also classify some deaths from cancer in which the hormone dependant effects of the malignancy could have led to its progress being hastened or modified by pregnancy as Indirect although these also do not accord with international definitions. Only *Direct* and *Indirect* deaths are counted for statistical purposes as discussed later in the section on measuring maternal mortality rates.

ICD-10 also introduced two new terms related to maternal deaths. One of them is **pregnancy related death**, defined as the death of a woman while pregnant or within 42 days of the end of her pregnancy, *irrespective* of cause. These deaths include deaths from *all* causes, including accidental and incidental causes. Although the latter deaths, which would have occurred even if the woman had not been pregnant, are not considered true maternal deaths, they often contain valuable lessons for this Enquiry. For example they provide messages and recommendations about domestic abuse or the correct use of seat belts. From the assessments of these cases it is often possible to make important recommendations. The ICD coding classifies these cases as fortuitous maternal deaths. However, in the opinion of the UK assessors, the use of the term fortuitous could imply a happier event and this Report, as did the last, names these deaths as **Coincidental**.

The other new term introduced in ICD-10 is **Late** maternal death, defined as the death of a woman from *Direct* or *Indirect* causes more than 42 days but less than one completed year after the end of the pregnancy. Identifying *Late* maternal deaths enables lessons to be learnt from those deaths in which a woman had problems that began with her pregnancy, even if she survived for more than 42 days after its end. However, although this category has only been recently recognised in the ICD 10 codes, and then only for deaths from *Direct* or *Indirect* causes, the previous three UK Enquiry Reports had already included all *Late* deaths notified to the assessors (including *Coincidental* deaths) occurring up to one year after delivery or abortion, as does this.

Table 1
Definitions of maternal deaths

*Maternal deaths**	Deaths of women while pregnant or within 42 days of the end of the pregnancy† from any cause related to or aggravated by the pregnancy or its management, but not from accidental or incidental causes.
*Direct**	Deaths resulting from obstetric complications of the pregnant state (pregnancy, labour and puerperium), from interventions, omissions, incorrect treatment, or from a chain of events resulting from any of the above.
*Indirect**	Deaths resulting from previous existing disease, or disease that developed during pregnancy and which was not due to direct obstetric causes, but which was aggravated by the physiologic effects of pregnancy.
*Late***	Deaths occurring between 42 days and one year after abortion, miscarriage or delivery that are due to *Direct* or *Indirect* maternal causes.
Coincidental **(Fortuitous)***	Deaths from unrelated causes which happen to occur in pregnancy or the puerperium.
Pregnancy-related deaths*	Deaths occurring in women while pregnant or within 42 days of termination of pregnancy, irrespective of the cause of the death.

† This term includes delivery, ectopic pregnancy, miscarriage or termination of pregnancy.

* ICD 9

** ICD 10

*** ICD 9/10 classifies these deaths as *Fortuitous* but the Enquiry prefers to use the term *Coincidental* as it is a more accurate description. The Enquiry also considers deaths from *Late Coincidental* causes.

Estimating maternal mortality ratios and rates

The international definition of the maternal mortality ratio (MMR) is the number of *Direct* and *Indirect* deaths per 100,000 live births. In many countries of the world this is difficult to measure due to the lack of death certificate data (should it exist at all) as well as a lack of basic denominator data, as baseline vital statistics are also not available or unreliable. The recent World Health Organisation publication "Beyond The Numbers; reviewing maternal deaths and disabilities to make pregnancy safer"[4] contains a more detailed examination and evaluation of the problems in both determining a baseline MMR or interpreting what it actually means in helping to address the problems facing pregnant women in most developing countries.

Conversely the UK has the advantage of accurate denominator data, including both live and still births and has defined its maternal mortality rate as the number of *Direct* and *Indirect* deaths per 100,000 maternities. Maternities are defined as the number of pregnancies that result in a live birth at any gestation or stillbirths occurring at or after 24 weeks' completed gestation and are required to be notified by law. This enables a more detailed picture of maternal death rates to be established and is used for the comparison of trends over time.

Furthermore, in the United Kingdom maternal mortality rates can be calculated in two ways:

- Through official death certification to the Registrars General (the Office for National Statistics (ONS) and its equivalents), or

- Through deaths known to this Enquiry. The overall maternal death rate is calculated from the number of *Direct* and *Indirect* deaths.

ONS data are based on death certificates where the cause of death is directly or secondarily coded for a pregnancy-related condition such as postpartum haemorrhage, eclampsia etc.

For the past 50 years the Enquiry has calculated its own maternal mortality rate as the overall number of maternal deaths identified by the proactive case finding methodology used by this Enquiry has always exceeded those officially reported. This is because not all maternal deaths are recorded as such on death certificates. For example, a large proportion of women known to the Enquiry who died of pre-existing medical conditions influenced by their pregnancy, for example cardiac disorders, epilepsy and some malignancies, were excluded from the official statistics. Other women excluded in official data are those who required long term intensive care and whose final cause of death was registered as a non pregnancy condition such as multiple organ failure even though the initiating cause was an obstetric event. Conversely, the maternal deaths known to the Registrars General may include *Late* deaths as it is not possible to identify from the death certificate when the delivery or termination occurred.

In order to aid the international comparison of the UK data with those from other countries calculated by using the ICD defined Maternal Mortality Ratio, this Report has also calculated the overall UK MMR as well as the more complete Enquiry maternal mortality rate. These are shown in Chapter 1. However, when making such comparisons, it is important to note two points:

- The criteria used by the UK assessors for *Indirect* deaths are far more inclusive than those used in other countries. For example in this Enquiry all cases of cardiac disease, asthma and epilepsy are coded as *Indirect*, as are cases of suicide unless obviously occurring in women with a longstanding previous psychiatric history.

- Case ascertainment is lower in the vast majority of other countries because they do not undertake such comprehensive enquiries.

Case ascertainment

The role of the Office for National Statistics

Since the introduction of a new Office for National Statistics (ONS) computer programme in 1993, all conditions given anywhere on the death certificate are now coded enabling a more extensive search of death entry information to identify all conditions listed which suggest a maternal death. In the past this has helped in improving case ascertainment, with a number of previously unreported deaths being identified. Fortunately for this Report the ONS record linkage study described below has identified very few additional cases of *Direct* or *Indirect* deaths. This is a reduction in the already small degree of under-ascertainment calculated for previous Reports.

For the past nine years, ONS have been able to match death records of women of fertile age living in England and Wales with birth registrations up to one year previously. The aim is to identify deaths of all women in England and Wales who died within one year of giving birth and to see how many additional cases can be found. The methodology, used in the past two triennia, was again applied for this Report and again shows that the majority of these deaths occurred *Late*, i.e. some months after delivery. The vast majority of these *Late* deaths were due to *Coincidental Late* causes and these are shown in Chapter 14.

Denominator data used for calculating mortality rates

Number of maternities

It is impossible to know the exact number of pregnancies which occurred during this or any preceding triennium since not all pregnancies result in a registered live or still birth. Because of the unreliability of these data, due to the lack of appropriate denominators, the most common denominator used throughout this and previous Reports is the number of maternities rather than the total number of pregnancies. Maternities are the number of pregnancies that result in a live birth at any gestation or stillbirths occurring at or after 24 weeks' completed gestation and are required to be notified by law. The total number of maternities for the United Kingdom for 2003-05 was 2,113, 831.

Estimated pregnancies

This denominator is used for calculating the rate of early pregnancy deaths. It is a combination of the number of maternities, together with legal terminations, hospital admissions for spontaneous miscarriages (at less than 24 weeks' gestation) and ectopic pregnancies with an adjustment to allow for the period of gestation and maternal ages at conception. The estimate for the United Kingdom 2003-05 was 2,898,400. However, the resulting total is still an underestimate of the actual number of pregnancies since these figures do not include other pregnancies which miscarry early, those where the woman is not admitted to hospital, or indeed those where the woman herself may not even know she is pregnant.

Table 2

Maternal mortality definitions used in this Report

Maternal mortality definitions	Reasons for use
UK Enquiry maternal mortality rates; *Direct* and *Indirect* deaths per 100,000 maternities.	The most robust figures available for the UK and used for 50 years trend data in this Report.
The internationally defined Maternal Mortality Ratio (MMR); *Direct* and *Indirect* deaths per 100,000 live births.	For international comparison although care needs to be taken in its interpretation due to the more accurate case ascertainment in the UK though the use of this Enquiry.
Deaths from obstetric causes per 100,000 estimated pregnancies.	Because the data from spontaneous abortions and ectopic pregnancies are unreliable this denominator is only used when calculating rates of death in early pregnancy.

References

1 Department of Health, England. *Maternity Services*. Standard 11 of the National Service Framework for Children, Young People and Maternity Services. London; Department of Health 2004. www.dh.gov.uk

2 Department of Health. *"Maternity matters: choice, access and continuity of care in a safe service"*. Department of Health, London, April 2007. www.dh.gov.uk

3 National Service Framework for Children, Young People and Maternity Services in Wales. Cardiff. 2005. www.wales.nhs.uk

4 World Health Organisation. *Beyond the Numbers - Reviewing maternal deaths and complications to make pregnancy safer*. WHO; Geneva: 2004.: www.who.int/reproductive-health

5 Lewis G, in British Medical Bulletin. *Pregnancy: Reducing maternal death and disability*. British Council. Oxford University Press.2003. www.bmb.oupjournals.org

6 Ministry of Health. *Report of the Confidential Enquiry into Maternal Deaths in England and Wales, 1952-1954*. Reports on Public Health and Medical Subjects No.97: HMSO. 1954.

7 Ruststein D, Berenberg W, Chalmers T, Child C, Fishman A et al. *Measuring the quality of care; a clinical method*. New England Journal of Medicine, March 11 1976, 582-588.

8 Scottish Programme for Clinical Effectiveness in Reproductive Health. *Confidential Audit of Severe Maternal Morbidity*. 2nd Annual Report. SPCERCH December 2005. ISBN 1-902076

9 Knight M, Kurinczuk JJ, Tuffnell D, Brocklehust P. *The UK Obseteric Suveillance System for rare disorders of pregnancy*. BJOG 2005: 112(3);263-5.

10 Knight M, Kurinczuk JJ, Spark P and Brocklehurst P. *United Kingdom Obstetric Surveillance System (UKOSS) Annual Report 2007*. National Perinatal Epidemiology Unit, Oxford.

Chapter 1 Which mothers died, and why

Gwyneth Lewis • Statistical analysis by Alison Macfarlane

Summary of key points

- Maternal deaths are extremely rare in the United Kingdom. The maternal mortality rate for 2003-05 calculated from all maternal deaths directly or indirectly due to pregnancy identified by this Enquiry was 14 per 100,000 maternities. Although this is a slight increase from the last Report, it is not statistically significant.

- If, as is the case in other countries, the numbers of maternal deaths are restricted to those identified by the underlying cause of death given on death certificates alone, the UK maternal death rate was 7 per 100,000 maternities, half that identified by this much more in-depth Enquiry.

- The maternal mortality rate for those mothers' deaths that could only be due to pregnancy e.g. haemorrhage or eclampsia, i.e. *Direct* deaths, showed a slight increase for this triennium compared to the last Report. This is not statistically significant.

- The mortality rate for mothers' deaths from *Indirect* causes, i.e. from pre-existing or new medical or mental health conditions aggravated by pregnancy such as heart disease, has not changed since the last Report. Although the maternal death rate from *Indirect* causes was still higher than for deaths from *Direct* causes, the gap between them was smaller.

- Many possible factors lie behind the lack of decline in the maternal mortality rate. They include rising numbers of older or obese mothers, women whose lifestyles put them at risk of poorer health and a growing proportion of women with medically complex pregnancies. Because of the rising numbers of births to women born outside the UK, the rate may also be influenced by the increasing number of deaths of migrant women. These mothers often have more complicated pregnancies, more serious underlying medical conditions or may be in poorer general health. They can also experience difficulties in accessing maternity care.

- More than half of all the women who died from *Direct* or *Indirect* causes, for whom information was available, were either overweight or obese. More than 15% of all women who died from *Direct* or *Indirect* causes were morbidly or super morbidly obese.

- The commonest cause of *Direct* death was again thromboembolism. Despite apparent slight rises in rates of death from thromboembolism, pre-eclampsia/ eclampsia and genital tract sepsis and apparent slight declines in rates of death from haemorrhage and direct uterine trauma, none of these differences were statistically significant. There has also been an apparently inexplicable rise in deaths from amniotic fluid embolism, a rare and largely unavoidable condition.

- Cardiac disease was the most common cause of *Indirect* deaths as well as of maternal deaths overall. In the main this reflects the growing incidence of acquired heart disease in younger women related to less healthy diets, smoking, alcohol and the growing epidemic of obesity.

- There has been a decrease in the rate of suicide, the overall leading cause of death in the last Report. If sustained in the next Report, this decline may indicate that the recommendations made in previous Reports concerning identifying women at potential risk in the antenatal period, and developing management plans for them, are having a beneficial effect.

- Whilst there has been no increase in the number of cases associated with sub-standard care, or avoidable factors, a number of health care professionals failed to identify and manage common medical conditions or potential emergencies outside their immediate area of expertise. Resuscitation skills were also considered poor in some cases.

- In many cases the care provided was hampered by a lack of cross-disciplinary or cross-agency working and problems with communication. This included:

  - poor or non existent team working

  - inappropriate or too short consultations by phone

  - the lack of sharing of relevant information between health professionals, including between GPs and the maternity team

  - poor interpersonal skills.

There were also a number of cases where significant information, particularly regarding a risk of self-harm and child safety, was not shared between the health and social services, and an assumption by social services that their pregnant clients were attending for maternity care.

Vulnerability and other risk factors for maternal deaths

- Vulnerable women with socially complex lives who died were far less likely to seek antenatal care early in pregnancy or to stay in regular contact with maternity services. Overall 17% of the women who died from *Direct* or *Indirect* causes booked for maternity care after 22 weeks of gestational age or had missed over four routine antenatal visits compared to 5% of women who were employed themselves, or who had a partner in employment. Of the women who died from any cause, including those unrelated to pregnancy:

  - 14% self-declared that they were subject to domestic abuse

  - 11% had problems with substance abuse, 60% of whom were registered addicts

  - 10% lived in families known to the child protection services.

- A third of all women who died were either single and unemployed or in a relationship where both partners were unemployed.

- Women with partners who were unemployed, many of whom had features of social exclusion, were up to seven times more likely to die than women with partners who were employed. In England, women who lived in the most deprived areas were five times more likely to die than women living in the least deprived areas.

- Black African women, including asylum seekers and newly arrived refugees have a mortality rate nearly six times higher than White women. To a lesser extent, Black Caribbean and Middle Eastern women also had a significantly higher mortality rate.

Key findings for 2003-05

Maternal deaths related to pregnancy

Maternal deaths are extremely rare in the United Kingdom. This Confidential Enquiry identified only 295 women who died from causes directly or indirectly related to their pregnancy, out of more than two million mothers who gave birth in the United Kingdom (UK) between the years 2003-05.

Of these, 132 mothers died of conditions that could only occur in relation to pregnancy (*Direct* deaths), and 163 died of underlying medical or psychiatric causes, such as heart disease or severe depression, aggravated by their pregnancy (*Indirect* deaths) as shown in Table 1.1[i].

The overall UK maternal mortality rate for this triennium, as calculated by this Enquiry, i.e. total number of *Indirect* and *Direct* deaths combined per 100,000 maternities, was 13.95 deaths per 100,000 maternities. As shown in Table 1.1, the difference between this and the rate of 13.07 for the previous Report[1] is not statistically significant. Changes in the rates of *Direct* and *Indirect* deaths since 1985 are shown in Figure 1.1. This figure also demonstrates the impact of improved methods of case ascertainment especially for death from *Indirect* causes.

The mortality rate for maternal deaths from *Direct* causes of death was 6.24 per 100,000 maternities compared to 5.31 in 2000-02. Although the numbers of *Direct* deaths rose from 106 in 2000-02 to 132 in 2003-05 but the numbers of maternities also rose from 1,997,472 to 2,114,004. The key comparison is between the mortality rates and not the actual numbers of deaths. As the confidence interval in Table 1.1 shows, this difference is not statistically significant.

Due to the constraints of the international definition of maternal deaths[i], which place a cut off point for inclusion in the statistics of 42 days after birth, the deaths of eleven further women died of *Direct* causes later than this are not included in these figures. However, the lessons to be learnt from them are discussed in the relevant Chapters of this Report.

Table 1.1
Direct and *Indirect* maternal deaths and mortality rates per 100,000 maternities* as reported to the Enquiry; United Kingdom: 1985-2005.

Triennium	Direct deaths known to the Enquiry			Indirect deaths known to the Enquiry			Total Direct and Indirect deaths known to the Enquiry		
	Number	Rate	*95 per cent CI*	Number	Rate	*95 per cent CI*	Number	Rate	*95 per cent CI*
1985-1987	139	6.13	*5.19* *7.23*	84	3.70	*2.99* *4.58*	223	9.83	*8.62* *11.21*
1988-1990	145	6.14	*5.22* *7.23*	93	3.94	*3.22* *4.83*	238	10.08	*8.88* *11.45*
1991-1993	128	5.53	*4.65* *6.57*	100	4.32	*3.55* *5.25*	228	9.85	*8.65* *11.21*
1994-1996	134	6.10	*5.15* *7.22*	134	6.10	*5.15* *7.22*	268	12.19	*10.82* *13.74*
1997-1999	106	4.99	*4.13* *6.04*	136	6.40	*5.41* *7.57*	242	11.40	*10.05* *12.92*
2000-2002	106	5.31	*4.39* *6.42*	155	7.76	*6.63* *9.08*	261	13.07	*11.57* *14.75*
2003-2005	132	6.24	*5.27* *7.40*	163	7.71	*6.61* *8.99*	295	13.95	*12.45* *15.64*
Change in rate 2000-02 to 2003-05		0.94	*-0.54* *2.42*		0.05	*-1.66* *1.77*		0.89	*-1.37* *3.14*

* Numbers of maternities are given in Table 1.2.

[i] The Introduction to this Report provides detailed descriptions of the definitions of maternal deaths used throughout the Report.

Indirect deaths

The rate of *Indirect* maternal deaths, 7.71 per 100,000 maternities, remains virtually unchanged from the 7.76 per 100,000 maternities cited in the last Report. The numbers of maternal deaths from *Indirect* causes still continue to outnumber *Direct* deaths, as has been seen in the past three Reports and in the rates shown in Figure 1.2.

International comparisons

In the United Kingdom maternal mortality rates can be calculated in two different ways:

1. Through deaths proactively reported to this Enquiry. The overall maternal death rate for the Enquiry is calculated from the number of deaths assessed as being due to *Direct* and *Indirect* deaths. This is the rate generally used by the Departments of Health in their reports.

2. Through coding the underlying cause of death using the information on death certificates. These are the data used in official death statistics published by the Registrars General at the Office for National Statistics (ONS) and its Scottish and Northern Irish counterparts. This method is used by most other countries.

Because of the proactive case-finding methodology of this Enquiry, described in Appendix 1, the numbers of *Direct* and *Indirect* deaths identified in this manner always exceeds those identified through the rate from data certificate data alone. In this, the UK is unusual since most other countries currently derive their official maternal mortality rate from death certificate data alone. For international comparisons therefore, the equivalent UK rate, is given in Table 1.2. This shows that, using death certificates alone, 149 maternal deaths were identified in 2003-05, giving a maternal death rate of 7.05 per 100,000 maternities, just over half that found by this Enquiry. The corresponding maternal mortality ratio, where live birth rather than maternities are used as the denominator[ii], as used in international comparisons, was 6.98 per 100,000 live births.

The numbers of maternities shown in Table 1.2 are also those used as denominators for all the tables in this Report, apart from those relating to early pregnancy deaths.

Table 1.2
Registered maternal deaths using death certificate data alone, and mortality rates per 100,000 maternities; United Kingdom: 1985-2005.

Triennium	Number with underlying cause given as *Direct* or *Indirect* maternal death, ICD9 600-676, ICD10 O00-O99				Number of maternities
	Number	Rate	*95 per cent CI*		
1985-1987	159	7.01	*6.00*	*8.19*	2,268,766
1988-1990	171	7.24	*6.24*	*8.42*	2,360,309
1991-1993	150	6.48	*5.52*	*7.60*	2,315,204
1994-1996	158	7.19	*6.15*	*8.40*	2,197,640
1997-1999	128	6.03	*5.07*	*7.17*	2,123,614
2000-2002	136	6.81	*5.76*	*8.05*	1,997,472
2003-2005	149	7.05	*6.00*	*8.27*	2,114,004

Source: Office for National Statistics, General Register Office, Scotland, General Register Office, Northern Ireland.

[ii] The Introduction to this Report provides detailed descriptions of the definitions of maternal deaths used throughout the Report.

Figure 1.1: Overall maternal mortality rate (deaths from *Direct* and *Indirect* causes combined) per 100,000 maternities; United Kingdom: 1985-2005.

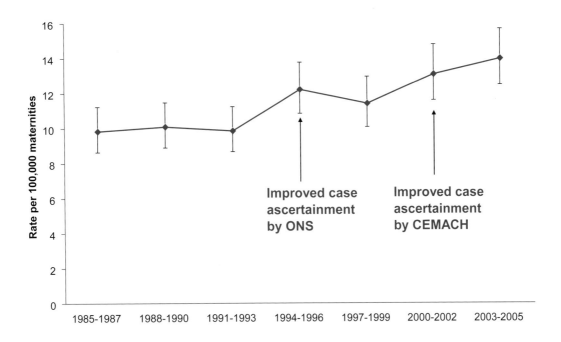

Figure 1.2a: *Direct* maternal mortality rates per 100,000 maternities; United Kingdom: 1985-2005.

Figure 1.2b: *Indirect* maternal mortality rates per 100,000 maternities; United Kingdom: 1985-2005.

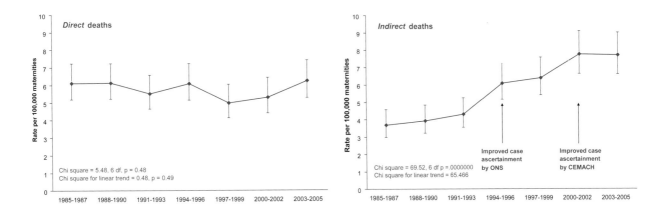

Interpreting trends in maternal mortality

The mortality rate for *Direct* deaths since the mid 1980s has remained at a relatively constant level with small random fluctuations, as Table 1.1 and Figure 1.2a show. The differences between triennia are compatible with random variation and no linear trend can be detected. This contrasts with the significant decline from the mid 1930s to the mid 1980s discussed in the previous Report[1].

A number of factors, individually or combined, may account for the lack of any further decline since the mid 1980s. These include newly emerging risk factors and changes in the population of women of childbearing age. These are also discussed in Annex 1 to this Chapter – The changing face of motherhood in the UK. The fact that the rate is not falling means that there are no grounds for complacency and highlights the necessity for further vigilance and the need for these Reports to continue.

Improved case ascertainment

A cross check between death certificates and the Office for National Statistics (ONS) record linkage study, described in the introduction of this Report, shows that virtually all *Direct* and *Indirect* maternal deaths were identified and assessed. Improved case ascertainment, therefore, is unlikely to account for the lack of decline.

Older mothers with health problems

As discussed in more detail in Annex 1 to this Chapter, factors such as an increase in the mean age of childbirth and a rise in risk factors such as obesity means more mothers are likely to have complicated pregnancies than in the past. Anecdotally obstetricians and midwives are regularly reporting they are seeing larger numbers of, older and less healthy mothers.

Increases in numbers of births to migrant women

Since the previous triennium the percentage of births which were to mothers born outside the UK has increased. There has been a corresponding increase in deaths amongst women arriving in the UK in poor health. Compared to the last Report an additional 19 *Direct* maternal deaths occurred in recently arrived women who were either new migrants, refugees, asylum seekers or 'health tourists' who had travelled to the UK specifically to seek maternity care. For the first time several maternal deaths occurred amongst recently arrived women from the new member states of the European Union; these women too tended to be in poorer general health.

Excluding refugees and asylum seekers from the numbers of maternal deaths, as shown in Table A1.3 in the Annex to this Chapter, the mortality rate for 2003-05 was 12.25 per 100,000 maternities, compared with 12.47 per 100,000 maternities in 2000-02. This difference is not statistically significant.

Changes in standards of clinical care

Since the last Report there has been no appreciable increase, or decrease, in the proportion of maternal deaths assessed as having avoidable factors. However, the assessors were struck by the lack of some health professionals' skills in identifying and managing common medical conditions or potential emergencies outside their immediate area of expertise. Resuscitation skills were also considered poor in quite a few cases. Although these messages were identified in the last Report, this lack of knowledge and skills seemed more prevalent in this Report.

Deaths in pregnant women or new mothers up to one year after delivery which were not due to, or affected by, pregnancy

In order to ascertain which deaths that occurred in pregnant or recently delivered women were directly or indirectly related to their pregnancy, and thus are of importance to this Enquiry, it was necessary to first assess the cases of all mothers who died whilst pregnant or within a year of their delivery, from whatever cause. The majority of deaths, once assessed, were found to be unrelated to pregnancy e.g. road traffic accidents or deaths from cancers. These fall into two broad categories; *Coincidental* and *Late*[ii]. By international convention these do not contribute to the statistics used to calculate the UK maternal mortality rate determined by this Enquiry.

Coincidental deaths

The deaths of 55 women who died of *Coincidental* causes, meaning their deaths were linked to pregnancy only by a temporal association in that they occurred during pregnancy or within six weeks of birth, were assessed this triennium. This was a similar number to the last Report. However, whilst apparently unrelated to pregnancy, these deaths often contain important public health messages such as domestic abuse and the use of seat belts and are discussed in Chapter 14.

Late deaths

In this triennium the CEMACH regional managers were able to proactively collect data on many more, but not all, deaths from any cause, which occurred amongst all women later in their first postnatal year. These are classified as *Late* deaths which occurred in women between six weeks and one year after delivery and were notified to the Enquiry through the record linkage system developed by the Office for National Statistics (ONS) which has been described in detail in earlier Reports.

The ONS linkage system identifies all women who have died within a year of giving birth from whatever cause. Whilst this has meant an increase in the number of deaths identified and identified and assessed, it does not reflect an increase in actual maternal death rates whatsoever. This too, is discussed in more detail in Chapter 14.

Whilst it has never been possible to determine overall trends from the *Late* deaths assessed in this or earlier Reports, some cases do contain lessons for the management of women with complex underlying medical, mental health or social problems and these are classified as either *Late Direct* or *Late Indirect* deaths and discussed in the relevant Chapters of this Report. However, the majority of later deaths are unrelated to pregnancy, *Late Coincidental* deaths, and because of a lack of comparability and consistency, and the experience of this triennium which has shown that there are very few additional lessons that can be drawn from the majority of these cases, such detailed assessments will not be routinely undertaken in future. The exception to this will be those few *Late Direct* and *Late Indirect* deaths due to causes from which important lessons for maternity care can still be drawn.

The children left behind

In the period of this Report it is estimated that at least 360 existing children and 160 live newborn babies lost their mother to a reported *Direct* or *Indirect* death. Of the existing children, 112, or nearly a third, were already in the care of social services. Any child whose mother dies faces a far poorer start to family life and the fact that so many of the children were already living in complex and excluded families, or were in care, underscores the important public health dimension of this Enquiry.

The clinical reasons why mothers died

Table 1.3 gives the numbers and maternal death rates per 100,000 maternities by specific cause of death for this triennium and since 1985-87.

The numbers of deaths have been checked for consistency and some therefore differ slightly from those in earlier Reports. This data should therefore be used as a baseline for future analyses. The numbers of maternities shown in Table 1.2 have been used to calculate the rates given in this and subsequent tables. For reasons of space, the 95 % confidence intervals for the rates given in Table 1.3 are shown in the relevant Chapters.

---

ii The Introduction to this Report provides detailed descriptions of the definitions of maternal deaths used throughout this Report.

Table 1.3
Numbers and rates per 100,000 maternities of maternal deaths reported to the Enquiry by cause;
United Kingdom: 1985-2005.

Cause of death	1985-87	1988-90	1991-93	1994-96	1997-99	2000-02	2003-05	1985-87	1988-90	1991-93	1994-96	1997-99	2000-02	2003-05
	Numbers							Rates per 100,000 maternities						
Direct deaths														
Thrombosis and thromboembolism	32	33	35	48	35	30	**41**	1.41	1.40	1.51	2.18	1.65	1.50	1.94
Pre-eclampsia and eclampsia*	27	27	20	20	16	14	**18**	1.19	1.14	0.86	0.91	0.75	0.70	0.85
Haemorrhage*	10	22	15	12	7	17	**14**	0.44	0.93	0.65	0.55	0.33	0.85	0.66
Amniotic fluid embolism	9	11	10	17	8	5	**17**	0.40	0.47	0.43	0.77	0.38	0.25	0.80
Early pregnancy deaths	16	24	17	15	17	15	**14**	0.71	1.02	0.73	0.68	0.80	0.75	0.66
Ectopic	11	15	9	12	13	11	**10**	0.48	0.64	0.39	0.55	0.61	0.55	0.47
Spontaneous miscarriage	4	6	3	2	2	1	**1**	0.18	0.25	0.13	0.09	0.09	0.05	0.05
Legal termination	1	3	5	1	2	3	**2**	0.04	0.13	0.22	0.05	0.09	0.15	0.09
Other	0	0	2	0	0	0	**3**	0.00	0.00	0.09	0.00	0.00	0.00	0.14
Genital tract sepsis**	9	17	15	16	18	13	**18**	0.40	0.72	0.65	0.73	0.85	0.65	0.85
Other *Direct*	27	17	14	7	7	8	**4**	1.19	0.72	0.60	0.32	0.33	0.40	0.19
Genital tract trauma	6	3	4	5	2	1	**3***	0.26	0.13	0.17	0.23	0.09	0.05	0.14
Fatty liver	6	5	2	2	4	3	**1***	0.26	0.21	0.09	0.09	0.19	0.15	0.05
Other causes	15	9	8	0	1	4	**0**	0.66	0.38	0.35	0.00	0.05	0.20	0.00
Anaesthetic	6	4	8	1	3	6	**6**	0.26	0.17	0.35	0.05	0.14	0.30	0.28
All *Direct*	**139**	**145**	**128**	**134**	**106**	**106**	**132**	*6.13*	*6.14*	*5.53*	*6.10*	*4.99*	*5.31*	*6.24*
Indirect														
Cardiac	23	18	37	39	35	44	**48**	1.01	0.76	1.60	1.77	1.65	2.20	2.27
Psychiatric *Indirect*	-	-	-	9	15	16	**18**	-	-	-	0.41	0.71	0.80	0.85
Other *Indirect*	62	75	63	86	75	90	**87**	2.73	3.18	2.72	3.91	3.53	4.51	4.12
Indirect malignancies	-	-	-	-	11	5	**10***	-	-	-	-	0.52	0.25	0.47
All *Indirect*	**84**	**93**	**100**	**134**	**136**	**155**	**163**	*3.70*	*3.94*	*4.32*	*6.10*	*6.40*	*7.76*	*7.71*
Coincidental	**26**	**39**	**46**	**36**	**29**	**36**	**55**	*1.15*	*1.65*	*1.99*	*1.64*	*1.37*	*1.80*	*2.60*
Late														
Direct	-	13	10	4	7	4	**11**							
Indirect	-	10	23	32	39	45	**71*****							

* Three cases of uterine rupture are counted in Chapter 4, haemorrhage and one of fatty liver in Chapter 3, pre-eclampsia and eclampsia.
** Including early pregnancy deaths due to sepsis.
*** Includes one death from choriocarninoma which ideally should be regarded as a *Direct* death.
**** Rise due to improved case ascertainment.
- Data not previously collected separately.

Leading causes of maternal deaths: 2003-05

Direct deaths

The commonest cause of *Direct* maternal deaths was again thromboembolism. Although the rates appear to have risen slightly, this is compatible with random variation. Similarly, although there appears to be a three-fold increase in the number of deaths due to Amniotic Fluid Embolism (AFE), these were largely concentrated in the first two years of the triennium and were largely unavoidable. The small variation in rates of deaths from sepsis, pre-eclampsia/eclampsia, haemorrhage, anaesthesia and direct uterine trauma are no greater than would be expected by chance. There was no under-reporting of any of these deaths.

Indirect deaths

Cardiac disease was the commonest cause of maternal death overall, and was more common than the most frequent *Direct* cause of maternal death, thromboembolism. It also outnumbers deaths from suicide, which was the leading overall cause of maternal death in the last Report.

The care the mothers received

Antenatal care

Table 1.4 shows the type of antenatal care provided for the mothers who died.

Table 1.4
Maternal deaths by type of antenatal care; United Kingdom: 2003-05.

	Type of Death							
	Direct	*Indirect*	*Direct* and *Indirect*		*Coincidental*	*Late Direct*	All deaths	
	n	n	n	(%)	n	n	n	(%)
Team-based or "shared" care	54	60	**114**	*(39)*	17	6	**137**	*(33)*
Consultant led unit only	15	39	**54**	*(18)*	9	1	**64**	*(15)*
Midwife only	11	16	**27**	*(9)*	8	0	**35**	*(8)*
Midwife and GP	5	4	**9**	*(3)*	6	3	**18**	*(4)*
Death before booking or after miscarriages or TOP	22	9	**31**	*(11)*	5	0	**36**	*(9)*
Unaware of pregnancy	5	1	**6**	*(2)*	1	0	**7**	*(2)*
Suboptimal antenatal care:								
Concealed pregnancy	3	2	**5**	*(2)*	0	0	**5**	*(1)*
No antenatal care	4	6	**10**	*(3)*	4	0	**14**	*(3)*
Late booker/poor attender	11	24	**35**	*(12)*	5	1	**41**	*(10)*
Not stated	2	2	**4**	*(1)*	55	0	**59**	*(14)*
All deaths	**132**	**163**	**295**	*(100)*	**110**	**11**	**416**	*(100)***

* Booked after 22 weeks gestation or had missed over four antenatal appointments.
** Percentages have been rounded to the nearest whole percentage.

The women who did not come for care

Fifty women, 17% of those who died from *Direct* or *Indirect* causes, first booked for maternity care after 22 weeks of gestational age, missed over four routine antenatal visits, did not seek care at all or actively concealed their pregnancies. This compares to 20% in the last Report. The 83% of the women who died and who had sought maternity care at an appropriate time in early pregnancy contrasts with the 98% of women overall who reported having "booked" with NHS maternity services by 18 weeks of gestation in a recent study undertaken by the National Perinatal Epidemiology Unit (NPEU)[2]. The possible reasons for this difference are varied and complex and are explored in depth throughout this Report. Identifying and overcoming the barriers to care these women faced in reaching maternity services will help improve the accessibility of local maternity services as well as the outcomes for maternal and newborn health. However, even when mothers seek care early the system can let them down. There were several instances of women not receiving appointments once referred for maternity care until several months into their pregnancy.

Maternity team and consultant led care

For the majority of women who died antenatal care was shared between their GP, midwife and obstetrician; so-called traditional "shared care" or, as described in the recent maternity services implementation strategy for England, "Maternity Matters", "team-based care"[3]. Many of these women saw a member of the obstetric staff once or twice, just to check all was well, and in the main their care was managed by a midwife. 18% of the mothers who died were already known or perceived to have been at higher risk of complications and their care was provided by the consultant-led maternity team, including midwives, obstetricians and anaesthetists. As a reflection of the changing nature of maternity service provision, only 3% of women had their care shared between midwives and their GPs.

Midwifery care

A renewed emphasis is being placed on midwives being the experts in the management of normal pregnancy and birth, as envisaged both in the National Services Framework for Maternity Care in England (NSF)[4] and "Maternity Matters[3]. In future it is likely that the majority of women with no known risk factors will have midwifery led care throughout pregnancy, delivery and after birth. This change is already happening. The recent NPEU study[2] demonstrated that around 50% of women surveyed reported having midwifery only antenatal care. For this Report, 27 (9%) of the mothers who died received midwifery care only throughout their antenatal period compared to 16 women who died from either *Direct* or *Indirect* causes in the previous triennium. Another six women who died of *Coincidental* causes, including murder in cases of known domestic abuse, had midwifery led care. For most of the women who died, their midwifery led care was both appropriate for their circumstances and of high quality, and they died of unforeseen catastrophic events during delivery or after childbirth. However, in a few cases discussed in the midwifery Chapter, this type of care was inappropriate.

The women who died before delivery

As shown in Table 1.5, 100 women died before delivery, 18 from *Coincidental* causes. For women dying of *Direct* causes, the largest numbers were from ectopic pregnancy and pulmonary thromboembolism. There were a wide variety of causes of *Indirect* deaths amongst undelivered women, with deaths from cardiac disease amongst the largest group.

Table 1.5
Maternal deaths by gestation, type of death and neonatal outcome; United Kingdom: 2003-05.

	Direct	Indirect	Direct and Indirect		Coincidental	Late Direct	All	
	n	n	n	(%)	n	n	n	(%)
Undelivered								
Less than 24 weeks'*	43	39	82	(28)	18	-	100	(28)
24 weeks or more	-	21	21	(7)	10	-	31	(9)
Delivered at 24 or more weeks of gestation								
Live birth**	64	83	147	(50)	16	7	170	(47)
Stillbirth**	17	10	27	(9)	6	2	35	(10)
Early Neonatal Death**	8	10	18	(6)	5	2	25	(7)
All	132	163	295	(100)	55	11	361	(100)

* Includes all ectopic pregnancies, miscarriages and termination of pregnancy.
** Twin pregnancies are counted as one birth event or maternity. There were five sets of twins in the *Direct* category, four in the *Indirect* category and one in the *Late Direct* group. There were no deaths of women with triplets or higher order pregnancies in this triennium.

The 10th revision of the International Classification of Diseases recommends that live and stillbirths at 22 weeks or more gestation should be included in all perinatal statistics. To date, this Report has used the UK definition of stillbirth, i.e. deaths at 24 weeks or more completed gestation, the numbers for which are given in Table 1.5. If the UK stillbirth definition were extended to 22 weeks there would have been an additional four women who died from *Indirect* causes and one from *Coincidental* causes who were delivered between 22-23 completed weeks of gestation. In each case the baby was stillborn.

Place of delivery

The majority of the 230 women who died from *Direct* or *Indirect* maternal causes and who gave birth at 24 or more completed weeks of gestation delivered in a consultant led maternity unit, as shown in Table 1.6.

Table 1.6
Maternal deaths by place of delivery at 24 or more completed weeks of gestation; United Kingdom: 2003-05.

	Type of Death							
	Direct	*Indirect*	*Direct* and *Indirect*		*Coincidental*	*Late Direct*		**All**
	n	n	n	(%)	n	n	n	(%)
Delivery suite in an obstetric unit	81	89	**170**	*(89)*	22	10	**202**	*(88)*
Midwife led birth centre	0	1	**1**	*(1)*	0	1	**2**	*(1)*
Emergency department	3	6	**9**	*(5)*	5	0	**14**	*(6)*
ICU	2	2	**4**	*(2)*	0	0	**4**	*(2)*
Hospital other	2	3	**5**	*(3)*	0	0	**5**	*(2)*
Home	1	2	**3**	*(2)*	0	0	**3**	*(1)*
Total	**89**	**103**	**192**	*(100)*	**27**	**11**	**230**	*(100)*

Midwifery led birth at home or in midwifery birth centres

Two women who died of causes directly or indirectly related to pregnancy had a planned home birth. A third woman who delivered at home had actively avoided maternity care. The third woman was one who actively avoided maternity care. One of the two women who had a planned home birth was morbidly obese and, although it did not directly contribute to her death, it was inappropriate for her to deliver in such a setting. A further six women who died of *Coincidental* causes had home births, one as a result of being kept prisoner and subject to domestic abuse. None were associated with sub-standard care at the time of delivery.

Type of delivery

The majority of the 230 women who died at 24 or more completed weeks of gestation were delivered by caesarean section, as shown in Table 1.7. A further three women who died of *Indirect* causes delivered between 22 and 23 completed weeks of gestation; two were delivered by a perimortem and one by an emergency caesarean section.

Table 1.7
Number of maternal deaths by mode of delivery at 24 or more completed weeks of gestation;
United Kingdom 2003-05.

	Type of Death							
	Direct	*Indirect*	*Direct* and *Indirect*		*Coincidental*	*Late Direct*		**All**
	n	n	n	(%)	n	n	n	(%)
Unassisted vaginal	24	33	57	(30)	8	5	70	(30)
Ventouse	3	3	6	(3)	0	0	6	(3)
Forceps	7	3	10	(5)	1	0	11	(5)
Vaginal breech	0	2	2	(1)	0	0	2	(1)
Caesarean section	55	62	117	(61)	18	6	141	(61)
Emergency	28	23	51	(27)	2	1	54	(23)
Urgent	3	3	6	(3)	1	3	10	(4)
Scheduled	2	5	7	(4)	5	1	13	(6)
Elective	4	9	13	(7)	2	0	15	(7)
Peri or postmortem	18	22	40	(21)	8	1	49	(21)*
Total delivered	89	103	192	(100)	27	11	230	(100)

*Twin pregnancies are counted as one event in this table.

Caesarean section

This Enquiry uses the classification of types of caesarean section according to the definitions from the Royal College of Obstetrics and Gynaecology (RCOG) as shown in Box 1.1[5].

Box 1.1
RCOG Definition of type of caesarean section.

Type	Definition
Emergency	Immediate threat to life of woman or fetus
Urgent	Maternal or fetal compromise which is not immediately life threatening
Scheduled	Needing early delivery but no maternal or fetal compromise
Elective	At a time to suit the patient and the maternity team
Perimortem	Carried out in extremis while the mother is undergoing active resuscitation
Postmortem	Carried out after the death of the mother in order to try to save the fetus.

The balance of maternal and fetal risks between caesarean section and vaginal delivery is a controversial topic and in considering the maternal deaths in which a caesarean section was performed, it is almost impossible to disentangle the consequences of caesarean section from the indication for the operation. Table 1.8 shows the underlying reason/s for the caesarean section, by type, for *Direct* and *Indirect* deaths respectively. Only one was performed for these women for maternal request and the remaining cases had serious prenatal or intrapartum complications or illness that required a caesarean section. Perimortem caesarean section is the starkest example of this. Six of the eleven women who died from *Late Direct* causes had a caesarean delivery, all for serious maternal and/or fetal complications.

Table 1.8
Indication and type of caesarean section for *Direct* and *Indirect* deaths; United Kingdom: 2003-05.

Indication*	Direct				Indirect				Total
	Elective or Scheduled	Urgent or Emergency	Peri/Post mortem	**All**	Elective or Scheduled	Urgent or Emergency	Peri/Post mortem	**All**	
Maternal health									
Failure to progress	1	4	0	**5**	0	3	0	**3**	**8**
Maternal medical condition	4	7	15	**26**	9	16	22	**47**	**73**
Pre-eclampsia	0	9	0	**9**	1	3	2	**6**	**15**
Placenta praevia	0	1	0	**1**	0	0	0	**0**	**1**
Placental abruption	0	2	1	**3**	0	2	0	**2**	**5**
Chorioamnionitis	0	2	0	**2**	0	0	0	**0**	**2**
Previous caesarean section	0	0	0	**0**	1	0	0	**1**	**1**
Failed induction of labour	0	0	0	**0**	0	1	0	**1**	**1**
Maternal request	0	0	0	**0**	1	0	0	**1**	**1**
Fetal health									
Presumed fetal compromise	0	1	0	**1**	1	0	0	**1**	**2**
Unstable lie	0	5	0	**5**	0	5	0	**5**	**10**
Breech	0	0	0	**0**	2	0	0	**2**	**2**
Multiple pregnancy	0	0	0	**0**	1	0	0	**1**	**1**
Other	1	0	0	**1**	0	0	0	**0**	**1**
Not known	0	0	2	**2**	0	0	0	**0**	**2**
All caesarean sections	**6**	**31**	**18**	**55**	**14**	**26**	**22**	**62**	**117**

* In some cases there was more than one indication for caesarean section.

Peri or post mortem caesarean section

Table 1.9 shows the fetal outcomes for peri or post mortem caesarean sections by place of operation. These procedures were carried out either whilst the mother was undergoing active cardio-pulmonary resuscitation (CPR) or after her death had been confirmed. As it has been difficult to ascertain the precise distinction between whether the intervention was actually peri or post mortem the two have been counted together. There has been a large increase in the numbers of these procedures this triennium, and also of note is that every women who died of *Direct* causes with a gestational age of 24 weeks or more was delivered, many having a perimortem section carried out at the time of their collapse. Table 1.10 describes the fetal outcomes by gestational age. The figures include two cases where perimortem sections were undertaken for women whose pregnancies were no more than 20 weeks' gestation.

The number of perimortem caesarean sections has almost doubled compared with the last Report, in which eight babies survived, including five delivered in an Emergency Department (ED). In this Report, twenty babies survived, including one set of twins, but their chances of survival were greatly improved with advanced gestational age and maternal collapse in, or near, a delivery suite or operating theatre. These findings indicate that with improved resuscitation techniques more babies are surviving perimortem caesarean sections, particularly where the women collapsed in an already well-staffed and equipped delivery room or operating theatre. However, they also highlight the very poor outcome for babies delivered in Emergency Departments, especially for women who arrive after having undergone CPR for a considerable length of time. The babies who survived were born to mothers who were near or at term, and who suffered a cardiac arrest whilst already undergoing active treatment in the ED.

Table 1.9
Outcome of perimortem and post-mortem caesarean sections by place of delivery; United Kingdom: 2003-05*.

Place of delivery	Live birth	Stillbirth	Early neonatal death	Total
Emergency Department	3	18	2	23
Delivery room or operating theatre	15	5	6	26
Critical Care or other hospital department	2	1	0	3
Total	**20**	**24**	**8**	**52***

* Twin pregnancies counted as two births in this table but as one delivery in Table 1.7.

Table 1.10
Outcome of perimortem caesarean sections by gestational age (completed weeks); United Kingdom: 2003-05.

	Live births		Stillbirths and neonatal deaths		All	
	n	(%)	n	(%)	n	(%)
20-23	0	*(0)*	2	*(6)*	2	*(4)*
24-27	5	*(25)*	8	*(25)*	13	*(25)*
28-31	3	*(15)*	3	*(9)*	6	*(12)*
32-35	2	*(10)*	6	*(19)*	8	*(15)*
36 and over	10	*(50)*	13	*(41)*	23	*(44)*
All	**20**	**(100)**	**32**	**(100)**	**52**	**(100)**

The quality of care the women received

Sub-standard care remained very difficult to evaluate in many of the cases in this Report due to the lack of key data from some records and case notes. Whilst it is clear that many of the cases received less than optimum care, it has not always been possible to quantify these with certainty. Box 1.2 gives the definitions of sub-standard care used in this Report.

Box 1.2 Definitions of sub-standard care used in this Report	
Type	**Definition**
Major	Contributed significantly to the death of the mother. In many, but not all cases different treatment may have altered the outcome.
Minor	It was a relevant contributory factor. Different management might have made a difference but the mother's survival was unlikely in any case.

Despite the limitations, the assessors classified 64 % of *Direct* deaths and 40% of *Indirect* deaths as shown in Table 1.11 as having some degree of substandard care. Table 1.12 gives the degree of substandard care compared to the previous two Reports. The overall rate of sub-standard care for women dying of *Direct* causes has fallen a little compared to the 67% reported for the last triennium whilst there has been a very small rise in the rate for *Indirect* deaths. By contrast, only about 10 % of both *Coincidental* and *Late* deaths had elements of sub-standard care. The major concerns about the care provided for these groups of women were a lack of liaison and communication between the health and social services in providing support for vulnerable young girls and a lack of multidisciplinary or co-ordinated care.

Table 1.11
Numbers and percentage of *Direct* and *Indirect* deaths assessed as having substandard care by cause of death; United Kingdom: 2003-05.

Cause of death	Numbers with substandard care			Total number of cases	*Percentage of all cases with substandard care*
	Major	Minor	**Major and Minor**		
Direct					
2. Thromboembolism	19	4	23	41	*56*
Pulmonary embolism	18	4	22	33	*67*
Cerebral thrombosis	1	0	1	8	*13*
3. Pre-eclampsia/eclampsia*	9	4	13	18	*72*
4. Haemorrhage**	10	0	10	17	*59*
5. Amniotic fluid embolism	6	1	7	17	*41*
6. Early pregnancy	10	1	11	14	*79*
7. Sepsis	12	2	14	18	*78*
8. Anaesthetic	6	0	6	6	*100*
All Direct	**72**	**12**	**84**	**132**	**64**
Late Direct	**6**	**0**	**6**	**11**	**55**
Indirect					
9. Cardiac	15	7	22	48	*46*
10. Other *Indirect*	25	5	30	86	*35*
11. Psychiatric***	3	5	8	19	*42*
12. Cancer****	2	3	5	10	*50*
All Indirect	**45**	**20**	**65**	**163**	**40**

* Including one case of fatty liver.
** Including three cases of uterine rupture.
*** Includes only deaths from suicide and drug overdose classified as *Indirect* .i.e. up to and including six completed postnatal weeks.
**** Includes only deaths from cancer classified as *Indirect*.

Table 1.12
Numbers and percentages of *Direct* and *Indirect* deaths by degree of substandard care;
United Kingdom: 1997-2005.

	Numbers of all deaths with substandard care			Total number of cases by type of death (optimal and substandard care)
	Major	Minor	Major and Minor	
	n (%)	n (%)	n (%)	n (%)
Direct				
1997-99	53 *(50)*	11 *(10)*	**64 *(60)***	106 *(100)*
2000-02	50 (47)	21 (20)	**71 (67)**	106 *(100)*
2003-05	72 (55)	12 (9)	**84 (64)**	132 *(100)*
Indirect				
1997-99	26 (13)	20 (10)	**46 (22)**	205 *(100)*
2000-02	31 (20)	25 (16)	**56 (36)**	155 *(100)*
2003-05	45 (28)	20 (12)	**65 (40)**	163 *(100)*

Northwick Park Hospital

The investigation into the 10 maternal deaths which occurred between 2002 and 2005 at Northwick Park Hospital[6], some of which happened during this triennium and are included here, identified a number of underlying factors many of which are mirrored in this Report. These were a failure of staff to recognise deviation of progress from the norm, delays in seeking medical advice and a lack of a management plan for high-risk women. The investigation also identified issues around communication and team working and a lack of learning lessons from any internal reviews. These, too, are seen in a number of other vignettes in this Report.

Lack of clinical knowledge and skills

Whilst the overall level of sub-optimal care remains broadly similar to the previous Report, for this triennium the assessors were particularly struck by the number of health care professionals who failed to identify and manage common medical conditions or potential emergencies outside their immediate area of expertise. Resuscitation skills were also considered poor in quite a few cases. Although these messages were identified in the last Report, this lack of knowledge and skills seemed more prevalent in this Report.

Identifying and managing maternal collapse

In other cases, the early warning signs of impending maternal collapse also went unrecognised. The early detection of severe illness in mothers remains a challenge to all involved in their care. The relative rarity of such events combined with the normal changes in physiology associated with pregnancy and childbirth compounds the problem. Modified early warning scoring systems have been successfully introduced into other areas of clinical practice and systems appropriately modified for obstetric mothers are discussed in Chapter 19, together with a suggested chart.

These messages are repeated in many Chapters in this Report, as well as under-pinning three of the top ten key recommendations of this Report:

- *Service providers and clinical directors must ensure that all clinical staff caring for pregnant women actually learn from any critical events and serious untoward incidents (SUIs) occurring in their Trust or practice. How this is planned to be achieved should be documented at the end of each incident report form.*

- *All clinical staff must undertake regular, written, documented and audited training for:*

  - *the identification and management of serious medical and mental health conditions which, although unrelated to pregnancy, may affect pregnant women or recently delivered mothers*

  - *the early recognition and management of severely ill pregnant women and impending maternal collapse*

  - *the improvement of basic, immediate and advanced life support skills. A number of courses provide additional training for staff caring for pregnant women*

  - *staff also need to recognise their limitations and to know when, how and whom to call when assistance is required.*

- *Trusts should adopt one of the existing modified early warning scoring systems of the type described in Chapter 19 which will help in the more timely recognition of woman who have, or are developing, critical illness. It is important these charts also be used for pregnant women being cared for outside the obstetric setting for example in gynaecology, Emergency Departments and in Critical Care.*

Lack of senior support

Many women were not seen by an appropriately trained senior or consultant doctor in time, and a few never saw a consultant doctor at all, despite, in some cases, being in a Critical Care unit. The reasons for this were, generally, a lack of awareness of the severity of the woman's illness by more junior or locum maternity staff, both doctors and midwives. In a few cases, but in smaller numbers than in previous Reports, the consultant(s) did not attend in person until too late and relied on giving advice over the phone.

One of the learning points in the midwifery Chapter highlights the problems some midwives faced in either feeling able to refer directly to a consultant or to ask for a second medical option. If a midwife remains worried following a medical opinion, s/he should have no qualms about contacting relevant senior medical personnel directly, such as the obstetric consultant on call.

Poor management of higher risk women

Another recurrent feature of these Reports is the lack of multidisciplinary care for women with pregnancies complicated by existing, or new, medical or psychiatric problems. Whilst there has been a growth of multidisciplinary clinics for the management of the commoner medical conditions that might affect pregnant women such as epilepsy, diabetes and cardiac disease, some of the women who died still did not receive such care. The number of deaths from neurological causes, point to the need to establish more combined neurology or general medical / obstetric clinics in order to improve the care for these pregnant women.

However, even though a far larger proportion of women with medically complex pregnancies than previously had care provided by a multidisciplinary team, they did not always have a clear management plan. As such, some did not receive the additional services they required and others had significant problems when they ran into difficulties and required emergency treatment.

Only a third of the ninety or so substance abusing women known to the Enquiry had care from a combined specialist substance abuse maternity service which would most probably have improved their attendance and the quality of their care. Virtually none of the mothers with problems with substance misuse or other difficulties necessitating their child being taken into care had adequate follow-up in the postnatal period. It seemed as if once the child was removed the care for the mother diminished at the very time when they were at their most vulnerable.

And, regrettably, despite previous recommendations, there was a lack of active follow-up of women who consistently failed to attend antenatal care, particularly for those women with known high risk conditions.

Lack of communication or communication skills

- Poor communications used as a generic term, which covers:

  - poor or non existent team working

  - inappropriate or too short consultations by phone

  - the lack of sharing of relevant information between health professionals, including between GPs and the maternity team

  - poor interpersonal skills.

Deficiencies in all of these areas featured in many cases in this Report, as demonstrated in the vignettes described in each Chapter. Although issues around poor team working and the lack of sharing of information are addressed throughout this Report, there are two new areas of concern; telephone consultations and interpersonal skills, which are discussed further here.

Telephone consultations

Telephone consultations are increasingly being used in medical and midwifery contacts, including the triage of acute illnesses, as was the case for a number of women described in this Report. Whilst broadly acceptable to patients, clinicians also value them but have anxieties about missing serious conditions[7]. There are cases described in this Report which underline this concern. Whilst there is evidence that telephone consultations are shorter than face-to-face consultations[8] there is little evidence about the quality of care. Telephone consultations require an additional range of skills since the importance of verbal cues and focussed history-taking need to compensate for the inability to examine the woman. The BMA recommends that:

> *"Consulting over the telephone should normally be modified to allow the patient greater time to explain their problem. The doctor should also take a detailed history and seek the answers to all the relevant direct questions. There should be a summation and agreement with the caller/patient as to what exactly the problem is that the doctor is attempting to solve. The doctor should explain their assessment and detail the action he intends to take. If it is not possible to safely manage the patient over the telephone, the doctor should arrange a face-to-face consultation and make an appropriate referral.[9]"*

Doctors may need specific training in telephone consultations, an area that is currently neglected in the training and professional development, particularly for GPs[10].

Referral letters; providing complete information

General practitioners (GPs) are the only professionals who have access to a woman's complete medical history and as such are the only health professionals able to provide a complete medical, psychiatric and social history. It is therefore crucial that all relevant information is included in referral letters to enable appropriate and planned care. These Reports have regularly highlighted examples of where inadequate information in referral letters led to adverse consequences for pregnant women and this triennium is no exception. A GP has a responsibility to ensure that any relevant history is conveyed in as much detail as possible to the midwife or obstetric team who will be caring for the woman during pregnancy.

Compassionate care

Although there were many examples of excellent care provided by health care staff this triennium, there were also a few examples of what the assessors described as "breathtaking" "callous" and "dreadful" behaviour on the part of some other health care workers. The following case displays the best and the worst:

> *A pregnant woman of around five months' gestation was admitted with a life threatening illness. In addition, she started to miscarry. The staff nurse on the Early Pregnancy Assessment Unit (EPU) who had seen the woman earlier, suggested that she would need extra care as this was going to be extremely traumatic for everyone concerned. The Critical Care staff thus called the obstetric Senior House Officer (SHO) who declined to attend because s/he had never delivered a baby and the locum obstetric registrar said the staff should "just get on with it as the baby was dead". No midwives could be spared from the delivery suite and the consultant obstetrician was not informed. Eventually the EPU nurse managed to find cover, attended and delivered a dead baby. She then stayed to comfort and support both the woman, her partner and the nursing staff, who had been very traumatised by the events. The mother died shortly afterwards.*

The staff nurse who determinedly cared for this woman despite indifference from her medical colleagues, is to be commended. She took it on herself to obtain senior nursing support to cover her whilst she attended the mother. Not only did she appreciate the need to be present to deliver the baby and comfort and support the parents but she correctly anticipated that this was going to be extremely traumatic for the Critical Care staff as well. However, the "shocking aspects" of this case include indifference, poor decision-making, a lack of consultant input into any aspects of her care and an absence of appropriately trained obstetric staff. One assessor said "I find it extraordinary that an extremely ill pregnant woman can be transferred to Critical Care without being seen either by a consultant in obstetrics or gynaecology, internal medicine or Critical Care." Worse, it appears that there was no critical incident report; neither does an internal review appear to have been carried out so no lessons were learnt. However, perhaps the saddest aspect of all was the attitude of the obstetric registrar who showed no insight or compassion for a terminally ill woman and her partner; they were both losing their baby and the mother was losing her life.

Critical incident reports and internal reviews

The above vignette highlights another area of poor practice, that of not providing a critical incident report or undertaking an internal review after any serious untoward incident, or death. This was not the only case. Without such reviews lessons cannot be learnt and practice cannot improve.

Even when the reviews were carried out their quality was extremely variable. Although there were many examples of very good internal reviews following a maternal death, this was not always the case. It was also not always evident who was involved in such reviews. In some cases it was clear the review only involved those directly associated with the woman's care and lessons may not have been widely disseminated to others in the maternity service. If lessons are to be learnt it is important that all clinical staff are aware of the findings of such reviews, particularly those who may not have ready access e.g. GPs and community midwives. The Supervisor of Midwives network is an opportunity to disseminate findings to midwives.

Underlying health status

Age

Maternal mortality is closely associated with mothers' ages, as shown in Table 1.13. The highest rates are among the oldest women, although differentials have changed over time and *Indirect* deaths have made an increasing contribution. The linear trend by age was statistically significant in 2003-2005. As discussed in the Annex to this Chapter the average age at childbirth has risen, with increases in the proportions of women who have babies in their thirties and forties. In the 2003-05 triennium, the youngest mother who died was a girl of 14 and the oldest was 46 years of age.

Table 1.13
Total number of *Direct* and *Indirect* deaths age of the women who died and rate per 100,000 maternities;
United Kingdom: 1985-2005*.

	Age (years)						Not stated	All ages
	Under 20	20-24	25-29	30-34	35-39	40 and over		
Numbers								
1985-87	15	47	53	60	35	13	0	223
1988-90	17	38	74	57	31	18	3	238
1991-93	7	30	87	61	36	7	1	229
1994-96	15	40	71	70	53	11	8	268
1997-99	19	34	60	66	50	13	0	242
2000-02	16	30	70	79	47	19	0	261
2003-05	15	39	66	91	64	20	0	295
Rates per 100,000 maternities								
1985-87	7.6	7.1	6.7	13.6	22.8	48.4		9.8
1988-90	8.8	6.0	8.9	11.5	18.7	57.4		10.1
1991-93	4.2	5.5	10.6	10.9	19.1	20.6		9.9
1994-96	10.2	9.0	9.6	11.5	24.1	29.1		12.2
1997-99	11.7	8.9	9.3	10.5	19.2	29.0		11.4
2000-02	10.6	8.2	13.0	13.2	16.2	35.6		13.1
2003-05	9.9	9.8	12.4	14.5	19.1	29.4		14.0

* Chi squared for trend = 21.0, p = 0.00000.

Parity

Just under half of the 64 women who died from *Direct* and the 30 who died from *Coincidental* causes were primiparous, compared to 34% of the 55 women who died from *Indirect* causes. Twenty women who died of *Direct* or *Indirect* causes had four or more previous live births; one having eleven previous living children. Maternal mortality rates by parity have not been estimated for this triennium. Parity is recorded at birth registration only for births within marriage.

Multiple pregnancies

Eleven women who died had twin pregnancies; six deaths were due to *Direct* or *Late Direct* causes and five were *Indirect*. Four other mothers of twins died of *Late Coincidental* causes. Table 1.14 shows that in 2003-05 the difference between the rates for multiple and singleton maternities was greater than would be expected by chance and the risk of death associated with multiple birth varies around twice that associated with singleton birth.

Table 1.14
Direct (including *Late Direct*) and *Indirect* deaths and rates per 100,000 maternities for singleton and multiple births; United Kingdom: 1997-2005.

	Direct and *Indirect* deaths				Relative risk of death associated with multiple birth			Maternities
	Numbers	Rate	95 per cent CI (for rate)		Relative risk	95 per cent CI (for risk)		Numbers
Singleton								
1997-99	234	11.17	9.83	12.70	1.0			2,093,965
2000-02	255	12.96	11.46	14.65	1.0			1,967,834
2003-05	295	14.17	12.64	15.88	1.0			2,082,429
Multiple								
1997-99	8	26.16	13.26	51.62	2.3	1.2	4.7	30,578
2000-02	6	20.24	9.28	44.17	1.6	0.7	3.5	29,638
2003-05	11	34.84	19.45	62.38	2.5	1.4	4.5	31,575

Assisted conception

As Table 1.15 shows, twelve women were known to have undergone In-Vitro Fertilisation (IVF) for infertility, three resulting in a multiple pregnancy. Eight of the deaths were from *Direct* causes, four of which were due to ovarian hyperstimulation syndrome (OHSS). The other four *Direct* deaths were from sepsis, embolism and bleeding and were not related to IVF. There was one *Indirect* and three *Late* deaths from unrelated causes.

The numbers of treatment cycles shown in Table 1.15 come from a reanalysis of data by the Human Fertilisation and Fertilisation Authority (HFEA)[11] based on year of procedure. These differ from analyses in previous Reports which were based on IVF data which were published on a financial year basis. The data in Table 1.15 also relate to procedures undertaken in clinics in the United Kingdom during a calendar year, rather than maternities in the year to women who had undergone assisted conception. There are other uncertainties in the data as some of the women were resident outside the United Kingdom and may have returned home to give birth. Information about this has not been consistently recorded in the records sent by clinics to the Human Fertilisation and Embryology Authority. There are also anecdotal accounts of United Kingdom residents having assisted conception abroad, but no data on the subject.

Table 1.15
Maternal deaths and rates per 100,000 assisted reproductive technology (ART) procedures, including IVF; United Kingdom: 1997-2005.

	Deaths				Numbers of treatment cycles
	Number	Rate	95 per cent CI		
1997-99	20	19.17	12.41	29.61	104,320
2000-02	8	7.32	3.71	14.44	109,308
2003-05	12	10.08	5.76	17.61	119,080

* Source Human Fertilisation and Embryology Authority[11].

Ovarian hyperstimulation syndrome (OHSS)

Of the four known deaths from OHSS assessed in this triennium, three women were pregnant and the fourth had undergone ovarian hyperstimulation and intrauterine insemination although there are conflicting reports about whether or not her pregnancy test was positive at the time of her death. The four women died from different sequelae of OHSS and their deaths are counted in the Chapters relating to the eventual cause of death. The general lessons are briefly discussed here.

Two of these women were known to have had OHSS in the past but had subsequent repeated IVF cycles with many eggs being retrieved in the final cycle, indicating a risk of OHSS. Despite this, embryo transfer was carried out. One of these women was found unconscious a few weeks later and her brain scan showed a large cerebral infarct. There was delay in recognising her OHSS and in getting the brain scan. Earlier recognition of OHSS might have allowed effective treatment with fluids and thromboprophylaxis. The other woman with a known past history of OHSS also had a large number of eggs collected and embryo transfer performed. She subsequently developed abdominal pain, collapsed within a few weeks of the procedure and died of thromboembolism. In both cases embryo transfer should not have been performed because of the high risk of OHSS. Neither of these women received thromboprophylaxis, nor did a woman who died of pulmonary embolism associated with OHSS or a woman who was admitted with OHSS and deteriorated before being transferred to Critical Care. The last woman's autopsy showed patchy infarction throughout the body. Women admitted to hospital with severe OHSS should receive thromboprophylaxis[12].

In view of the four deaths from OHSS, which would have gone unnoticed unless considered by this Enquiry, in future this Enquiry will seek to assess all deaths from OHSS and others associated with IVF and other Assisted Reproduction Technology procedures. This is because these deaths occurred as a direct result of interventions to aid conception and pregnancy.

Obesity

The National Institute for Health and Clinical Excellence (NICE) has recommended that the Body Mass Index (BMI) which is the person's weight in kilograms divided by the square of their height in metres (kg/m^2), is used to classify obesity[13]. Box 1.3 shows how it has been classified by NICE and the terms widely used elsewhere, for example in the Health Survey for England[14].

Box 1.3 Classifications of Body Mass Index[13]		
Body Mass Index, kg/m^2	**NICE classification[13]**	**Body Mass Index classification[14]**
Under 18.5		Underweight
18.5-24.9	Healthy weight	Normal
25.0-29.9	Overweight	Overweight
30.0-34.9	Obesity I	Obese
35.0-39.9	Obesity II	
40 or over	Obesity III	Morbidly obese

Obesity in pregnancy is usually defined as a Body Mass Index of 30 or greater at booking. In the UK there are no national statistics about the prevalence of obesity in pregnancy. The Health Survey for England has shown a steady increase among the general population of childbearing age since the mid 1990s and a study of pregnant women in Glasgow showed a significant increase over a recent decade[15]. Prevalence figures in cross-sectional research studies have varied from 11% to 20%[14, 16, 17].

Obesity in pregnancy is associated with increased risks of complications for both mother and baby and a summary of these is given in Box 1.4. Obese women are more likely than non-obese women to experience spontaneous first trimester miscarriage[18] and to develop gestational diabetes[19], pre-eclampsia[18] and thromboembolism during pregnancy[15]. In this triennium, 14 (nearly half) of the 31 women with a known BMI who died of a thromboembolic event were obese.

Women with obesity in pregnancy also have higher rates of induction of labour, caesarean section and postpartum haemorrhage[15,20] and there is an increased risk of post-caesarean wound infection[21].

There is also evidence that babies of obese women have significantly increased risks of adverse outcomes, including fetal congenital anomaly, prematurity, stillbirth and neonatal death[22-27].

Box 1.4
Risks related to obesity in pregnancy

For the mother
Increased risks include

- Maternal death or severe morbidity

- Cardiac disease

- Spontaneous first trimester and recurrent miscarriage

- Pre-eclampsia

- Gestational diabetes

- Thromboembolism

- Post caesarean wound infection

- Infection from other causes

- Post partum haemorrhage

- Low breast feeding rates.

For the baby
Increased risks include

- Stillbirth and neonatal death

- Congenital abnormalities

- Prematurity.

The obese women who died

From the notes available to the Enquiry, the BMI was available for all but 18 of the women who died after 22 weeks' gestation from *Direct* or *Indirect* causes. It was not recorded for 46 women who died earlier than this either due to complications in early pregnancy such as ectopic pregnancies and miscarriages, or following a termination of pregnancy.

As can be seen from Table 1.16, 15% of women who died from *Direct* or *Indirect* causes and who had a BMI recorded had BMIs of 35 or over, with half of these having BMIs exceeding 40. A further 12% of women had BMIs in the range 30-34 and and 24% had BMIs of 25-29. In all, 27% of these women had BMIs of 30 or more and overall 52% had BMIs of 25 or more.

The causes of death for overweight or obese women are shown in Table 1.17.

Table 1.16
Body Mass Index by *Direct* and *Indirect* maternal death for women who had a BMI recorded;
United Kingdom: 2003-05.

	BMI						Total with known BMI		Total with BMI of 25 or over		Not stated or recorded
	Less than 20	20-24	25-29	30-34	35-39	40 or over					
	n (%)	n (%)	n (%)	n (%)	n (%)	n (%)	n (%)		n (%)		
Direct	9 (9)	36 (36)	23 (23)	12 (12)	9 (9)	10 (10)	**99 (100)**		54 (55)		33
Indirect	17 (13)	50 (38)	32 (24)	16 (12)	8 (6)	9 (7)	**132 (100)**		65 (49)		31
Total	26 (11)	86 (37)	55 (24)	28 (12)	17 (7)	19 (8)	**231 (100)**		119 (52)		64

Table 1.17
Numbers of maternal deaths from *Direct* and *Indirect* causes by BMI and percentages overweight or obese; United Kingdom: 2003-05.

BMI	Less than 20	20-24	25-29	30-34	35-39	40-60	Total with BMI 25 or over	Total number with known BMI	Not stated or recorded
	n	n	n	n	n	n	n (%)	n (%)	
Direct									
Thromboembolism	3	8	6	6	2	6	20 (65)	31 (100)	10
Pre-clampsia / eclampsia	1	8	6	0	1	2	9 (50)	18 (100)	1
Haemorrhage	2	6	2	3	2	0	7 (47)	15 (100)	2
AFE	2	6	4	0	2	0	6 (43)	14 (100)	3
Early pregnancy	0	4	0	1	1	0	2 (33)	6 (100)	8
Sepsis	1	2	5	2	0	1	8 (73)	11 (100)	7
Anaesthetic	0	2	0	0	1	1	2 (50)	4 (100)	2
All *Direct*	9	36	23	12	9	10	54 (55)	99 (100)	33
Indirect									
Cardiac	4	9	14	6	4	5	29 (69)	42 (100)	6
Other Indirect	8	35	12	10	4	1	27 (39)	70 (100)	17
Psychiatric	3	4	4	0	0	2	6 (46)	13 (100)	5
Malignancies	2	2	2	0	0	1	3 (43)	7 (100)	3
All *Indirect*	17	50	32	16	8	9	65 (49)	132 (100)	31
All	26	86	55	28	17	19	119 (52)	231 (100)	64

Six women who died from *Direct* or *Indirect* causes had a BMI greater than 45 and for two it exceeded 60. Such severe obesity not only compromises a mother's underlying general health but also causes logistical problems. Resuscitation was delayed in one case because the ambulance services were unable to remove the woman from her house and for another woman, a lack of suitably sized blood pressure cuffs led to delayed diagnosis of pre-eclampsia. In others, the mothers size masked clinical symptoms or caused problems with access at operation. And, as in previous Reports, there were a few cases where caesarean sections had to be performed on two beds pushed together as the weight of the woman exceeded the maximum safe weight for the operating table.

The fact that obesity appears to carry a greater risk of death will probably come as no surprise to those who have viewed the increasing weight of the maternity population with concern. However, the magnitude of this risk means that obesity represents one of the greatest and growing overall threats to the childbearing population of the UK. The predominance of obese women among those who died from thromboembolism, sepsis and cardiac disease means that early multidisciplinary planning regarding mode of delivery and use of thromboprophylaxis for these women is essential.

Pre-pregnancy counselling and weight loss, together with wider public health messages about optimum weight should help to reduce the number of obese women who become pregnant.

There are currently no national statistics on the prevalence of maternal obesity and only limited information regarding the provision of maternity services for obese women in the UK[28]. Whilst there are National Institute for Health and Clinical Excellence (NICE) guidelines for the management of obesity in children and adults[13], there is no specific guideline for the management of obesity in pregnancy; a key recommendation in this Report.

CEMACH is developing a national programme on obesity in pregnancy to commence in 2008, which will include a survey of the provision of maternity services for obese women, development of consensus standards, information on national and regional prevalence figures and pregnancy outcomes, and an audit of clinical care. The UK Obstetric Surveillance System (UKOSS) is also planning to collect information on the most morbidly obese pregnant women.

Smoking

The 2005 Infant Feeding Survey[29] found that 33% of all women in the United Kingdom smoked at some time in the year before or during pregnancy. These included 16% who smoked before pregnancy but gave up, mainly on confirmation of pregnancy and 17% who smoked throughout pregnancy. This was a slight decrease from 2000 when 35% smoked at some time in the year before pregnancy and 20% smoked during pregnancy.

The percentage who smoked at some time in the year before pregnancy ranged from 20% of women in managerial and professional occupations to 48% of those in routine and manual occupations and 35% of those who had never worked. Linked to this were differences by age. The percentage of women smoking before or during pregnancy ranged from 68% of women aged under 20 to 21% of those aged 35 or over.

A smoking history was not documented for 67% of the women who died which makes further analysis of the increased contribution of smoking in pregnancy to maternal mortality impossible. It also highlights the need for better awareness amongst health professionals as well as better record keeping.

Vulnerability

Ethnicity

The ethnic groups of all women who died were reported to the Enquiry, but the ethnic group of mothers in general is recorded only in England and not in the other countries of the United Kingdom. Since 1995, ethnic group information has been recorded in the Hospital Maternity Episode Statistics (HES) System for England, but coverage is still not complete. By the financial year 2004-05, ethnic group was recorded for 75% of deliveries in England for the years covered by this Report. A comparison of maternity HES data for 2000-01 with data about children under the age of one recorded in the 2001 census showed that the ethnic group distribution in HES delivery data was broadly comparable as long as maternities to women whose ethnic group was not stated are grouped with those to women whose ethnic group was recorded as White[30]. Maternity HES data for the financial years 2003-04 and 2004-05 have been grossed up to the total numbers of registered maternities in England in the 2003-05 triennium to produce the estimated maternities in Table 1.18. These have been used to produce estimated mortality rates and relative risks by ethnic group for England.

Table 1.18
Numbers and estimated rates of maternal death by type and ethnic group per 100,000 maternities;
England only: 2003-05.

Ethnic group	Direct deaths	Indirect deaths	Total Direct and Indirect deaths						Estimated number of maternities
	Numbers	Numbers	Numbers	Rate	95 per cent CI for rate		Relative risk compared with white	95 per cent CI for relative risk	
White	71	91	162	11.1	9.5	12.9	1.0	- -	1,462,537
Mixed	0	1	1	5.2	0.9	29.5	0.5	0.1 3.4	19,232
Black African	15	15	30	62.4	43.7	89.0	5.6	3.8 8.3	48,103
Black Caribbean	7	2	9	41.1	21.6	78.1	3.7	1.9 7.3	21,910
Indian	2	7	9	20.3	10.7	38.6	1.9	0.9 3.6	44,288
Pakistani	3	3	6	9.2	4.1	20.1	0.8	0.4 1.9	64,993
Bangladeshi	3	3	6	23.6	10.8	51.4	2.1	0.9 4.8	25,455
Chinese and other Asian	1	0	1	14.0	2.5	79.2	1.3	0.2 9.0	7,146
Middle east	4	3	7	32.0	15.5	66.1	2.9	1.4 6.2	21,845
Other	1	1	2	28.0	7.7	10.2	2.5	0.6 10.2	7,146
Total	**107**	**126**	**233**	**13.5**	**11.9**	**15.4**			**1,722,655**

These rates and relative risks are based on small numbers and the coding of ethnicity may be problematic so they should be interpreted with caution. Nevertheless, analysis of the English data suggests that for Black African women and, to a lesser extent Black Caribbean and Middle Eastern women, the mortality rate is significantly higher than that for White women. This may not only reflect the cultural factors implied in ethnicity but their social circumstances and the fact that some of them may have recently migrated to the United Kingdom under less than optimal circumstances. Table 1.19 shows the main causes of death by ethnic group, and Table 1.20 their access to care.

Table 1.19
Direct and *Indirect* maternal deaths by major ethnic group; England: 2003-05.

	White	Black African	Black Caribbean	Indian	Pakistani	Bangla-deshi	Chinese and Asian	Middle Eastern	Other	Not stated	Total
Direct											
Thromboembolism	30	3	3	0	2	0	1	1	1	0	41
Pre-eclampsia/ eclampsia	12	2	2	0	0	1	1	1	0	0	19
Haemorrhage	7	2	1	1	2	1	1	1	1	0	17
AFE	11	4	0	1	0	1	0	0	0	0	17
Early pregnancy	12	2	0	0	0	0	0	0	0	0	14
Sepsis	14	3	1	0	0	0	0	0	0	0	18
Anaesthetic	5	0	0	0	0	0	1	0	0	0	6
All Direct	**91**	**16**	**7**	**2**	**4**	**3**	**4**	**3**	**2**	**0**	**132**
Indirect											
Cardiac	33	6	1	4	0	1	2	0	1	0	48
Other *Indirect*	59	10	1	3	3	4	3	2	1	1	87
Psychiatric *Indirect*	16	2	0	0	0	0	0	0	0	0	18
Indirect malignancies	8	1	0	1	0	0	0	0	0	0	10
All Indirect	**116**	**19**	**2**	**8**	**3**	**5**	**5**	**2**	**2**	**1**	**163**
Total	**207**	**35**	**9**	**10**	**7**	**8**	**9**	**5**	**4**	**1**	**295**

Table 1.20
Characteristics of antenatal care sought by pregnant or recently delivered women by ethnic group and knowledge of English. Deaths from *Direct* and *Indirect* causes after 12 weeks or more weeks of gestation; United Kingdom: 2003-05.

Ethnic group	Late or non attenders for antenatal care (ANC)				Number of deaths after 12 or more weeks of gestation	
	Booked 22 weeks or missed more than four visits	No ANC	Subtotal			
	n	n	n	(%)	n	(%)
White	25	6	31	(17)	183	(100)
Black African	9	3	12	(40)	30	(100)
Black Caribbean	3	1	4	(57)	7	(100)
Indian	1	0	1	(11)	9	(100)
Pakistani	0	0	0	(0)	5	(100)
Bangladeshi	0	1	1	(13)	8	(100)
Chinese and Asian	1	0	1	(11)	9	(100)
Middle Eastern	1	0	1	(25)	4	(100)
Other	0	0	0	(0)	3	(100)
Total	**40**	**11**	**51**	**(20)**	**258**	**(100)**
Women who did not speak English	**6**	**3**	**9**	**(35)**	**26**	**(100)**

Newly arrived migrants, refugees and asylum seeking women

Women who have recently arrived into the UK, whatever their immigration status, bring new challenges for maternity services, some of which are seen in the UK for the first time in this Report. The key issues include poor overall health status, underlying and possible unrecognised medical conditions including congenital cardiac disease, and, increasingly HIV/AIDS and TB, all of which are classified as maternal deaths. Some suffered the consequences of genital mutilation. Others suffered the psychological and medical effects of fleeing war torn countries; four women raped by soldiers were too ashamed to admit to being pregnant or to seek maternity care on arrival in the UK. One other woman, who spoke no English, was kidnapped, raped and trafficked into the country to work as a prostitute then left on the street when her pregnancy became too advanced. Women who have been trafficked have fears about their status, language difficulties and do not know where to turn for help. Trafficked women also feel ashamed of being forced into sex work which transgresses their own cultural values and beliefs and make it difficult for them to reveal their situation[31].

African migrant women

Of the 35 Black African women who suffered a maternal death, 16 died from *Direct* and 19 from *Indirect* causes, as shown in Table 1.21. Only four of the Black African women were UK citizens. Of the remaining 31, most were either recently arrived new immigrants, refugees or asylum seekers. In some cases their immigration status was not clear so these women are grouped together as "new arrivals". This is more than double the number of cases in the last Report. There were an additional five women who appeared to have come to the UK to have NHS care for their pregnancy and childbirth. A further seven Black African women died within a year of childbirth, the majority from *Late Indirect* causes.

Apart from the five women who appeared to have come late in pregnancy expressly to have their baby in the UK, who came mainly from Nigeria, the African countries with the greatest representation of women were Somalia and Ethiopia, but a wide range of other countries were also represented including, for the first time, Francophone African countries.

Female Genital Cutting or Mutilation (FGC/M)

Although it is illegal to perform female circumcision, a procedure more commonly known as Female Genital Cutting (FGC[iv]) or Mutilation (FGC/M), in the UK it is likely that its prevalence amongst the pregnant population is increasing[32]. This is largely due to inward migration from countries or cultures where it is still routine practice, despite almost universal international condemnation at Government level. As well as being illegal to perform it in the UK, it is also illegal to perform it in any other country on UK citizens or permanent residents.

Estimates of prevalence in England and Wales have been derived by analysing births in England and Wales by the mother's country of birth and applying estimates based on surveys to the prevalence of FGC/M in the country of origin. The estimated percentages of all maternities in England and Wales which were to women with FGC/M increased from 1.06 per cent in 2001 to 1.43 per cent in 2004. The latest study showed considerable geographical variation. In some major cities and other conurbations with large populations of Somali or Kenyan women, the estimated percentages of maternities affected by FGC/M had already exceeded two per cent by 2004[28].

FGC can affect women's pregnancies in a number of ways[33]. This Report considered the deaths of at least four women known to have been cut in this way, three of whom did not disclose their condition until very late in pregnancy or in early labour. For one woman, her late disclosure may have directly contributed to her death following an unnecessary caesarean section because staff were not aware that a corrective procedure could have been performed during her antenatal period. For another, her condition was not apparent until she was first examined in established labour yet the obstetrician was not informed until her labour stalled some hours later. There are a growing number and variety of educational materials and sources of help available for both health professionals and women themselves.

In response to the increasing prevalence of women living with FGC/M in the UK, there are an increasing number of midwives and obstetricians and specialist services able to advise, help and support pregnant women living with FGC/M. As a result, women from counties where this is likely to be practiced should be sensitively asked about this during pregnancy and management plans agreed during the antenatal period.

[iv]Women who have been cut generally do not like the term mutilation and prefer to the practice as genital cutting.

Other migrant women

Although Black African women formed the majority of recently arrived women who died from maternal causes, there were also increases in, or lessons to be learnt from, other groups of new migrants.

Women who contract to marry UK men

Previous Reports have commented on how some women who contract to marry UK men in order to build a better life for themselves, who are sometimes demeaningly referred to as "mail order" brides, died because they were not helped by their husbands to seek the care they needed once pregnant. Language difficulties and cultural and geographical isolation meant they were also probably unaware of the maternity services available and where and how to access them. In this triennium at least one other such woman appears to have died for the same reasons. In previous Reports the majority of these women came from Thailand, but in this triennium three Vietnamese women also died.

New countries of the European Union (EU)

There were several maternal deaths of women who had recently arrived from countries newly admitted to the European Union. This reflects the experiences of the maternity services in general who report rising numbers of women from the expanded EU, many of whom do not speak English. As there are now 49 countries in Europe, with some of the best and poorest maternal health outcomes in the world, providing translation services is an ever increasing challenge. For the first time in this Report, there were a few maternal deaths in women from Turkey, an EU accession country.

"Health tourism"

Deaths amongst pregnant women who had specifically travelled to the UK for NHS health care is a new category for this Enquiry. There were at least five cases where women with pre-existing or past medical or obstetric complications came to the UK for NHS treatment. From the case details provided it is also possible six other women, who claimed to be refugees, may have entered the UK in order to obtain medical assistance. One European holiday maker, early in pregnancy, died of a pulmonary embolism shortly after her arrival.

Translation

Thirty-four women who died from maternal causes, another six who died from *Coincidental* causes, and eight who died some months after childbirth spoke little or no English. Very few had access to translation services and in most cases family members or friends were used as interpreters. Several of these were the woman's own children, who may have been the only family members who could speak English. The use of family members or friends as translators causes concern because:

- The woman may be too embarassed to seek help for intimate concerns or discuss her past history

- It is not clear how much correct information was conveyed to the woman as the person who was interpreting did not have a good grasp of the language, or may have withheld information. In some cases the woman's pre-existing medical condition meant she was at considerable risk

- In some cases the translator was a perpetrator of domestic abuse against his partner, thus not enabling her to ask for advice or help

- It is not appropriate for a child to translate intimate details about his or her mother and unfair on both the woman and child.

Cultural practices and /or attitudes of male partners

Some women who died seemed to have been denied access to care because of cultural beliefs and practices where the responsibility for decision-making fell to their husbands or other family members. This was especially true for women who could not speak English. For example:

> *A pregnant woman who spoke no English had a port of arrival chest x-ray which was indicative of cardiac disease. Her English speaking husband was told by the port authorities that she*

was ill and he should take her to a doctor immediately. They had no means of communicating this directly to the woman who had, in any event, just landed in a strange airport in a distant country. Her husband did not tell her she was ill and she had no antenatal care at all. Her first contact with maternity services was when she was admitted in labour. She died of a post partum haemorrhage apparently still unaware of her possible cardiac disease.

For others, the actions of their partner may have been fatal:

> *Another non-English speaking woman had recurrent vaginal bleeding and was known to have a cervical fibroid. Heavy bleeding occurred in her second trimester and, although her husband said he would take her to hospital, he didn't. She collapsed at home the next day and required emergency admission. At this point she was unconscious, her wrists were found to have been grazed and bandaged, her haemoglobin was 7g and there was an intrauterine death. At hysterotomy a partially organised retroplacental clot was found. She had severe disseminated intravascular coagulation (DIC) and a CT scan showed contusions associated with small undisplaced fractures of her temporal and frontal bones. She died despite neurosurgical intervention for subdural haematoma.*

In the autopsy report there was no mention of her wrist injuries, no reference to the DIC or its possible causes, and no examination of her skull. The report then identified a swollen brain with no signs of intracranial pressure.

There were instances when both partners and families were obstructive:

> *An extremely young, underage, bride who appears to have been brought into the country under false pretences became pregnant but had no antenatal care. She spoke no English and was not allowed out of her parents' in-laws' house. Her 'husband' eventually took her to see the GP in mid pregnancy, moribund from tuberculosis. Her in-laws lied about her age and showed no concern for her obvious ill-health or pregnancy and her "husband" told the GP he was not at all interested in obtaining antenatal care but wanted her treated because she was now too ill for sex. She died, in a caring hospital, alone in a strange country, only a few days later.*

Socio-economic classification and employment

Since 2001, the National Statistics Socio-Economic Classification (NS SEC) has been used to classify social class in all official statistics in the United Kingdom. Because women's occupations are missing from so many birth registration records, the NS SEC of the women's husband or partner derived from his occupational code, is used in published tabulations of birth statistics for England and Wales. These are the data available for use as denominators for stillbirth, infant and maternal mortality rates. Therefore in order to calculate maternal mortality rates by NS SEC, the women's husbands' or partners' occupations, where available, were used, irrespective of whether the woman's own occupations were recorded. As numbers were small, the 3-class version of NS SEC was used. Where women were identified from their case notes as having no partner, this may have not been clear cut. For these women, the denominator used was sole registration by the mother alone, but it cannot be guaranteed that these women's births would have been sole registrations had they survived.

Table 1.21
Numbers of maternal deaths by National Statistics Socio-Economic Classification (NS SEC) and rates per 100,000 estimated maternities; England and Wales: 2003-05.

Social class of husband or partner and partnership status	Direct	Indirect	Direct and indirect	Rate	95 per cent CI for rate		Relative risk	95 per cent CI for relative risk		Estimated maternities*
	n	n	n (%)	Rate						
				Compared with managerial and professional						
Managerial and professional	27	25	52 (19)	8.8	6.7	11.5	1.0			590,780
Intermediate	16	20	36 (13)	9.0	6.5	12.4	1.0	0.7	1.6	401,520
Routine and manual	29	35	64 (23)	9.7	7.6	12.4	1.1	0.8	1.6	659,310
				Compared with women with employed partners						
All employed	72	80	152 (55)	9.2	7.8	10.8	1.0			1,651,610
Unemployed, unclassifiable or not stated	31	39	70 (26)	68.5	54.2	86.6	7.4	5.6	9.9	102,150
All women with partners	103	119	222 (81)	12.7	11.1	14.4				1,753,760
Women without partners	20	32	52 (19)	38.6	29.4	50.6	4.2	3.1	5.7	134,743
Employed	11	4	15 (5)							
Unemployed	9	28	37 (14)							
All women	123	151	274 (100)	14.5	12.9	16.3				1,888,487

*Numbers of maternities by class are estimated from a 10 per cent sample and so do not necessarily add up to the total for all women.

For women with a husband or partner in employment, the social class differences in mortality were small and were no bigger than would be expected by chance, as shown in Table 1.21. In contrast, the rate for women whose partners were unemployed or whose occupations were unclassifiable was over seven times higher than that for all women with partners in employment. This group of women made up just over a quarter of the women in England and Wales who died, while only 55 per cent had partners in employment. Nearly a fifth of the women appeared to have no partner. Based on the tentative assumptions in the previous paragraph, their mortality rate was over four times that of women who had partners in employment.

Table 1.22 shows access to antenatal care by employment and partnership status.

Table 1.22

Characteristics of the antenatal care sought by pregnant or recently delivered women by employment and partnership. *Direct* and *Indirect* causes and gestation of 12 weeks of more; United Kingdom: 2003-05.

Employment and relationship	Late or non attenders for antenatal care (ANC)				Number of deaths after 12 or more weeks of gestation	
	Booked after 22 weeks or missed more than four visits	No ANC	Subtotal			
	n	n	n	(%)	n	(%)
In partnership with at least one partner in employment	8	1	9	(5)	165	(100)
In partnership with neither partner in employment	10	4	14	(47)	30	(100)
Single woman in employment	0	0	0	(0)	14	(100)
Single woman unemployed	16	3	19	(56)	34	(100)
Total	**34**	**8**	**42**	**(17)**	**243**	**(100)**

Area deprivation scores

As in the last Report, maternal deaths that occurred to residents of England have been analysed using the English Indices of Multiple Deprivation 2004. This is a score based on data for each small local area, known as a super output area, within electoral wards in England[v]. Postcodes are used to code addresses to super output areas and derive the scores. These are then ranked in to order and according to the score, and then grouped into quintiles. Of the 235 *Direct* and *Indirect* maternal deaths of women resident in England, 211 had a valid postcode at the time of death, and could therefore be included in the analysis in Table 1.23. Mortality rates and confidence intervals for each quintile are shown in Figure 1.3 and Table 1.23. This shows a clear gradient between the mortality rates for the least and most deprived areas and that mortality rates in the most deprived quintile were around five times higher than in the least deprived quintile. This was true for both *Direct* and *Indirect* causes of death independently.

Figure 1.3: *Direct* and *Indirect* maternal mortality rates and 95 per cent confidence intervals by deprivation quintile of place of residence; England: 2003-05.

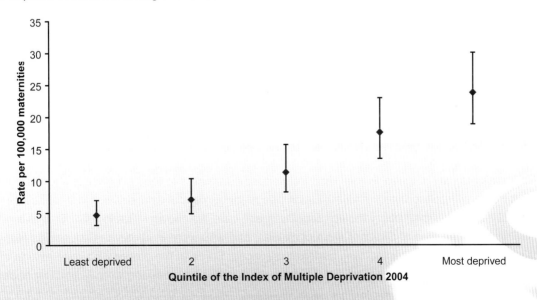

[v] See www.odpm.gov.uk/stellent/groups/odpm_urbanpolicy/documents/page/odpm_urbpol_029534.pdf

Table 1.23
Direct and *Indirect* deaths, rates per 100,000 maternities and relative risks by quintiles of place of residence of the Index of Multiple Deprivation 2004; England: 2003-05.

Quintile	Number	Rate	95 per cent CI for rate		Relative risk	95 per cent CI for relative risk		Number of maternities
Direct								
Least deprived (1)	10	2.0	1.1	3.8	1.0	-	-	490,102
2	17	4.5	2.8	7.2	2.2	1.0	4.8	378,896
3	20	6.2	4.0	9.5	3.0	1.4	6.4	325,057
4	24	8.0	5.4	11.9	3.9	1.9	8.2	301,043
Most deprived (5)	28	9.4	6.5	13.6	4.6	2.2	9.5	297,908
All *Direct*	**99**	**5.5**	**4.5**	**6.7**				**1,793,006**
Indirect								
Least deprived (1)	13	2.7	1.6	4.5	1.0	-	-	490,102
2	10	2.6	1.4	4.9	1.0	0.4	2.3	378,896
3	17	5.2	3.3	8.4	2.0	1.0	4.1	325,057
4	29	9.6	6.7	13.8	3.6	1.9	7.0	301,043
Most deprived (5)	43	14.4	10.7	19.4	5.4	2.9	10.1	297,908
All *Indirect*	**112**	**6.2**	**5.2**	**7.5**				**1,793,006**
Direct and Indirect								
Least deprived (1)	23	4.7	3.1	7.0	1.0	-	-	490,102
2	27	7.1	4.9	10.4	1.5	0.9	2.7	378,896
3	37	11.4	8.3	15.7	2.4	1.4	4.1	325,057
4	53	17.6	13.5	23.0	3.8	2.3	6.1	301,043
Most deprived (5)	71	23.8	18.9	30.1	5.1	3.2	8.1	297,908
All	**211**	**11.8**	**10.3**	**13.5**				**1,793,006**

Domestic abuse

Chapter 13 addresses the general issue of domestic abuse in pregnancy and how it affected the 70 women who were abused and whose deaths were considered by this Enquiry. For 19 women this abuse was fatal. The majority of the woman who suffered abuse during pregnancy had reported this to a maternity health professional. No woman appeared to have been routinely asked about abuse, a recent recommendation in these Reports, although the new national programme in England is only just being introduced. Eight women were living in a refuge having fled from abuse at home.

Even though the majority of these women died from causes unrelated to their pregnancy, there are lessons to be learnt from them concerning the identification and management of women living with abuse as well as the impact it is has on their ability to seek regular health care, as shown in Table 1.24. This shows that 81% of the women who died of *Direct* or *Indirect* causes, and who were in abusive relationships found it difficult to access or maintain contact with maternity services. Some of the others who were able to attend regularly had domineering partners who disrupted the relationship between the woman and her health care provider. Further, 77% of these women were in contact with their local social services and the child protection services were involved with 64% of the mothers and their children.

Table 1.24
Characteristics of the antenatal care sought by pregnant or recently delivered women who were murdered or known to be suffering domestic abuse; United Kingdom: 2003-05.

Type of death	Death in early pregnancy	Late or non attenders for antenatal care (ANC)			Total number of deaths of women*
		Booked after 22 weeks or missed more than four visits	No ANC	Subtotal	
	n	n	n	n (%)	n (%)
Direct	3	0	0	3 (75)	4 (100)
Indirect	1	6	3	10 (83)	12 (100)
All	**4**	**6**	**3**	**13 (81)**	**16 (100)**
Coincidental	2	4	3	9 (69)	13 (100)
Late deaths	0	15	2	17 (41)	41 (100)
Total	**6**	**25**	**8**	**39 (56)**	**70 (100)**

* Total number of deaths of women who were murdered or known to be suffering domestic abuse same as Table 13.1.

Child protection issues

Sixty-nine of the women whose deaths were reviewed this triennium were known to social services and /or child protection services (CPS), the vast majority of whom had previous children in care. Thirty women died from complications related to their pregnancy, i.e. from *Direct* or *Indirect* conditions, and half of the women who were murdered were also known by the CPS and/or social services.

As shown in Table 1.25, more than 80% of the women who died from *Direct* or *Indirect* did not seek care at all, booked late or failed to maintain regular contact with the maternity services, in the main because of fear that their unborn child might be removed at birth.

In forty-one cases a child protection case conference was held, 23 after the removal of the infant into care. Five women committed suicide shortly before or after their child's case conference and another 18 women died from an apparent accidental overdose of a drug of abuse. Many of these women were late in booking and often defaulted from maternity care because of fear of social services involvement. In most cases, it appears that upon removal of the child the level of support and care from both maternity and social services fell or ceased. For example, in two such cases where an overdose of street drugs may have masked a suicide and a murder by a known abusive partner, the assessors said:

> "Despite intensive support during pregnancy her care stopped in the post natal period. As soon as the baby was removed her care plans stopped, 24 hours after delivery.

> "Once again it appears the care for the mother stops at the point at which the safety of the child is secured."

Of all of the women who died and whose cases were assessed, 112 of their previous living children had already been adopted or placed in care. Several mothers had more than six previous children in care, the highest number being eight.

Table 1.25
Characteristics of the antenatal care sought by pregnant or recently delivered women who were known to the child protection services; United Kingdom: 2003-05.

Type of death	Death in early pregnancy	Late or non attenders for antenatal care (ANC)			Total number of deaths in women known to social services or the child protection services
		Booked after 22 weeks or missed more than four visits	No ANC	Subtotal	
	n	n (%)	n	n (%)	n (%)
Direct	3	3	2	8 *(100)*	8 *(100)*
Indirect	2	13	3	18 *(75)*	24 *(100)*
All	**5**	**16**	**5**	**26 *(81)***	**32 *(100)***
Coincidental	0	3	2	5 *(45)*	11 *(100)*
Late Direct deaths	0	1	0	1 *(10)*	10 *(100)*
Total	**5**	**20**	**7**	**32 *(60)***	**53 *(100)***

Characteristics of the antenatal care sought by pregnant or recently delivered women who were known to the child protection services; United Kingdom: 2003-05.

Substance misuse

Ninety-three of the women whose deaths were assessed this triennium had problems with substance misuse. Of these, 52 were drug addicts, another 32 women were occasional drug users and the remaining women were alcohol dependent. Seven died in very early pregnancy before they could access maternity care.

As seen in Table 1.26, as with domestic abuse and child protection, the majority of these women found it difficult to maintain contact with maternity services. However, for those who did, there was increasing evidence of a greater emphasis on planned multidisciplinary and multi-agency care, and in some cases the care they received was outstanding. Many of the women who received good or excellent care were in touch with their local Sure Start or Children's Centre. Issues relating to substance misuse and pregnancy are discussed in Chapter 12.

Table 1.26

Characteristics of the antenatal care sought by pregnant or recently delivered women who were known substance misusers and whose pregnancy exceeded 12 weeks' gestation; United Kingdom: 2003-05.

Type of death	Late or non attenders for antenatal care (ANC)			Total number of deaths of substance misusers after 12 or more weeks of gestation
	Booked after 22 weeks or missed more than four visits	No ANC	Subtotal	
	n	n	n (%)	n (%)
Direct	3	2	5 (100)	5 (100)
Indirect	13	3	16 (73)	22 (100)
All	**16**	**5**	**21 (78)**	**27 (100)**
Coincidental	1	3	4 (33)	12 (100)
Late deaths	27	2	29 (62)	47 (100)
Total	**44**	**10**	**54 (63)**	**86 (100)**

Six women with substance abuse problems died early in pregnancy from *Direct* or *Indirect* causes, and there was one other *Coincidental* death. However, as shown in Table 1.26, 21 of the other 27 women whose pregnancies were advanced enough to require care, accessed maternity services less than optimally, or not at all. None of the women who died from *Direct* causes regularly attended care, and only 22% of those women who suffered an *Indirect* death attended for optimal antenatal care. By comparison, two thirds of the twelve women who died from *Coincidental* causes regularly attended for care.

Risk factors and barriers to care

Many of the women who died found it difficult to seek, or to maintain contact with, maternity and/or other health services. The many possible reasons for this have been discussed throughout this Chapter and the main characteristics of the women who found it difficult to attend are summarised in Table 1.27. Understanding what the barriers were that prevented these women from feeling able to access maternity care will help future services to develop in response to these needs. One of the key issues addressed in "Maternity Matters", the modernisation agenda for maternity services in England[3], is developing services that encourage and support all women, but particularly the most vulnerable, to access care early and stay in touch with it thereafter.

Table 1.27
Characteristics of the women who were poor or non attenders for antenatal care and whose pregnancy was 12 weeks of gestation or more; *Direct* and *Indirect* deaths; United Kingdom: 2003-05.

Characteristic*	Women who were poor or non-attenders at antenatal care	Overall number of women
	n (%)	n (%)
Domestic abuse	13 (81)	16 (100)
Known to child protection services or social services	26 (81)	32 (100)
Substance misuse	21 (78)	27 (100)
Black Caribbean	4 (57)	7 (100)
Single unemployed	19 (56)	34 (100)
Both partners unemployed	14 (47)	30 (100)
Black African	12 (40)	30 (100)
No English	9 (35)	26 (100)
White	31 (17)	183 (100)
At least one partner in employment	9 (5)	165 (100)

* Some women had more than one characteristic recorded.

Characteristics of the women who were poor or non attenders for antenatal care and whose pregnancy was 12 weeks of gestation or more; *Direct* and *Indirect* deaths; United Kingdom: 2003-05

What did you learn from this case and how has it changed your practice?

> *"I remember her lying in bed huddled up and crying and feeling frightened. In future I would like to believe that if I see this again I would drop everything and sit, listen and offer support."*

It is easy to forget that, apart from the partners, families and the communities of the women who died, every health care worker who knew or was involved in providing care for them was affected by their death. These rare events have a huge and long lasting impact on the staff involved. As part of participating in this Enquiry, every health care professional who was involved is asked "what did you learn from this case and how has it changed your practice?". Many had never come across a maternal death before and all hope they would not do so again. A very few had to manage more than one, due entirely to the play of chance, and the impact of several deaths in a short period of time was immensely distressing for them.

Many thoughtful answers were provided, in general revealing the huge depth of caring and respect the staff had for the women who died, the babies and families who survived and the pain they themselves suffered as a result:

> *"The midwifery report made me cry."* (Central assessor)

> *"We all attended the funeral, even though she died some months after she left our care."* (A midwife who had cared for a terminally ill mother during her pregnancy).

Most staff reported learning clinical lessons which, in many cases, led to a change in personal or Trust based practice. Other staff were more reflective and philosophical:

> *Even though she was a mother she was still a child herself." (In relation to a young schoolgirl).*

> *"How inspiring the human spirit can be in the face of insuperable odds."*
> *(For a woman dying of cancer).*

On the other hand a few professionals seemed oblivious to the poor quality of care they had provided, or to have had any understanding of the wider circumstances that may have affected a mother's life and death. The assessors were also concerned by the apparently culturally dismissive or insensitive remarks made by a few professionals during the course of the reviews.

In some cases staff appeared to take the blame upon themselves despite providing the best possible care. In these cases the Enquiry assessors were saddened as they considered the care these professionals had provided was exemplary and that the failings in the system were totally outside the control of these workers. Some staff who cared for women who declined help, or who had to watch a woman bleed to death while refusing blood products, reported significant personal distress. It is important that all staff affected by a maternal death should be offered support and counselling to help them come to terms with their own reactions.

Discussion and conclusions

Although it is disappointing that the UK maternal mortality rate identified by this Enquiry has failed to decline there are a number of changing demographic and public health factors which may explain this lack of progress. The Annex to this Chapter demonstrates the rapidly changing nature of motherhood in the UK, with more than 20% of women having babies in the UK themselves having being been born elsewhere. In addition, women who have just recently arrived in the UK from every part of the world present new, but often differing, challenges for maternity services.

Maternal deaths are extremely rare, and the proportion of the very small number of mothers whose care was less than optimal has not increased for many years. In fact there were many instances of exemplary care provided for extremely sick women. However there is always room for improvement and high quality clinical care cannot, and should not, be taken for granted. When reviewing the cases for this triennium, the apparent lack of basic clinical knowledge and skills amongst some doctors, midwives and other health professionals, senior or junior, was one of the leading causes of potentially avoidable mortality. The Enquiry assessors were also struck by the number of health care professionals who failed to identify and manage common medical conditions or potential emergencies outside their immediate area of expertise. Resuscitation skills were also considered poor in an unacceptably high number of cases. As a result, several of the top ten recommendations of this Report address these critical areas.

This Chapter and its Annex has shown that women are starting motherhood later in life which may have consequences for their pregnancy. Mothers also tend to be less healthy than in the past and embark on pregnancy in poorer overall general health. Over half of the women who died were overweight or obese, and the fact that cardiac disease is now the leading cause of maternal death demonstrates the growing impact of less than healthy lifestyle choices. What has been noticeable over the past few Reports is the steady increase in deaths in young mothers in what should be the prime of their lives from diseases such as lung cancer and myocardial infarction, conditions never seen in earlier triennia.

However, as the global safe motherhood movement has long pointed out, the underlying root causes of maternal deaths are often underlying social and other non-clinical factors. The link between adverse pregnancy outcomes and vulnerability and social exclusion are nowhere more starkly demonstrated than by this Enquiry. Children born to women from the more vulnerable groups also experience a higher risk of death or morbidity and face problems with pre-term labour, intrauterine growth restriction, low birth weight, low levels of breast-feeding and higher levels of neonatal complications. The findings of this Report demonstrate yet again that those women who need maternity services most use them the least. The stark inequalities demonstrated by the identified risk factors for maternal deaths highlight that a disproportionate number of the women who died were from the vulnerable and more excluded groups of our society. These women also tend to have a multiplicity of problems in conjunction with their pregnancies and are the very women who are less likely to access or continue to remain in contact with maternity services. More than 17% of the women who died had not sought care until they were at least five months pregnant, or had four or less antenatal visits.

Due in part as a response to similar findings in earlier Reports, many maternity services have, or are in the process of, developing strategies designed to provide more locally accessible, flexible and individualised care for these women. By providing a modern maternity service that responds to each woman's needs by providing a choice of acceptable and accessible services for all women, the needs of the most vulnerable are now being treated with equal importance. If women are happy with the care provided early in pregnancy then they are more likely to continue to maintain regular contact throughout pregnancy. Examples of some of the innovative responses to these findings, which now provide midwifery services in easy to reach, community based, facilities at times that suit the women best, are contained within the midwifery Chapter.

However, whilst welcome action is now being taken with respect to addressing inequalities in maternal and infant health through maternity service design, this Report has identified a number of new issues that also require urgent attention. In terms of women with socially complex pregnancies, it was evident that many who were known to social services, and in particular the child protection services, were extremely vulnerable. Not only did they often hide their pregnancies from social services but also many also actively avoided maternity care despite being at high risk of medical or mental health problems. Even when social services knew a woman was pregnant it was assumed, usually erroneously, that she was receiving maternity care. Her risks were further compounded by the stress of child protection case conferences and the removal of infants into care. Whilst the needs of the child must remain paramount, the medical and social support and vigilance needed for the mother at such a distressing time was generally lacking, and any communication that there had been between the agencies involved in her care ceased once the baby was removed. It is therefore crucially important that social workers should liaise with and refer pregnant women in their care to the local maternity services if necessary, and that support and care for these women is stepped up rather then decreased or stopped, particularly if her child is removed.

Another factor which has affected the maternal mortality rate is the increasing number of migrant women who are seeking maternity care in the UK. Women who have recently arrived from countries around the world, particularly those from Africa and the Indian sub-continent, but also increasingly from central Europe and the Middle East, may have relatively poor overall general health and are at risk from illnesses that have largely disappeared from the UK, such as TB and rheumatic heart disease. Many are also more likely to be at risk of HIV infection. All of these conditions, alone or in combination, contributed to a number of the maternal deaths identified in this Report. None of the recently arrived women who died had had a routine medical examination during their pregnancy and the opportunity for remedial treatment was lost.

The overwhelming strength of successive Enquiry Reports has been the impact their findings have had on maternal and newborn health in the United Kingdom and further afield. Over the years there have been many impressive examples of how the implementation of their recommendations and guidelines have improved policies, procedures and practice and saved more mothers and babies lives. This Report is no exception. The health service has already responded by addressing the recommendations for helping to improve access for the most vulnerable women by already developing more localised and flexible antenatal care services. And, if the reduction in maternal suicides shown in this Report is sustained in the next, this may indicate that the recommendations made in previous Reports about identifying women at potential risk in the antenatal period are having a beneficial effect.

However, although there have been successes, some old problems still remain and new challenges continue to emerge. Some have questioned the need for such Reports in the future but the fact that the maternal mortality rate is not falling means that there can be no grounds for complacency and highlights the necessity for further vigilance and for these Reports to continue.

Acknowledgements

This Chapter would not have been possible without the help and advice from a number of people including Nirupa Dattani and Nigel Physick at the Office for National Statistics, Naufil Alam at CEMACH and Jo Modder and David Bogod in relation to their work and observation on the section on obesity.

References

1 Lewis G (ed). Confidential Enquiries into Maternal and Child Health. *Why Mothers Die.* The Sixth Report of the United Kingdom Confidential Enquiries into Maternal Deaths in the United Kingdom. London. RCOG Press. 2004. www.cemach.org.uk

2 Redshaw M, Rowe R, Hockley C, Brocklehurst, P. *Recorded delivery: a national survey of women's experience of maternity care 2006.* National Perinatal Epidemiology Unit. Oxford; NPEU; 2007. ISBN 978 0 9735860 8 0. www.npeu.ac.uk

3 Department of Health. *Maternity Matters: choice, access and continuity of care in a safe service.* Department of Health. April 2007. www.dh.gov.uk/publications

4 Department of Health, England. *Maternity Services.* Standard 11 of the National Service Framework for Children, Young People and Maternity Services. London; Department of Health 2004. www.dh.gov.uk

5 National Centre for Clinical Excellence. National Collaborating Centre for Women's and Children's Health. *Caesarean section: clinical guideline.* Royal College of Obstetricians and Gynaecologist Press. April 2004. www.nice.org.uk or www.rcog.org.uk

6 Health Care Commission. *Investigation into 10 maternal deaths at, or following delivery at, Northwick Park Hospital, North West London Hospitals NHS Trust, between April 2002 and April 2005.* Health Care Commission. London, August 2006. www.healthcarecommission.org.uk

7 Car J, and Sheikh A. *Information in practice: Telephone consultations.* BMJ, 2003, 326: 966-969

8 McKinstry B and Sheihk A. *Unresolved questions in telephone consultations.* J R Soc Med 2006: 99: 2-3

9 BMA. *Consulting in the modern world.* London, BMA, 2001.
http://www.bma.org.uk/guidance

10 Car et al. *Improving quality and safety of telephone based delivery of care: teaching telephone consultation skills.* Qual Saf Health Care 2004; 13: 2-3.

11 Human Fertilisation and Embryology Authority. *A long term analysis of the HFEA Register data, 1991-2006.* London: HFEA, 2007

12 Royal College of Obstetricians and Gynaecologists. *Thromboprophylaxis during pregnancy, labour and after normal vaginal delivery.* Guideline no.37. London: RCOG Press; 2004. Available at www.rcog.org.uk

13 National Institute for Health and Clinical Excellence . *Obesity: the prevention, identification, assessment and management of overweight and obesity in adults and children.* National Institute for Health and Clinical Excellence (NICE), 2006. http://www.nice.org.uk/guidance/CG43

14 Information Centre for Health and Social Care. *Statistics on obesity, physical activity and diet: England, 2006.* Leeds: Information Centre, 2006

15 Kanagalingam MG, Forouhi NG, Greer IA, Sattar N. *Changes in booking body mass index over a decade: retrospective analysis from a Glasgow Maternity Hospital.* BJOG 2005: 112: :1431-3.

16 Sebire NJ, Jolly M, Harris JP, Wadsworth J, Joffe M, Beard RW, et al. *Maternal obesity and pregnancy outcome: a study of 287,213 pregnancies in London.* Int J Obes Relat Metab Disord 2001;25:1175-82.

17 Shah A, Sands J, Kenny L. *Maternal obesity and the risk of stillbirth and neonatal death.* J Obstet Gynaecol 2006:26 I (Suppl 1)S19. 2005

18 Lashen H, Fear K, Sturdee DW. *Obesity is associated with increased risk of first trimester and recurrent miscarriage: matched case control study.* Hum Reprod 2004: 19: 1644-6.

19 Weiss JL, Malone FD, Emig D, Ball RH, Nyberg DA, Comstock CH, et al. *Obesity, obstetric complications and cesarean delivery rate – a population based screening study.* Am J Obstet Gynecol 2004: 190: 1091-7.

20 Usha KTS, Hemmadi J, Bethel J, Evans J. *Outcome of pregnancy in women with an increased body mass index.* BJOG 2005; 112: 768-72.

21 Myles TD, Gooch J, Santolaya J. *Obesity is an independent risk factor for infectious morbidity in patients who undergo caesarean delivery.* Obstet Gynecol 2002:100; 959-64.

22 Ray JG, Wyatt PR, Vermuelen MJ, Meier C, Cole DE. *Greater maternal weight and the ongoing risk of neural tube defects after folic acid flour fortificaton.* Obstet Gynecol 2005; 105: 261-5.

23 Watkins ML, Rasmussen SA, Honein MA, Botto LD, Moore CA. *Maternal obesity and risk for birth defects.* Paediatrics 2003: 111: 1152-8.

24 Cedegran MI, Kallen BA. *Maternal obesity and the risk of orofacial clefts in the offspring.* Cleft Palate Craniofac J 2005; 42: 367-71.

25 Cedegran MI, Kallen BA. *Maternal obesity and infant heart defects.* Obes Res 2003; 11: 1065-71.

26 Stephansson O, Dickman PW, Johansson A, Cnattingius S. *maternal weight, pregnancy weight gain, and the risk of antepartum stillbirth.* Am J Obstet Gynecol 2001; 184: 463-9.

27 Kristensen J, Vestergaard M, Wisborg K, Kesmodel U, Secher NJ. *Pre-pregnancy weight and the risk of stillbirth and neonatal death.* BJOG 2005; 112: 403-8.

28 Heslehurst N, Lang R, Rankin J, Wilkinson JR, Summerbell CD. *Obesity in pregnancy: a study of the impact of maternal obesity on NHS maternity services.* BJOG 2007; 114: 334-42.

29 Bolling K, Grant C, Hamlyn B, Thornton A. *Infant Feeding Survey 2005.* Leeds: The Information Centre for Health and Social Care, 2007.

30 NHS Maternity Statistics, England 2005-06. *Statistical Bulletin 2006/08.* Leeds: Information Centre for Health and Social Care, 2006.

31 Department of Health. Responding to domestic abuse. *A handbook for health professionals.* London: Department of Health, 2006. www.dh.gov.uk/publications

32 Dorkenoo E, Morison L, Macfarlane AJ. *A study to estimate the prevalence of female genital mutilation (FGM) in England and Wales. Initial report December 2006.* London: Foundation for Women's Health, Research and Development (FORWARD), 2006).

33 World Health Organization (2000) *A systematic Review of the Health Complications of Female Genital Mutilation including Sequelae.* WHO.

Annex 1.1 The changing face of motherhood in the UK

Alison Macfarlane

Since the beginning of the twenty first century, there have been major changes in the patterns of birth in the countries of the United Kingdom and in the population of women of childbearing age. The trends in maternal mortality described in this Chapter should therefore be interpreted in the light of these changes.

Birth rates and age of mother

Throughout the 1990s, birth rates fell in all the countries of the United Kingdom. Within age groups, live births per thousand women fell among women in their twenties and rose among women in their thirties and forties. This was a consequence of the rising average age at childbirth as women, particularly those in professional occupations, have postponed childbearing.

In the United Kingdom as a whole, numbers and rates of birth started to rise in 2003, but the increase started in Scotland, the country with the lowest fertility rate, from 2002 onwards. Birth rates began to rise among women in their twenties as well as continuing to rise among older women. Although the rise among women aged 20-24 was small and showed signs of levelling off, rates continued to rise among women aged 25-29.

The numbers of maternities in each age group, shown in Table A1.1, reflect these changes, but also changes in numbers of women of childbearing age in the population. Thus in 2003-05, compared with 2000-02, the increase in the numbers and proportion of maternities which were to women aged 35 and over continued, but a smaller increase had become apparent in the number and proportion of maternities to women aged 20-24.

Table A1.1
Numbers and percentages of maternities by age of mother; United Kingdom: 1985-2005.

	Under 20	20-24	25-29	30-34	35-39	40 and over	All ages
	Numbers						
1985-87	197,277	660,523	788,931	441,792	153,399	26,844	2,268,766
1988-90	193,102	629,748	831,630	495,732	165,931	31,385	2,347,529
1991-93	166,091	549,527	820,616	558,902	188,251	33,940	2,317,328
1994-96	146,410	444,058	738,467	610,782	220,090	37,833	2,197,640
1997-99	162,643	383,129	646,967	625,608	260,390	44,876	2,123,614
2000-02	151,329	364,400	538,853	600,016	289,449	53,425	1,997,472
2003-05	151,052	398,847	533,754	626,676	335,505	67,997	2,114,004
	Percentages						
1985-87	8.70	29.11	34.77	19.47	6.76	1.18	100.00
1988-90	8.23	26.83	35.43	21.12	7.07	1.34	100.00
1991-93	7.17	23.71	35.41	24.12	8.12	1.46	100.00
1994-96	6.66	20.21	33.60	27.79	10.01	1.72	100.00
1997-99	7.66	18.04	30.47	29.46	12.26	2.11	100.00
2000-02	7.58	18.24	26.98	30.04	14.49	2.67	100.00
2003-05	7.15	18.87	25.25	29.64	15.87	3.22	100.00

Source: ONS, General Register Office, Scotland, General Register Office, Northern Ireland.

Country of birth and migration

A factor which is likely to have contributed to rising numbers of births is increasing numbers of births which were to women who were themselves born outside the United Kingdom. As Table A1.2 shows, this has led to increases throughout the United Kingdom in the proportions of births to mothers born outside the United Kingdom.

Table A1.2
Percentages of live births which were to mothers born outside the United Kingdom: 2001-05.

	England and Wales	Scotland	Northern Ireland
2001	16.5	6.3	6.4
2002	17.6	7.2	6.6
2003	18.6	7.6	7.3
2004	19.5	7.8	8.3
2005	20.8	8.6	8.2

Source: ONS, General Register Office, Scotland, General Register Office, Northern Ireland.

Data about mothers' countries of birth for live births in England and Wales are shown in fuller detail in Table A1.3 The corresponding data published for live births in Scotland and Northern Ireland are not so detailed, but they also show increasing numbers of births to women born in other parts of Europe, both in the countries of the European Union and those in other parts of Europe, as well as countries of the 'New Commonwealth' and the 'Rest of the World'. Among the 'New Commonwealth' countries, there were marked increases in births to women from India and Pakistan and from Southern and Western Africa, including Nigeria and Ghana. There were also considerable increases in numbers from the 'Rest of the World'.

Table A1.3
Live births by country of birth of mother; England and Wales: 1995, 2000-05.

Country of birth of mother	1995	2000	2001	2002	2003	2004	2005	1995	2000	2001	2002	2003	2004	2005
	Numbers							*Percentage of all live births*						
Total	**648,138**	**604,441**	**594,634**	**596,122**	**621,469**	**639,721**	**645,835**	*100.0*	*100.0*	*100.0*	*100.0*	*100.0*	*100.0*	*100.0*
United Kingdom[1]	566,452	510,835	496,713	490,711	506,076	515,144	511,624	*87.4*	*84.5*	*83.5*	*82.3*	*81.4*	*80.5*	*79.2*
Total outside United Kingdom	81,677	93,588	97,895	105,381	115,360	124,563	134,189	*12.6*	*15.5*	*16.5*	*17.7*	*18.6*	*19.5*	*20.8*
Irish Republic	5,167	4,050	3,843	3,708	3,734	3,597	3,463	*0.8*	*0.7*	*0.6*	*0.6*	*0.6*	*0.6*	*0.5*
Australia, Canada and New Zealand	3,051	3,635	3,695	3,885	4,132	4,152	4,217	*0.5*	*0.6*	*0.6*	*0.7*	*0.7*	*0.6*	*0.7*
New Commonwealth	**44,103**	**45,348**	**47,963**	**51,500**	**54,983**	**59,199**	**62,404**	*6.8*	*7.5*	*8.1*	*8.6*	*8.8*	*9.3*	*9.7*
India	6,684	6,650	6,598	7,222	7,995	9,146	10,079	*1.0*	*1.1*	*1.1*	*1.2*	*1.3*	*1.4*	*1.6*
Pakistan	12,324	13,561	14,588	15,357	15,107	15,736	16,477	*1.9*	*2.2*	*2.5*	*2.6*	*2.4*	*2.5*	*2.6*
Bangladesh	6,783	7,482	8,164	8,486	8,898	8,857	8,217	*1.0*	*1.2*	*1.4*	*1.4*	*1.4*	*1.4*	*1.3*
East Africa	5,128	3,959	3,745	3,724	3,985	3,991	4,042	*0.8*	*0.7*	*0.6*	*0.6*	*0.6*	*0.6*	*0.6*
Southern Africa	1,010	1,907	2,236	2,654	3,149	3,722	4,122	*0.2*	*0.3*	*0.4*	*0.4*	*0.5*	*0.6*	*0.6*
Rest of Africa	5,934	5,646	5,857	6,445	7,456	9,264	11,029	*0.9*	*0.9*	*1.0*	*1.1*	*1.2*	*1.4*	*1.7*
Caribbean	2,912	2,681	3,085	3,598	3,984	3,816	3,733	*0.4*	*0.4*	*0.5*	*0.6*	*0.6*	*0.6*	*0.6*
Far East	1,996	1,538	1,365	1,351	1,433	1,439	1,341	*0.3*	*0.3*	*0.2*	*0.2*	*0.2*	*0.2*	*0.2*
Rest of New Commonwealth	1,332	1,924	2,325	2,663	2,976	3,228	3,364	*0.2*	*0.3*	*0.4*	*0.4*	*0.5*	*0.5*	*0.5*
Other European Union	11,113	13,829	13,840	14,576	15,830	17,290	20,420	*1.7*	*2.3*	*2.3*	*2.4*	*2.5*	*2.7*	*3.2*
Rest of Europe	2,360	5,468	5,467	5,662	6,249	7,072	7,504	*0.4*	*0.9*	*0.9*	*0.9*	*1.0*	*1.1*	*1.2*
United States of America	2,641	2,895	2,878	2,828	3,037	2,916	2,930	*0.4*	*0.5*	*0.5*	*0.5*	*0.5*	*0.5*	*0.5*
Rest of the World	13,242	18,363	20,209	23,222	27,395	30,337	33,251	*2.0*	*3.0*	*3.4*	*3.9*	*4.4*	*4.7*	*5.1*
Not stated	9	18	26	30	33	14	22	*0.0*	*0.0*	*0.0*	*0.0*	*0.0*	*0.0*	*0.0*

Note: For comparability, the births data for all years for mothers born outside the United Kingdom were reclassified according to the 2005 country classification list and the definition of the European Union (EU25), as constituted in 2005, was used for all years' data.
[1] Including Isle of Man and Channel Islands.
Source: ONS Birth Statistics, England and Wales, 2005, Series FM1, Table 9.1.

The data in Tables A1.2 and A1.3 are derived from birth registration which gives the mother's country of birth, but not the length of time she has been in the United Kingdom. Migration and asylum statistics are not currently collected in sufficient detail to record how long women of childbearing age have been in the United Kingdom or the circumstances in which they arrived and there is no link to subsequent pregnancies.

This is an important gap in our knowledge in relation to maternal deaths as the numbers of *Direct* and *Indirect* deaths which were of women who were refugees and asylum seekers has risen over the past three triennia, as Table A1.4 shows. There were four in 1997-99, 12 in 2000-02 and 36 in 2003-05, when they accounted for 12 % of *Direct* and *Indirect* deaths.

Table A1.4
Direct and *Indirect* deaths, numbers and rates, excluding refugees and asylum seekers;
United Kingdom: 1997-2005.

Triennium	Total *Direct* and *Indirect* deaths known to the Enquiry						
	Number			Rate			
	Total	Refugees and asylum seekers	Excluding refugees and asylum seekers	Total	Excluding refugees and asylum seekers	*95 per cent CI*	
1997-1999	242	4	238	11.40	11.21	*9.87*	*12.72*
2000-2002	261	12	249	13.07	12.47	*11.01*	*14.11*
2003-2005	295	36	259	13.95	12.25	*10.85*	*13.84*
Change in rate 2000-02 to 2003-05					-0.21	*-2.38*	*1.94*

Excluding refugees and asylum seekers from the numerators in the mortality rates shows that the rate for 2003-05 now appears to be slightly lower rather than slightly higher than for 2000-02, although once again, the decrease was not statistically significant. As there were no national statistics about the numbers of maternities to refugees and asylum seekers, it was not possible to exclude them from the denominators.

Some idea of the extent of changes in numbers of live births to women born in selected countries of the 'Rest of the World', from which women may come as refugees or asylum seekers is shown in Table A1.5. This shows numbers of maternities in England and Wales by mother's country of birth for selected countries, and the percentage increase from 2000-02 to 2003-05. It shows substantial increases in the considerable numbers of maternities to women born in Iraq and countries in the Horn of Africa and Central Africa which have been the scene of recent and current conflicts.

Table A1.5
Maternities by mother's country of birth, selected countries, numbers and percentage increase: 2000-2005.

	2000	2001	2002	2000-02	2003	2004	2005	2003-05	*Percentage increase 2000-02 to 2003-05*
Afghanistan	495	556	895	**1,946**	941	1,202	1,296	**3,439**	*77*
Angola	309	370	491	**1,170**	580	553	634	**1,767**	*51*
Burundi	89	122	152	**363**	211	165	208	**584**	*61*
Congo	230	250	288	**768**	481	567	509	**1,557**	*103*
Congo (Democratic Republic)	557	609	681	**1,847**	770	829	981	**2,580**	*40*
Eritrea	205	231	266	**702**	293	332	366	**991**	*41*
Ethiopia	208	239	289	**736**	382	419	515	**1,316**	*79*
Iraq	599	703	754	**2,056**	874	1,044	1,291	**3,209**	*56*
Ivory Coast	160	206	224	**590**	287	300	365	**952**	*61*
Libya	336	460	538	**1,334**	495	555	551	**1,601**	*20*
Rwanda	83	114	152	**349**	165	158	165	**488**	*40*
Sierra Leone	448	529	552	**1,529**	668	634	689	**1,991**	*30*
Somalia	2,718	3,168	3,792	**9,678**	4,318	4,877	5,438	**14,633**	*51*

Source: Office for National Statistics, unpublished data.

Multiple births

As shown earlier, women with multiple pregnancies had higher rates of death than women who had singleton pregnancies. The percentages of maternities which are multiple have risen since the mid 1970s in the four countries of the United Kingdom, although the rate of increase has slowed in recent years. The two main factors which have led to the rise in multiple pregnancy rates have been the rising age at childbirth, because older women are more likely than younger women to have a multiple pregnancy and the use of ovarian stimulation and assisted conception. Guidelines issued by the RCOG and then by the Human Fertilisation and Embryology Authority restricting the occasions when more than two embryos can be replaced in IVF and related procedures have had a clear impact on numbers of triplet and higher order maternities, even though the total number of ART procedures has continued to increase[1].

Health and lifestyle

Obesity

Obesity is increasingly a matter of concern both general and in relation to pregnancy. There are no national data about body mass indices of pregnant women. Data about obesity in the population in general are collected through the Health Surveys undertaken in each country of the United Kingdom. The longest series of data are those collected through the Health Survey for England[2], shown in Table A1.6. These relate to all women and show a rise in the portion of women who are obese, with BMIs of 30.1 to 40.0, and a particular rise in proportions with BMIs over 40.

Table A1.6
Trends in Body Mass Index, women; England: 1993-2005[1].

| | BMI | | | | | |
	18.5 or under	18.6-25.0	25.1-30.0	30.1-40.0	Over 40	All
	Percentages					
1993	1.9	49.5	32.2	15.0	1.4	100.0
1994	2.2	49.1	31.4	15.7	1.6	100.0
1995	2.2	47.4	32.9	16.1	1.4	100.0
1996	2.0	46.0	33.6	17.0	1.4	100.0
1997	1.9	45.6	32.8	17.4	2.3	100.0
1998	2.1	44.6	32.1	19.3	1.9	100.0
1999	1.8	44.3	32.8	19.2	1.9	100.0
2000	1.8	43.1	33.8	19.1	2.3	100.0
2001	1.6	41.9	32.9	21.0	2.5	100.0
2002	1.9	41.6	33.7	20.2	2.6	100.0
2003	1.9	41.3	33.4	20.6	2.9	100.0
2004	1.7	39.8	34.7	21.3	2.6	100.0
2005	1.6	40.7	32.9	19.0	2.9	100.0

Source: Health Survey for England.

Body mass index varies with age, being higher on average for older women, with trends being apparent through the child bearing years, as Table A1.7 shows.

Table A1.7
Percentage distribution of Body Mass Index by age, women aged 16-24; England: 2003.

BMI	Percentage in each age group		
	16-24	25-34	35-44
18.5 or under	7.4	1.0	1.0
18.6-25.0	61.2	51.8	43.5
25.1-30.0	18.3	28.3	33.3
30.1-40.0	11.1	15.1	18.6
Over 40	2.00	3.00	3.50
All	100	100	100

Source: Health Survey for England.

One factor which has changed for the better is smoking. As described earlier in Chapter 1, although substantial proportions of women still smoke in pregnancy, the 2005 Infant Feeding Survey showed a reduction compared with 2005[3].

Despite this, as this Annex shows, there are many adverse trends. Others cannot be assessed because of lack of data on the subject. Many like tuberculosis, are not recorded in relation to all pregnancies, although it is beginning to contribute to deaths. Although data are not explicitly collected on the subject, it has been estimated that the proportion of maternities to women with Female Genital Cutting / Mutilation (FGC/M) is rising[4]. In addition, advances in health care have enabled many women experiencing serious conditions in childhood which in the past would have been life threatening conditions to survive childhood into early adulthood, but few data are available to document their extent in the population or how many attempt to have children.

Conclusions

The failure of the maternal mortality rate to decline has to be viewed in the light of both documented and undocumented changes in the childbearing population. Although there have been positive changes, there have also been increases in the numbers of women whose social circumstances and health put them at risk of maternal death.

References

1   Human Fertilisation and Embryology Authority. *A long term analysis of the HFEA Register data, 1991-2006.* London: HFEA, 2007.

2   Information Centre for Health and Social Care. *Statistics on obesity, physical activity and diet: England, 2006.* Leeds: Information Centre, 2006.

3   Bolling K, Grant C, Hamlyn B, Thornton A. *Infant Feeding Survey 2005.* Leeds: The Information Centre for Health and Social Care, 2007.

4   Dorkenoo E, Morison L, Macfarlane AJ. *A study to estimate the prevalence of female genital mutilation (FGM) in England and Wales.* Initial report December 2006. London: Foundation for Women's Health, Research and Development (FORWARD), 2006.

2 Thrombosis and thromboembolism

James Drife

Summary of key findings for 2003-05

The deaths of 41 women who died from thrombosis and/or thromboembolism are counted in this Chapter. Of these, 33 deaths were attributed to pulmonary embolism and eight to cerebral vein thrombosis. Additionally, three *Late* deaths attributed to pulmonary embolism are counted in Chapter 15 but the lessons to be learnt from these cases are discussed here.

Pulmonary embolism still remains the leading *Direct* cause of maternal death in the United Kingdom with a mortality rate of 1.56 per 100,000 maternities. Although the numbers of deaths attributed to pulmonary embolism appear to be higher than the 25 cases identified in the previous Report for 2000-2002, the difference is not statistically significant as Table 2.1 shows.

Table 2.1
Direct deaths from thrombosis and thromboembolism and rates per 100,000 maternities; United Kingdom: 1985-2005.

	Pulmonary embolism			Cerebral vein thrombosis			Thrombosis and thromboembolism		
	Number	Rate	*95 per cent CI*	Number	Rate	*95 per cent CI*	Number	Rate	*95 per cent CI*
1985-87	30	1.32	*0.83* *1.89*	2	0.09	*0.02* *0.32*	32	1.41	*1.00* *1.99*
1988-90	24	1.02	*0.68* *1.51*	9	0.38	*0.20* *0.72*	33	1.40	*1.00* *1.96*
1991-93	30	1.30	*0.91* *1.85*	5	0.22	*0.09* *0.51*	35	1.51	*1.09* *2.10*
1994-96	46	2.09	*1.57* *2.79*	2	0.09	*0.02* *0.33*	48	2.18	*1.65* *2.90*
1997-99	31	1.46	*1.03* *2.07*	4	0.19	*0.07* *0.48*	35	1.65	*1.19* *2.29*
2000-02	25	1.25	*0.85* *1.85*	5	0.25	*0.11* *0.59*	30	1.50	*1.05* *2.14*
2003-05	33	1.56	*1.11* *2.19*	8	0.38	*0.19* *0.75*	41	1.94	*1.43* *2.63*

The apparent difference arose mainly from fluctuations in numbers of antepartum deaths, as Table 2.2 shows. Despite the rising caesarean section rate, the numbers of women dying from postpartum pulmonary embolism after caesarean section remains lower than in the early 1990s as thromboprophylaxis becomes routine.

Table 2.2
Timing of deaths from pulmonary embolism; United Kingdom: 1985-2005.

	Deaths after miscarriage/ ectopic	Antepartum deaths	Collapse before delivery followed by perimortem caesarean section	Deaths in labour	Death after caesarean section	Deaths after vaginal delivery	Not known	**Total** **_Direct_** **deaths**	_Late_ deaths
1985-87	1	16	0	0	7	6	0	**30**	*
1988-90	3	10	0	0	8	3	0	**24**	4
1991-93	0	12	0	1	13	4	0	**30**	5
1994-96	3	15	0	0	15	10	3	**46**	2
1997-99	1	13	3	0	4	10	0	**31**	9
2000-02	3	4	1	1	9	7	0	**25**	1
2003-05	3	11	4	0	7	8	0	**33**	3

* Most _Late_ deaths were not reported to enquiry in this triennium.

Cases counted in other Chapters

Pulmonary embolism also contributed to a few deaths from other causes which are counted and discussed in other chapters. These include a case where it was the terminal event for a woman with advanced cancer, discussed in Chapter 11, and two women who died of _Indirect_ causes including Budd-Chiari syndrome due to thrombosis obstructing the hepatic vein whose cases are counted in Chapter 10.

It must be remembered that not all cases of sudden collapse in the puerperium are due to pulmonary embolism. For example, a woman who suffered a sudden fall in blood pressure two days after delivery was initially investigated for pulmonary embolism. The actual cause of her death, haemorrhage from the internal iliac vessels, was a rarity but intra-peritoneal haemorrhage should have been suspected from her pallor and hypotension.

Incidence of antenatal pulmonary embolism

A prospective national case-control study of antenatal pulmonary embolism was undertaken through the United Kingdom Obstetric Surveillance System (UKOSS) between February 2005 and August 2006. UKOSS is discussed in fuller detail in the Introduction to this Report. Ninety-four incidents of antenatal pulmonary emboli, including several deaths, were reported over the first year, representing an estimated incidence of 13.1 per 100,000 maternities with a 95% confidence interval from 10.6 to 16.1. Seventy-three of the women had one or more identifiable risk factors for thromboembolic disease. The main risk factors for pulmonary embolism in this group were multiparity, with an adjusted odds ratio of 2.90 with a 95% confidence interval 1.37 to 6.13 and a Body Mass Index (BMI) over 30, with an adjusted odds ratio of 2.80 with a 95% confidence interval from 1.12 to 7.02.

Pulmonary embolism

Of the 33 women who died from pulmonary embolism, ten died during the first trimester of their pregnancy and one during the second trimester. A further three women died antenatally; two following terminations of pregnancy and one following an ectopic pregnancy. An additional four women who collapsed in late pregnancy from a pulmonary embolism were delivered by a peri or post mortem caesarean section; these are also classified as antepartum deaths. No women died during labour. In all, fifteen women died in the postpartum period, eight following a vaginal delivery and seven after a caesarean section.

The women who died

Risk factors for thromboembolism were identifiable in 26 of the 33 women. Sixteen were overweight and four women had a past or family history of venous thromboembolism (VTE). Two died after air travel in pregnancy, one had hyperemesis gravidarum and one had ovarian hyperstimulation syndrome (OHSS). Three women had a history of surgery unrelated to pregnancy and one underwent craniotomy in the puerperium. Seven had no recorded risk factors but in four of these cases details were inadequate.

Of the 21 women whose pregnancies exceeded 12 weeks' gestation, four did not attend for regular antenatal care. In one case, an asylum seeker saw her General Practitioner early in pregnancy but did not receive a booking appointment until after five months had elapsed. The other three women had complex lives and were known to either be substance misusers, have child protection issues, or both. Six of the 21 women were Black African or Caribbean and two were South Asian. Three women could not speak English.

Risk factors

Weight

The National Institute for Clinical Excellence (NICE) guideline on antenatal care recommends that every woman should have her BMI checked at the first antenatal visit and that women with a BMI over 35 are not suitable for routine midwifery led care[2]. The mother's weight was recorded in only 25 cases and the BMI could be calculated for only 21. Of these, sixteen were overweight, with a BMI of over 25. Twelve of these were classified as obese with a BMI over 30, including eight who were morbidly obese with a BMI over 35. The latter included two who died after caesarean section. The highest reported BMI was 62, and another five women had BMIs over 40. Two of the morbidly obese women inappropriately had midwife-only care. Two of the three women who suffered a *Late Direct* death from pulmonary embolism were also obese or morbidly obese.

Women with a BMI of 40 or above are at a high risk of VTE but current RCOG guidelines[3, 4, 5] recommend the same prophylactic doses of low molecular weight heparin (LMWH) for all women with a BMI over 30 or a weight exceeding 90Kg. The RCOG guideline on thromboprophylaxis during pregnancy, labour and after normal vaginal delivery[2] recommends that "one or two risk factors alone may be sufficient to justify antenatal thromboprophylaxis with LMWH, for example an extremely obese woman admitted to the antenatal ward." This advice relies on clinical judgement and was reinforced in the last Report, but of the eight morbidly obese women whose deaths are discussed in the present Report, six received no thromboprophylaxis, one received an inadequate dosage and one received the correct dose but not until some time after her caesarean section. A specific guideline is now required on thromboprophylaxis for morbidly obese women.

Age

The ages of the women ranged between 18 and 39 years with a median of 30 years. Their age distribution is shown in Table 2.3 together with mortality rates per 100,000 maternities. This suggests a shift to a younger age of death, despite an overall increase in age at childbearing. Although no difference was detected in the mortality rates overall, the rate increased significantly among women aged under 25 and decreased among those aged 40 and over.

Table 2.3
Numbers of deaths attributed to pulmonary embolism and rates per 100,000 maternities by age;
United Kingdom: 1985-90 and 1997-2005*.

	Under 25	25-29	30-34	35-39	40 and over	Total
Numbers						
1985-90	3	19	12	13	7	54
1997-99	5	6	11	8	1	31
2000-02	3	8	7	6	1	25
2003-05	9	8	10	5	1	33
1997-2005	17	22	28	19	3	89
Overall mortality rates						
1985-90	0.18	1.17	1.28	4.07	12.02	1.17
1997-2005	1.05	1.28	1.51	2.15	1.80	1.43
Difference	0.88	0.11	0.23	-1.92	-10.22	0.26
95 per cent CI	*0.35,1.52*	*-0.68, 0.89*	*-0.83,1.10*	*-4.92,0.15*	*1.80,12.02*	*-0.19, 0.69*

* Detailed analyses by age were not published for 1991-93 or 1994-96.

Air travel

Of the two women died after air travel, only one followed a long-haul flight. One occurred in the first trimester and one in the second, suggesting that the risk is related to prothrombotic changes and not venous stasis in late pregnancy. Unfortunately the RCOG has now withdrawn its advice for preventing deep vein thrombosis for pregnant women travelling by air from its website. The RCOG guideline on thromboprophylaxis[2], however, includes "long-haul travel" in its list of risk factors as shown in the Annex to this Chapter. The recommendation of the NICE guideline on antenatal care[1] is as follows: *"Pregnant women should be informed that long-haul air travel is associated with an increased risk of venous thrombosis, although whether or not there is additional risk during pregnancy is unclear. In the general population, wearing correctly fitted compression stockings is effective at reducing the risk."*

Family history

In two deaths there was a family history of thromboembolism and the woman's weight was an additional factor in both cases. In one *Late* death a woman had been diagnosed with thrombophilia after family screening when she was a child, but when she developed deep venous thrombosis after pregnancy she took her anticoagulant medication only intermittently and died of pulmonary embolism.

Previous history

Two women had had a previous VTE. One was very obese and also had a family history of VTE. Another had had thrombophilia screening after her previous VTE but the result was negative and this appears to have given false reassurance regarding her management in pregnancy. The current guideline is that if thrombophilia screening is negative and there are no other risk factors then LMWH is not recommended[2].

Immobility

One woman had been admitted to hospital with hyperemesis gravidarum and so had both immobility and dehydration as risk factors.

Surgery unrelated to pregnancy

Previous surgery may have been a factor in three cases. One woman had abdominal surgery during pregnancy and the other two had complex surgical histories and underwent caesarean section. All three received routine thromboprophylaxis.

Assisted conception

A woman known to be at risk of ovarian hyperstimulation syndrome (OHSS) underwent superovulation and had a large number of oocytes collected and embryo transfer performed. She subsequently developed abdominal pain, collapsed within two weeks of the procedure and died a few days later. She had been counselled about the risks of superovulation but embryo transfer should not be performed when there is a high risk of OHSS.

Antepartum deaths

Of the eighteen women had a pulmonary embolism in their antenatal period, thirteen died during the first trimester (up to and including 12 weeks of gestation). Six women appear to have suddenly collapsed without prior warning but five of the remaining eight women who complained of symptoms in early pregnancy, three to their GP and two to hospital doctors, did not have their complaints taken seriously and were not investigated. There is insufficient awareness that women are at risk of thromboembolism from the very beginning of pregnancy.

Of the two morbidly obese women who died in their first trimester, one actively avoided doctors and midwives completely. Morbid obesity is a distressing condition and sufferers may find it difficult to talk to clinicians for fear of stigmatisation. By contrast, the other woman, who besides her obesity had a history of thrombophilia, booked for antenatal care early and, although an appointment was made with a haematologist, died in the interim. Maybe such high-risk women should be treated as emergencies in future. It is clear that, wherever possible, obese women should have pre-pregnancy counselling about its associated risks.

Although pregnancy nowadays is often promptly diagnosed, and the NICE antenatal care guidelines recommend early booking[2], it is not always encouraged and early antenatal care may be uncoordinated:

> *An obese, parous woman was booked at home by a midwife in early pregnancy. A few days later she telephoned her General Practitioner (GP) because of mild breathlessness and was told to contact the practice again if it got worse. The next day a relative phoned and requested a home visit and was told that the doctor would attend after morning surgery. The woman died a few minutes later.*

There is no record of the recommended needs and risk assessment[2] being undertaken during the home booking, or of any communication between the midwife and the GP. The GP later commented that the relative did not convey a sense of urgency over the phone but it is unrealistic to expect a lay person to know that sudden and continuing breathlessness in an obese pregnant woman is a medical emergency. This fact should, however, be known by doctors and midwives.

Five women developed pulmonary embolism in later pregnancy and all underwent caesarean section. Four were perimortem but one was not:

> *A woman with a history of thromboembolism in her earlier life as well as previous pregnancies became pregnant again. She had also had a previous postpartum thromboembolism which required a thoracotomy and a filter in her inferior vena cava. Although her thrombophilia screen was negative she most probably had some as yet unidentified thrombophilia. Despite thromboprophylaxis and exemplary combined care she had a pulmonary embolism in mid-pregnancy. She underwent an elective caesarean section early in the third trimester. Her baby survived but she had further embolisms and died a few weeks after delivery.*

The staff are to be commended on their excellent care. One midwife commented: "I think she always knew how ill she was and all she wanted was a baby."

In the other four cases the pattern was of collapse in late pregnancy followed by a perimortem or postmortem caesarean section. Worryingly, the pattern was also that medical staff inappropriately reassured these women about their symptoms, which were often of dizziness, feeling flu-like and faint and having shortness of breath. One woman who returned from a holiday involving air travel and attended hospital feeling dizzy, faint and upset was told this was due to postural hypotension and sent home. She died the next day. The obstetrician commented that there were "no learning points" in this case but it illustrates the importance of taking these symptoms seriously. Although not many pregnant women who return from holiday have symptoms severe enough for them to attend hospital, in one case the woman's symptoms were severe enough for her GP to call the hospital:

> *A woman with marked varicose veins developed thrombophlebitis in her third trimester and was given graduated compression stockings. At term she complained of increasing breathlessness to her GP, who phoned the obstetric registrar and was reassured. She was asked to return for review but required urgent referral to hospital following a collapse the next day. She did not receive anticoagulant treatment until more than eight hours after admission and when she collapsed yet again a perimortem caesarean section was carried out. Her baby survived.*

Breathlessness severe enough to cause the GP to phone the hospital should be investigated. In this case the midwife later commented that thromboembolism had developed "in an otherwise low risk pregnancy". It is important to remember that labelling women as "low risk" does not preclude the need to maintain vigilance and take symptoms seriously. These lessons were reinforced in the other two deaths in early pregnancy. It is important also to remember that when breathlessness first appears in late pregnancy, pulmonary embolism should be considered.

In all four cases the women were inappropriately reassured by GPs and/or hospital staff including obstetricians, midwives and physicians. Of course clinical judgement is imperfect but these cases are a reminder of how subtle the symptoms of thromboembolism can be, and of how careful staff should be before offering reassurance.

Deaths after ectopic pregnancy or termination of pregnancy

One woman died after laparoscopic salpingectomy for early ectopic pregnancy despite the use of antiembolism boots and graduated compression stockings. Two other deaths in early pregnancy occurred after terminations of pregnancy and the lessons from these three cases suggest there is insufficient knowledge that such women are at risk. For example:

> *A young woman with complex social problems and a history of domestic abuse underwent a mid-trimester termination of pregnancy. Three weeks later she attended the Emergency Department (ED) with chest pain and a pulse rate of 120 bpm. A diagnosis of "urinary tract infection or pelvic inflammatory disease" was made, and she was referred to the gynaecological team but not admitted. She died a few days later.*

Chest pain and tachycardia in an apyrexial woman who has recently been pregnant are suggestive of pulmonary embolism or other serious cardiorespiratory pathology, as is sudden onset breathlessness, which was misattributed to anaemia in the other case.

Intrapartum deaths

There were no intrapartum deaths from pulmonary embolism in this triennium.

Deaths after vaginal delivery

Eight women died after vaginal delivery. Six women had delivered spontaneously and two by vacuum extraction. Known risk factors were present in seven of these cases; three were either overweight or obese, three were morbidly obese with BMIs exceeding 40 and one mother was aged over 40. In the remaining two cases the mothers' weight was not recorded. Five of the deaths were between postpartum days 8 and 28, as shown in Table 2.4.

Table 2.4
Time between delivery and death from pulmonary embolism; United Kingdom: 2003-05.

Time after delivery, days	Method of delivery		All
	Vaginal	Caesarean section	
0-7	1	1	2
8-14	2	2	4
15-28	3	2	5
29-42	2	1	3
42-365	2	2	4
Total	**11**	**6**	**18**

Two women were misdiagnosed in hospital as their breathlessness was attributed to chest infection. One had dyspnoea and haemoptysis eight days after delivery and was diagnosed with bronchopneumonia although she also received full heparinisation:

> *After an assisted vaginal delivery a woman complained of breathlessness for several days before calling her GP, who admitted her to hospital with a suspected pulmonary embolism. Her pulse rate was 130/minute, respiratory rate 30/bpm and her oxygen saturation was 92%. She was apyrexial. The medical registrar diagnosed pneumonia. She was transferred to the ward with a blood pressure of 84/48 mm/Hg and died a few hours after admission.*

Her care was sub-standard. Tachycardia and tachypnoea without pyrexia in a recently delivered woman strongly suggest thromboembolism. The internal hospital report stated that the ED was "busy". It is a pity that she was not promptly treated as the GP had made the correct diagnosis and had referred her appropriately. A GP with concerns about a patient being referred to the ED should contact the ED consultant directly.

Three morbidly obese women with a BMI over 40 did not receive thromboprophylaxis. For example:

> *An extremely obese woman was classed as a "low risk" case and received midwifery-only care. She underwent induction of labour, had three attempts at suturing a third-degree tear and was discharged home with a haemoglobin of less than 9.0g%. She collapsed and died some weeks after delivery.*

Her care was also sub-standard. Because of their co-morbidity, morbidly obese women are unsuitable for midwife-only care. As with the other two women, this mother should also have received thromboprophylaxis, particularly as additional risk factors developed. Another woman with a BMI over 40 was also classified as "low risk" and received inappropriate midwifery-only care. In her case she complained of pain in her leg a few days after delivery and her midwife reassured her and advised her to see her GP if the pain worsened. She died a few weeks later. In this case she was wrongly reassured about a symptom suggestive of deep venous thrombosis.

The third very obese woman with a BMI over 40 had a socially and psychologically complex pregnancy and was very anxious throughout. She had a difficult labour resulting in an instrumental delivery and went home a few days later. She collapsed a few days afterwards. In her case it is possible that thromboprophylaxis may have been overlooked because the staff were focussed on her psychological state. In all three cases a management protocol for the morbidly obese woman would have been helpful. Such a protocol should combine medical assessment with the sensitive midwifery and obstetric support these women require.

Deaths after caesarean section

Seven women died after caesarean section. Two others died later in the puerperium and are classified as *Late* deaths. The intervals between the delivery and death were shown in Table 2.4. All the women received thromboprophylaxis. In contrast to the women who died after vaginal delivery, only two of the women who died following a caesarean section were morbidly obese. Care, however, was sub-standard, for example:

> A morbidly obese woman required a wheelchair because she weighed almost 200Kg at the end of her pregnancy. Correctly she was assessed antenatally by the anaesthetist and excellent care was provided when fetal distress developed in labour and a caesarean section was required. She had thromboprophylaxis (tinzaparin 5000 units daily) and was discharged within a week of delivery. Shortly afterwards she complained of breathlessness but this was attributed to her obesity. She died a few days later.

Although the general care provided for this woman was excellent, she presented a very difficult problem and once again guidelines on the management of the morbidly obese woman may have been helpful. The prophylactic dose of tinzaparin was appropriate for normal body weight but the RCOG guideline recommends 4,500 units 12-hourly for a woman with a body weight over 90Kg. The other woman also required an urgent caesarean section which was complicated by bleeding from the uterine angle and blood transfusion was needed. Thromboprophylaxis, in her case 40mg enoxaparin, was given but not until well after the operation. She collapsed and died two days later. Her thromboprophylaxis was delayed and the caesarean section in such a difficult case should have been performed by a consultant.

An intravenous drug user also presented difficulty:

> A young woman who had used intravenous drugs and had suffered domestic and childhood abuse was classed as a low risk and received midwife-only care. Her membranes ruptured early and on admission a footling breech presentation was diagnosed. Preparations were made for a caesarean section but, due to sclerosis, peripheral venous access was impossible and a femoral central line was inserted. She was given thromboprophylaxis but she died a few days later.

Here too midwifery-only care was inappropriate. The state of her veins should have been noted and she should have been assessed in advance by an anaesthetist. Access via a neck vein may have been preferable to a femoral vein.

Late deaths

Three *Late Direct* maternal deaths from pulmonary thromboembolism are counted in Chapter 14. All the women had known risk factors. One had thrombophilia (protein S deficiency) and the other two were obese.

Cerebral vein thrombosis

Eight women died of cerebral venous thrombosis. Their ages ranged between 22 and 34 years, with a median age of 26 years. In the four cases where weight was recorded, two were obese, with a BMI over 30 and two were overweight, with a BMI over 25. Four women died in the first trimester, one in the second and two in the third, both requiring perimortem caesarean section. One died in the puerperium. There was one additional *Late* death, of an older woman, who was also obese, counted in Chapter 14.

There were was only one case of sub-standard care, where a woman died after developing ovarian hyperstimulation syndrome (OHSS) during assisted conception treatment. She had had superovulation followed by embryo transfer but no thromboprophylaxis. Thromboprophylaxis should always be given in OHSS. It is concerning that two deaths in this Chapter and one in Chapter 6 - Early pregnancy deaths, resulted from in vitro fertilisation procedures involving ovarian stimulation to produce large numbers of mature follicles.

The characteristic clinical picture of all of the women who died from central venous thrombosis was of a relatively short history of headache followed, sometimes very quickly, by neurological signs such as clouding of consciousness or confusion. One woman was an asylum seeker who did not speak English and psychiatric referral was considered but the correct diagnosis was quickly made. No woman was diagnosed at the stage of headache alone. A severe headache of new onset can be an indication for neuro-imaging in, or after pregnancy even in the absence of focal signs.

There is a striking similarity between cerebral and pulmonary thrombosis with regard to risk factors, including obesity. It is to be hoped that increasing application of thromboprophylaxis among at-risk women will reduce deaths from both forms of thromboembolism.

Sub-standard care overall

Care was judged to be sub-standard in only one case of cerebral vein thrombosis, but present in two-thirds (22 of the 33) cases of pulmonary embolism. The main reasons were inadequate risk assessment in early pregnancy compounded by a failure to recognise or act on risk factors and a failure to appreciate the significance of signs and symptoms in the light of known risk factors. There were also failures to initiate treatment promptly or in adequate dosages. Giving thromboprophylaxis to morbidly obese women in doses recommended by current guidelines was not judged to be sub-standard care provided that the higher recommended dose was given to women to women with body weight over 90kg.

There was poor risk assessment in early pregnancy (or before pregnancy in the case of morbidly obese women), and failure to recognise the significance of symptoms such as leg pain and breathlessness. Better awareness of symptoms among professionals and women themselves could reduce the number of deaths from this condition. New guidelines are needed on thromboprophylaxis for morbidly obese women, especially those with a BMI over 40. Current guidelines recommend that the prophylactic and therapeutic doses of low molecular weight heparin depend on the woman's weight. This was followed sometimes but not in all cases and a specific guideline on morbid obesity is needed.

Conclusions

With increasing rates of obesity, more and further air travel, a rise in the average age at childbearing and caesarean section rates of around 23%, it is pleasing that the number of maternal deaths from thromboembolism has hardly changed since 1985-87. This is almost certainly due to increasing vigilance among obstetricians and midwives and the careful application of thromboprophylaxis protocols. The fall in deaths from postpartum embolism after caesarean section shows the effectiveness of this strategy.

The same strategy should now be applied to prevent deaths in early pregnancy and postpartum deaths after vaginal delivery. Thromboembolism is not a "bolt from the blue". Risk factors were identified in 27 of the 41 women whose deaths are counted in this Chapter. Of the ten women who died in the first trimester of pregnancy, seven had identifiable risk factors. Four were obese or morbidly obese. We repeat our previous recommendation that public health education is necessary so that women at risk because of their weight, family history or past history can seek advice before becoming pregnant.

The inappropriate classification of obese women, and those with complex pregnancies and risky lifestyles, as "low risk" is a worrying trend. A full risk and needs assessment in early pregnancy must be undertaken before care plans are decided. Partly as a result of recommendations made in preceding Reports, and in Maternity Matters[6], NICE is in the process of developing such a risk assessment tool which should be used at all booking appointments as soon as it is available. Antenatal care must reflect clear and objective judgement and this point is also made in the midwifery Chapter (Chapter 16) of this Report. Again we repeat the recommendation that "All women should undergo an assessment of risk factors in early pregnancy or before pregnancy. This assessment should be repeated if the woman is admitted to hospital or develops other intercurrent problems."

False reassurance, including reassurance over the telephone when the woman has not even been examined, is another worrying trend which is also picked up in the new Chapter for GPs. Early symptoms of life-threatening embolism are generally mild and reassurance is too easy to give and accept.

Finally, our examination of these 41 cases reinforces our view that only a national survey such as this can draw useful conclusions about emerging trends. Reflection on individual cases in Trusts is necessary but local investigations may be insufficiently self-critical or indeed too self-critical, and may not reveal important new factors such as the high risks run by morbidly obese women. Our main recommendation for this triennium is that there is an urgent need for a guideline on management of obese pregnant women.

References

1 Knight M, Kurinczuk JJ, Spark P and Brocklehurst P. *United Kingdom Obstetric Surveillance System (UKOSS) Annual Report 2007*. National Perinatal Epidemiology Unit, Oxford.

2 National Collaborating Centre for Women's and Children's Health commissioned by the National Institute for Clinical Excellence. *Antenatal care: routine care for the healthy pregnant woman*. London: RCOG Press, 2003. Available at www.nice.org.uk

3 Royal College of Obstetricians and Gynaecologists. *Thromboprophylaxis during pregnancy, labour and after normal vaginal delivery*. Guideline no.37. London: RCOG Press; 2004. Available at www.rcog.org.uk

4 Royal College of Obstetricians and Gynaecologists. *Thromboembolic disease in pregnancy and the puerperium: acute management*. Guideline no.28. London: RCOG Press; 2001. Available at www.rcog.org.uk

5 Royal College of Obstetricians and Gynaecologists. *Report of the RCOG Working Party on prophylaxis against thromboembolism in gynaecology and obstetrics*. London: RCOG Press; 1995.

6 Department of Health. *Maternity Matters: choice, access and continuity of care in a safe service*. London: Department of Health; April 2007. www.dh.gov.uk

Annex 2.1

Summary of the key recommendations of the Royal College of Obstetricians and Gynaecologists (RCOG) guidelines for thromboprophylaxis in pregnancy, labour and after vaginal delivery and caesarean section.

Thromboprophylaxis during pregnancy, labour and after normal vaginal delivery[3].

Risk factors for venous thromboembolism in pregnancy and the puerperium[a]

Pre-existing	New onset or transient[b]
Previous VTE	Surgical procedure in pregnancy or puerperium
Thrombophilia	*eg. evacuation of retained products of conception, postpartum sterilisation*
Congenital	
Antithrombin deficiency	Hyperemesis
Protein C deficiency	Dehydration
Protein S deficiency	Ovarian hyperstimulation syndrome
Factor V Leiden	Severe infection e.g. pyelonephritis
Prothrombin gene variant	Immobility (>4 days' bed rest)
Acquired	Pre-eclampsia
(antiphospholipid syndrome)	Excessive blood loss
	Long-haul travel[c]
Lupus anticoagulant	Prolonged labour[c]
Anticardiolipin antibodies	Midcavity instrumental delivery[c]
Age over 35 years	Immobility after delivery[c]
Obesity	
(BMI >30kg/m2 either pre-pregnancy or in early pregnancy)	
Parity >4	
Gross varicose veins	
Paraplegia	
Sickle cell disease	
Inflammatory disorders	
e.g. inflammatory bowel disease	
Some medical disorders	
e.g. nephritic syndrome, certain cardiac diseases	
Myeloproliferative disorders	
eg. essential thrombocythaemia, polycythaemia vera.	

a   Although these are all accepted as thromboembolic risk factors, there are few data to support the degree of increased risk associated with many of them.

b   These risk factors are potentially reversible and may develop at later stages in gestation than the initial risk assessment or may resolve; an ongoing individual risk assessment is important.

c   Risk factors specific to postpartum VTE only.

Recommendations

All women should undergo an assessment of risk factors for VTE in early pregnancy or before pregnancy. This assessment should be repeated if the woman is admitted to hospital or develops other intercurrent problems. **(C)**

Women with previous VTE should be screened for inherited and acquired thrombophilia, ideally before pregnancy. **(B)**

Regardless of their risk of VTE, immobilisation of women during pregnancy, labour and the puerperium should be minimised and dehydration should be avoided. **(GPP)**

Women with previous VTE should be offered postpartum thromboprophylaxis with LMWH. It may be reasonable not to use antenatal thromboprophylaxis with heparin in women with a single previous VTE associated with a temporary risk factor that has now resolved. **(C)**

Women with previous recurrent VTE or a previous VTE and a family history of VTE in a first-degree relative should be offered thromboprophylaxis with LMWH antenatally, and for at least six weeks postpartum. **(C)**

Women with previous VTE and thrombophilia should be offered thromboprophylaxis with LMWH antenatally and for at least six weeks postpartum. **(B)**

Women with asymptomatic inherited or acquired thrombophilia may qualify for antenatal or postnatal thromboprophylaxis, depending on the specific thrombophilia and the presence of other risk factors. **(C)**

Women with three or more persisting risk factors should be considered for thromboprophylaxis with LMWH antenatally and for three to five days postpartum. **(*GPP)**

Women should be reassessed before or during labour for risk factors for VTE. Age over 35 years and BMI greater than 30 or a body weight greater than 90Kg are important independent risk factors for postpartum VTE even after vaginal delivery. The combination of either of these risk factors with any other risk factor for VTE (such as pre-eclampsia or immobility) or the presence of two other persisting risk factors should lead the clinician to consider the use of LMWH for three to five days postpartum. **(*GPP)**

Antenatal thromboprophylaxis should begin as early in pregnancy as practical. Postpartum prophylaxis should begin as soon as possible after. **(B)**

LMWHs are the agents of choice for antenatal thromboprophylaxis. They are as effective as and safer than unfractionated heparin in pregnancy. **(B)**

Warfarin should usually be avoided during pregnancy. It is safe after delivery and during breastfeeding. **(B)**

Once the woman is in labour or thinks she is in labour, she should be advised not to inject any further heparin. She should be reassessed on admission to hospital and further doses should be prescribed by medical staff. **(GPP)**

The grades of recommendations (B or C) are as follows:

B   Requires the availability of well controlled clinical studies but no randomised clinical trials on the topic of recommendations (Evidence levels IIa, IIb, III).

C   Requires evidence obtained from expert committee reports or opinions and/or clinical experiences of respected authorities. Indicates an absence of directly applicable clinical studies of good quality (Evidence level IV).

GPP   The other recommendations represent Good Practice Points (GPP), i.e. recommended best practice based on the clinical experience of the guideline development group.

For further details, see the full Report[3].

Prophylaxis against thromboembolism in caesarean section

The following recommendations, taken from the RCOG Working Party Report on prophylaxis against thromboembolism[5], are widely used for risk assessment and are of relevance to women requiring caesarean section. It is important to note that the 2004 guideline[3] updates and replaces previous guidance on dosage of thromboprophylaxis.

Box 2.1.1
RCOG Risk assessment profile for thromboembolism in caesarean section

Low risk - Early mobilisation and hydration

Elective caesarean section - uncomplicated pregnancy and no other risk factors

Moderate risk – Consider one of a variety of prophylactic measures

- Age >35 years
- Obesity (>80kg)
- Parity 4 or more
- Labour 12 hours or more
- Gross varicose veins
- Current infection
- Pre-eclampsia
- Immobility prior to surgery (>4 days)
- Major current illness, e.g. heart or lung disease, cancer, inflammatory bowel disease, nephrotic syndrome
- Emergency caesarean section in labour

High risk – Heparin prophylaxis +/- leg stockings

- A patient with three or more moderate risk factors from above
- Extended major pelvic or abdominal surgery, e.g. caesarean hysterectomy
- Patients with personal or family history of deep venous thrombosis, pulmonary embolism or thrombophilia paralysis of lower limbs
- Patients with antiphospholipid antibody (cardiolipin antibody or lupus anticoagulant)

Management of different risk groups

Low risk patients

Patients undergoing elective caesarean section with uncomplicated pregnancy and no other risk factors require only early mobilisation and attention to hydration.

Moderate risk patients

Patients assessed as of moderate risk should receive subcutaneous heparin (doses are higher during pregnancy) or mechanical methods. Dextran 70 is not recommended until after the delivery of the fetus and is probably best avoided in pregnant women.

High risk patients

Patients assessed as high risk should receive heparin prophylaxis and, in addition, leg stockings would be beneficial.

Prophylaxis until the fifth postoperative day is advised (or until fully mobilised if longer).

The use of subcutaneous heparin as prophylaxis in patients with an epidural or spinal block remains contentious. Evidence from general and orthopaedic surgery does not point to an increased risk of spinal haematoma.

3 Pre-eclampsia and eclampsia

James Neilson

Pre-eclampsia and eclampsia: Specific recommendations

Women with a systolic blood pressure of 160 mm/Hg or more need anti-hypertensive treatment. Consideration should be given to initiating treatment at lower pressures if the overall clinical picture suggests likely rapid deterioration with anticipation of severe hypertension.

Anaesthetists should anticipate an additional rise in blood pressure at intubation in women with severe pre-eclampsia who are undergoing caesarean section under general anaesthesia and take measures to avoid a speed that compromises maternal wellbeing, even when there are concerns about fetal wellbeing.

Syntometrine should not be given for the active management of the third stage if the mother is hypertensive, or if her blood pressure has not been checked.

Summary of key findings for 2003-05

The deaths of 18 women who died from eclampsia or pre-eclampsia are counted in this Chapter. The death of one additional woman from fatty liver of pregnancy is also counted here.

Of the women who died from eclampsia or pre-eclampsia, ten died from intracranial haemorrhage, two from cerebral infarction (one with secondary haemorrhage), two from multi-organ failure that included adult respiratory distress syndrome (ARDS), one from massive liver infarction, and three from other causes. The total number of deaths and the mortality rate are similar to those for the previous two triennia, as Table 3.1 shows.

Table 3.1
Numbers of *Direct* deaths attributed to eclampsia and pre-eclampsia and mortality rates per 100,000 maternities; United Kingdom: 1985-2005.

Triennium	Number	Rate	95 per cent CI	
1985-87	27	1.19	0.82	1.73
1988-90	27	1.14	0.79	1.66
1991-93	20	0.86	0.56	1.33
1994-96	20	0.91	0.59	1.41
1997-99	16	0.75	0.46	1.22
2000-02	14	0.70	0.42	1.18
2003-05	18	0.85	0.54	1.35

The causes of death are compared with figures from recent triennia in Table 3.2. There were no deaths from pulmonary causes alone. This is consistent with the trend of recent years and is assumed to reflect better fluid management in women with pre-eclampsia.

Table 3.2

Numbers of deaths from pre-eclampsia or eclampsia; United Kingdom 2003-05.

Triennium	Cerebral					Pulmonary				Hepatic				Total
	Intracranial haemorrhage	Subarachnoid	Infarct	Oedema	**All**	ARDS	Oedema	Other	**All**	Rupture	Failure/ necrosis	Other	**All**	
1985-87	11	0	0	0	**11**	9	1	2	**12**	0	1	3	**4**	27
1988-90	10	2	2	0	**14**	9	1	0	**10**	0	1	2	**3**	27
1991-93	5	0	0	0	**5**	8	3	0	**11**	0	0	4	**4**	20
1994-96	3	1	0	3	**7**	6	2	0	**8**	2	1	2	**5**	20
1997-99	7	0	0	0	**7**	2	0	0	**2**	2	0	5	**7**	16
2000-02	9	0	0	0	**9**	1	0	0	**1**	0	0	4	**4**	14
2003-05	10	0	2	0	**12**	0	0	0	**0**	0	2	4	**6**	18

Incidence of eclampsia in the United Kingdom

Cases of severe maternal morbidity and mortality from eclampsia were surveyed through the UKOSS system from February 2005 to February 2006[1]. Over the thirteen months of the study, 209 confirmed cases of eclampsia, including deaths, were reported. This represented an estimated incidence of 26.8 cases per 100,000 maternities with a 95% confidence interval from 23.3 to 30.7. This represents a significant decrease since an earlier national surveillance study, which found an incidence of 49 per 100,000 maternities, with a confidence interval from 45 to 54 per 100,000 maternities in 1992[2]. Ninety-nine per cent of women in the UKOSS study were treated with magnesium sulphate in accordance with national guidelines.

The women who died

The ages of the women ranged between 23 and 40 years, with a median age of 33 years. The gestational ages at delivery ranged from 21 to 42 weeks, with a median of 37 weeks. Nine women were at, or after, term (37 weeks of gestation or more) at the time of delivery and only two were less than 28 weeks' pregnant. Fulminating disease occurred throughout the gestational range. Their parity ranged between 0 and 5 previous pregnancies, with a median of one. Seven women were primigravid. All the pregnancies were singleton.

Twelve women were White, two each were Black Caribbean or Black African and the other two women had recently arrived from other parts of the world. Only one did not speak English. Two booked late for antenatal care despite problems in previous pregnancies and one woman appeared to be a health tourist arriving in the UK near term.

Six women had eclamptic fits, five in the antenatal period. HELLP syndrome was diagnosed in eight women.

Thirteen cases showed features of remediable factors, and in eight of these there was major sub-standard care.

As in the last Report, intracranial haemorrhage was the single most common cause of death, and failure of effective anti-hypertensive therapy the most common source of sub-standard care. Although most sub-standard care was seen in the hospital sector, there were examples in primary care of midwives failing to test urine for proteinuria in women who subsequently developed severe pre-eclampsia.

All of the women who died were in hospital. In one case, the first indication of clinical concern was the observation of fetal growth restriction, pre-dating signs of pre-eclampsia.

Women with pre-eclampsia but who died from other causes are counted and discussed in other Chapters, including cases of post caesarean section haemorrhage in Chapter 4, iatrogenic haemothorax in Chapter 8, and intracranial haemorrhage that was probably unrelated to pre-eclampsia in Chapter 10. Key learning points are shown in Box 3.1.

Box 3.1
Learning points: pre-eclampsia and eclampsia

Fulminating pre-eclampsia occurs at term and post term, as well as pre-term.

Systolic blood pressures over 160 mm/Hg must be treated.

Syntometrine should not be given for the active management of the third stage if the mother is hypertensive, or her blood pressure has not been checked.

The anaesthestist should be given as much time as possible to try to prevent the pressor effects of intubation in the pre-eclamptic woman, even when there are pressing fetal reasons for urgent caesarean section under general anaesthesia.

Systolic hypertension

The single major failing in clinical care in pre-eclampsia in the current triennium was inadequate treatment of systolic hypertension. The sequel, intracranial haemorrhage, occurred in several cases. The following description is illustrative:

> A woman whose early pregnancy blood pressure was 140/70 mm/Hg was normotensive until mid-third trimester when her blood pressure was found to be 180/100 mm/Hg, with proteinuria ++ and she was admitted for care. Labetalol was started and she was discharged but remained hypertensive. She was subsequently readmitted with a blood pressure of 160/100 mm/Hg and proteinuria +++. Over the next 48 hours, her blood pressure remained elevated and reached a maximum systolic pressure of 205 mm/Hg. The dose of oral labetalol was increased, and low molecular weight heparin thromboprophylaxis started. After a further 48 hours, she was still symptomatic and had a blood pressure of 220/110 mm/Hg with disordered liver function.

> Magnesium sulphate was started and a single oral dose of nifedipine given. Induction of labour was unsuccessful and caesarean section was performed. After delivery, her systolic blood pressure remained elevated between 190 and 205 mm/Hg, on oral labetalol. Neurological signs first appeared within a day of delivery. Her systolic pressure remained between 180-200 mm/Hg. She became unresponsive and a CT scan showed a cerebral haemorrhage. She died in the Critical Care unit. Autopsy showed dual intracranial pathology: cerebral sinus thrombosis as well as the haemorrhage.

This woman had prolonged hypertension with systolic pressures frequently above 200 mm/Hg, and no effective treatment. There was additional sub-standard care through inappropriate discharge, inappropriate referral to community midwifery care after discharge on anti-hypertensive medication and inappropriate delay in delivery.

There is incomplete understanding of the precise mechanisms that link hypertension and haemorrhagic stroke, both in pregnant and non-pregnant patients, but systolic hypertension is certainly important. With large pulse pressures, the mean arterial pressure (MAP) may not convey the real threat of a very high systolic pressure. In the last Report it was suggested that clinical guidelines should identify a systolic pressure above which urgent and effective anti-hypertensive treatment is required. Since then, a publication from the United States has presented a convincing case that the threshold should be 160 mm/Hg[3]. Clinically, it is also important to recognise the increase in, as well as the absolute values of, systolic hypertension. In severe and rapidly worsening pre-eclampsia early treatment, at less than 160 mm/Hg, is advisable if the trend points to the likely development of severe hypertension.

If automated systems are used to monitor blood pressure it is important to ensure that these have been validated for use in pregnancy as some systematically underestimate systolic pressure in pre-eclampsia.

There are clinical interventions that can increase blood pressure still further in women with pre-eclampsia. These include intubation, and active management of the third stage of labour.

Pressor effects:

> *A woman with a family history of pregnancy induced hypertension had a booking blood pressure of 100/55 mm/Hg. After an otherwise normal pregnancy she had a seizure at home during early labour at term. She was given rectal diazepam by the paramedics and transferred to hospital where her blood pressure was 120/96 mm/Hg, with proteinuria +++. Her eclamptic seizures continued despite treatment with magnesium sulphate and a fetal bradycardia occurred, leading to an emergency caesarean section. She had a further seizure during pre-oxygenation and her blood pressure rose to 209/120 mm/Hg after intubation, despite having been given alfentanil. After delivery she was found to have an intracranial haemorrhage.*

In this case, in which there was no sub-standard care, the clinicians found themselves in the very difficult situation of balancing the risks to a seriously ill woman of rapid anaesthesia and surgery, with the risks to a bradycardic fetus of delayed delivery. The pressor effects of laryngoscopy and intubation[4] were known to the anaesthetist, who administered alfentanil to try to attenuate the hypertensive response. These effects may be less well known to obstetricians, who need to be aware of the difficulties that these present to anaesthetists in such circumstances. However in a similar case, care was less than optimal:

> *A previously healthy woman had her induction of labour for post-term pregnancy delayed because of service pressures. She was normotensive at the time but her urine was not tested. She became unwell the next morning with epigastric pain and vomiting. Her blood pressure was 170/90 mm/Hg and cardiotocography showed repetitive heart rate decelerations. It was thought likely that she had had a placental abruption. A decision was made to perform an emergency caesarean section. Her blood pressure was 200/105 mm/Hg in the anaesthetic room prior to (standard) induction of anaesthesia. Intubation proved difficult and her systolic pressure lay between 195 and 210 mm/Hg for the first 15 minutes of the operation. The baby was delivered in reasonable condition but the mother could not be roused from general anaesthesia. A delayed CT scan showed massive intracranial haemorrhage. Hepatic haemorrhage was also seen at autopsy.*

Despite the fulminating progress of this woman's pre-eclampsia, there were possible missed opportunities to make an earlier diagnosis, with urine untested at the antenatal clinic at term and in hospital at the time of proposed induction of labour. A finding of proteinuria two days before delivery was not investigated. Unlike the previous case, no specific measures were taken to avoid the pressor effects of intubation. Like the previous case, the anaesthetist was placed in a very difficult position.

Syntometrine

Two women presented so late in labour that their blood pressures were not measured before delivery. One of the women had had a normal blood pressure recording and normal urinalysis at the antenatal clinic the previous day. Both women received intramuscular syntometrine for third stage prophylaxis, and both were found subsequently to be hypertensive. In both cases, by coincidence, the blood pressures rose to maxima of 210/115 mm/Hg. One woman remained hypertensive despite intravenous hydrallazine and experienced eclamptic seizures despite magnesium sulphate. She died from a large cerebral haemorrhage. The other woman had her hypertension treated aggressively, and improved for some time before becoming profoundly hypotensive. At laparotomy she was found to have a large haemoperitoneum from, in part, a tear of the liver capsule. She died, much later, of multi-organ failure in the intensive care unit. In both cases, the progress of pre-eclampsia was extremely rapid.

It is well recognised that syntometrine, which contains ergometrine, is contra-indicated in hypertensive women. It seems less well recognised that women should have their blood pressure checked before giving syntometrine, or alternatively, they should be given intramuscular oxytocin if time and circumstances do not permit blood pressure measurement.

Postnatal complications

Three women had later sequelae of pre-eclampsia after postnatal discharge from hospital. In one case the woman developed a cavernous sinus thrombosis (despite low molecular weight heparin while in hospital) with secondary haemorrhage from a venous infarct. In another, a woman had been in the UK for a short time and, as a result, had not had time to enable appropriate arrangements attended the Emergency Department with headache and epigastric pain. Her blood pressure was 155/95 mm/Hg, having previously been around 90-120/50-60 mm/Hg, and her urine seems not to have been tested. An obstetric trainee was consulted by phone but did not visit the woman. She was discharged home but collapsed the following day with a fatal massive intracranial haemorrhage. Her plasma urate was very high as were her liver enzymes. A third woman was very overweight, had diabetes and chronic hypertension, and was a heavy smoker. She was admitted with superimposed pre-eclampsia and had a fetal death in hospital due to placental abruption. Delivery was by caesarean section but, despite the risk factors, she was not given low molecular weight heparin. She was readmitted to hospital after discharge, comatose, with a massive cerebral infarct resulting from thromboses in internal carotid and middle cerebral arteries.

Acknowledgements

This Chapter has been seen and discussed with Professor Andrew Shennan (London). I thank Dr Rustam Al-Shahi Salman (Edinburgh) and Professors Philip Bath and Peter Rubin (Nottingham) for their advice about hypertension and haemorrhagic stroke.

References

1   Knight M, Kurinczuk JJ, Spark P and Brocklehurst P. *United Kingdom Obstetric Surveillance System (UKOSS) Annual Report 2007.* National Perinatal Epidemiology Unit, Oxford.

2   Douglas KA, Redman CW. *Eclampsia in the United Kingdom. BMJ* 1994; 309(6966):1395-400.

3   Martin Jr JN, Thigpen BD, Moore RC, Rose CH, Cushman J, May W. *Stroke and pre-eclampsia and eclampsia: a paradigm shift focusing on systolic blood pressure.* Obstet Gynecol 2005;105:246-54.

4   Allen RW, James MF, Uys PC. *Attenuation of the pressor response to tracheal intubation in hypertensive proteinuric pregnant patients by lignocaine, alfentanil and magnesium sulphate.* Br J Anaesth 1991;66:216-23.

4 Haemorrhage

William Liston

Obstetric haemorrhage: Specific recommendations

All staff require regular training on identification and management of maternal collapse, including the identification of hidden bleeding and the management of haemorrhage, which is also a key recommendation of this Report.

An early warning scoring system of the type described in the Chapter on Critical Care, another key recommendation of this Report, may help in the more timely recognition of cases of hidden bleeding.

When severe haemorrhage occurs it is good practice to call straight away for the aid of colleagues with greater gynaecological surgical experience.

The management of women with placenta percreta requires careful multidisciplinary planning in the antenatal period and the involvement of a consultant-led multidisciplinary team at delivery.

Guidelines for the management of women who refuse blood products must be made available to, and discussed with, all maternity staff as part of their routine training, postgraduate education, continuing professional development and practice.

Women should be advised that caesarean section is not an entirely risk-free procedure and can hold problems for current and future pregnancies.

All women who have had a previous caesarean section must have their placental site determined. This, too, is a key recommendation of this Report. If there is any doubt, magnetic resonance imaging (MRI) can be used along with ultrasound scanning in determining if the placenta is accreta or percreta.

Summary of key findings for 2003-2005

The last Report drew attention to the impressive decline in deaths from obstetric haemorrhage in the United Kingdom over the last 50 years and outlined some of the possible reasons for this. In this triennium, 2003-05, 14 women died from haemorrhage; a rate of 0.66 per 100,000 maternities, similar to the rate for the previous triennium. Three other cases of haemorrhage associated with uterine rupture or genital tract trauma are included here, which, in previous Reports were counted and discussed in a now defunct Chapter relating to other causes of *Direct* maternal deaths. This old Chapter is no longer required as the number of maternal deaths from these causes is now too small for them to require a specific Chapter of their own.

Overall in the United Kingdom (UK), the risk of a pregnant women dying from haemorrhage is very small. However, there are several points which are not immediately apparent from these few UK deaths:

- Ten of the 17 women, almost three-fifths, of those who died received less than optimal care. In particular, there were questions concerning the most appropriate management of women with placenta percreta, a problem likely to become more prevalent due to its emerging relationship with previous caesarean section scars. There were also apparent failures in recognising the signs and symptoms of intra-abdominal bleeding especially after caesarean section. Lastly, ergometrine often seems to have been forgotten as a useful oxytocic drug.

- At least two major surveys in developed countries[1, 2], have shown around two thirds of all cases of severe maternal morbidity, so called "near misses", are related to severe haemorrhage. Midwives, obstetricians and anaesthetists routinely working on labour wards already know that anticipating or dealing with maternal haemorrhage occupies a considerable proportion of their skill and time. The management of severe haemorrhage can not only provoke extreme anxiety for the woman and her relatives, but also causes a great deal of worry and stress for the attendant staff.

- In global terms, haemorrhage remains one of the most important causes of maternal mortality[3] and accounts for 11% of all maternal deaths. The World Health Organisation (WHO) estimates a 1% case fatality rate for the 14 million annual cases of obstetric haemorrhage[4]. As a conservative estimate, some 140,000 deaths each year could be prevented if the women themselves had been given an understanding of the possible warning signs of bleeding, the knowledge and ability to seek skilled maternity care, at least at delivery, and had access to functioning emergency obstetric services.

Table 4.1 shows the details of the 17 women who died directly from obstetric haemorrhage this triennium, including two deaths from genital tract trauma associated with severe bleeding and one from a ruptured uterus, causes of mortality which, in the past, merited a Chapter of their own. For the purposes of comparison with previous triennia, these three women have been omitted from the rates from haemorrhage shown in Table 4.1. They are shown in a separate column, together with the corresponding numbers from previous triennia. Haemorrhage was also a complicating factor in nine other maternal deaths which are counted and discussed in other Chapters, including amniotic fluid embolism, sepsis and pre-eclampsia.

Table 4.1
Direct deaths by type of obstetric haemorrhage and mortality rate per 100,000 maternities; United Kingdom: 1985-2005.

| Triennium | Cause of Haemorrhage | | | Total | | | | Genital tract trauma* | Overall total | |
| | Placental abruption | Placenta praevia | Postpartum haemorrhage | | | | | | | |
	Number	Number	Number	Number	Rate	95 per cent CI		Number	Number	Rate
1985-87	4	0	6	10	0.44	0.24	0.81	6	16	0.71
1985-87	6	5	11	22	0.93	0.62	1.41	3	25	1.06
1991-93	3	4	8	15	0.65	0.39	1.07	4	19	0.82
1994-96	4	3	5	12	0.55	0.31	0.95	5	17	0.77
1997-99	3	3	1	7	0.33	0.16	0.68	2	9	0.42
2000-02	3	4	10	17	0.85	0.53	1.36	1	18	0.90
2003-05	2	3	9	14	0.66	0.39	1.11	3	17	0.80

* Includes ruptured uterus. These deaths were discussed in a separate Chapter in previous Reports.

The women who died

The ages of the mothers who died from haemorrhage ranged between 25 and 44 years with a median age of 33 years. Five were primiparous, another five had one previous child and two had at least five children each. Six of these women had a body mass index (BMI) of greater than 30 and two were morbidly obese with a BMI over 35. Eleven were delivered by caesarean section.

More than half of the women were from ethnic minorities and several spoke no English. This extra barrier made the provision of care for these women more difficult. However, unusually, compared with most other causes of *Direct* maternal deaths, all but two of the women received regular and timely antenatal care and were also in stable relationships with at least one partner in full time employment. At least three of the women were professionally qualified health care workers.

In previous Reports some deaths from haemorrhage followed concealed pregnancies or a lack of engagement with the maternity services. This is also the case this triennium. For example:

> *A single woman whose previous children were in the care of social services concealed her pregnancy until she attended in spontaneous labour. She discharged herself almost immediately after an apparently uneventful delivery, leaving her baby behind. She died, alone, of a postpartum bleed several days later, having made herself impossible to trace for community midwifery follow-up.*

Although very little could have been done to help this woman, who seemed determined to avoid all contact with any heath or other agencies, there are lessons to be learnt from the care of another woman whose antenatal care was less than optimal:

> *A grand multiparous woman who spoke no English was referred to the local maternity services for booking by her General Practitioner (GP) in a timely manner. She did not receive a date for her first antenatal appointment, however, until she was more than five months pregnant. Her pregnancy proceeded well until labour was induced despite a clear history of precipitate labours. She suffered a massive postpartum haemorrhage and died, despite a hysterectomy, some days later.*

The health system let this woman down because, despite her prompt action when she discovered she was pregnant, she did not receive her booking appointment until well after the first trimester of her pregnancy, thus missing the benefits of early antenatal care and opportunities for screening. She was then further let down both by poor clinical decision-making and an additional lack of immediate access to Critical Care.

Women who refused blood products

Two women who died from haemorrhage declined blood transfusion due to their religious beliefs. This was their free choice. However, it is almost certain that if they had received blood products they would have survived. One other woman who refused blood products died of an amniotic fluid embolus and her case is counted and discussed in Chapter 5. Despite their care being generally of a high standard, there are some general points in the care of these women that need to be re-emphasised:

- Consultant obstetric and anaesthetic involvement is necessary during the antenatal period in order to develop a care plan together with the woman, her husband and family, and, if necessary, religious advisors, should any difficulty occur.

- Informed consent for red blood cell salvage during surgery and infusion of salvaged blood should be sought and clearly recorded in the case notes. This facility should be provided for all women who give consent for this procedure.

- All women who are known to have stated a wish not to receive blood products should be seen by a consultant obstetrician and anaesthetist at the onset of their labour and a final care plan developed. In the past some women who died of post-operative haemorrhage were delivered by caesarean sections carried out by trainee obstetricians. It is therefore important that, whenever possible, each woman in labour should be cared for by a consultant obstetrician and, should an elective caesarean section or other operative delivery be required, this should be conducted by a consultant obstetrician and anaesthetist.

Detailed guidelines for the management of women who refuse blood products were given in the last Report and can be easily downloaded from the CEMACH website www.cemach.org.uk. These guidelines must be made available to, and discussed with, all maternity staff as part of their routine training, postgraduate education, continuing professional development and practice.

Sub-standard care

In ten of the seventeen cases (58%), care was assessed as sub-standard. There are three main lessons to be learnt from the deaths this triennium; these relate to the identification and management of intra-abdominal bleeding, uterine atony and placenta percreta.

"Too little, too late": Failure to recognise signs of intra-abdominal bleeding.

There was, on occasion, a failure to recognise the clear signs and symptoms of intra-abdominal bleeding, especially after a caesarean section, in spite of what appears to be, at least in retrospect, very clear evidence that the woman was still bleeding. Perhaps shorter postgraduate training programmes and less practical experience in identifying and managing acutely ill women account for this. There were a few cases where it was difficult for the assessors to understand the clinical decision-making. For example:

> An African woman did not reveal her female genital mutilation (FGM) until late in pregnancy and was not referred to a specialist service for this. She had an elective caesarean section because it was considered that the consequences of her particular type of genital cutting would make vaginal delivery difficult. Although the operation was apparently straightforward, shortly afterwards she had a blood loss of several litres with a consequent fall in haemoglobin, which required transfusion. She continued to deteriorate with a steadily falling haemoglobin, rising pulse rate and falling blood pressure accompanied by poor urine output and increasing abdominal girth. Although she needed continual blood transfusion, an exploratory laparotomy was not performed until nearly two days later. By then she was in extremis, and several litres of blood were found in her abdomen. She sustained a cardiac arrest while still in theatre and could not be resuscitated.

Her death illustrates several important lessons. Firstly, elective caesarean sections are not without hazard. Here the mother died following an operation which was probably not necessary. The issues posed by the increasing numbers of women who have been genitally mutilated arriving in the United Kingdom, and their management, are discussed in Chapter 1.

It is also clear that in this case the obvious signs of sustained intra-abdominal bleeding were present for a very long time before appropriate action was taken. In four other cases intra-abdominal bleeding, usually following caesarean section, was also not recognised until too late and then resuscitative measures were inadequate, as demonstrated by the following case:

> An older parous woman with a high BMI and a multiple pregnancy correctly had consultant antenatal care. She went into spontaneous labour but vaginal manipulation of the transverse lie of the second baby failed and a caesarean section was carried out by an obstetric trainee, who had difficulty in delivering the baby. A uterine tear was repaired by the consultant who then left. Her recovery from the anaesthetic was prolonged and the consultant anaesthetist was called. Her blood pressure fell and despite transfusion she suffered a fatal cardiac arrest. At autopsy her abdominal cavity contained over four litres of blood from an inadequately sutured uterine vein.

The consultant obstetrician should have been called earlier and should have waited to check the woman's initial recovery. Major intra-abdominal bleeding should have been suspected when the blood pressure fell without obvious vaginal blood loss. "Too little, too late" was a frequent comment made by the assessors in relation to the resuscitation of these women. A scoring system of the type described in Chapter 19, Critical Care, may help in the more timely recognition of such cases in future.

Consultants have a duty to maintain their skills and recognise their limitations. Previous Reports have recommended that a consultant undertaking a caesarean hysterectomy should have support available from a colleague. Perhaps the lack of recognition of continuing intra-abdominal bleeding is due to a lack of experience by "obstetric only" consultants in dealing with surgical emergencies. The current tendency to divide obstetrics from gynaecology has led to a situation where some obstetric consultants have little surgical gynaecological experience and thus may not always be able to cope with procedures such as emergency hysterectomy in sick and bleeding women. It is good practice in such situations to call straight away for the aid of colleagues with greater gynaecological surgical experience. In the "lessons I have learned" section of the individual Enquiry report forms, several consultants have regretted not calling in additional, more skilled, consultant help sooner. In general terms it is a good idea to call for a consultant colleague to help, whether or not that consultant is on call. It is also essential to involve skilled consultant anaesthetists in these decisions.

It is interesting to recall that this Chapter of the last Report noted *"in several cases the consultant anaesthetist had to persuade the obstetrician that physical signs such as oliguria, tachycardia or hypotension were attributable to haemorrhage and further surgery was required"*.

Management of uterine atony

As every undergraduate midwifery and medical student should know, in many cases postpartum haemorrhage is caused by atony of the uterus. In treating atony it seems that the drug ergometrine, as first advocated by Chassar Moir in the 1930s[5], is frequently forgotten, despite the fact that in a European survey of policies undertaken in 2003 as part of the EUPHRATES project, 42 % of maternity units in the UK said that it was their drug of first choice for the immediate management of obstetric haemorrhage[6]. It is a very effective oxytocic agent and should be used except in cases of hypertension. The two drugs, syntocinon and ergometrine, should be the drugs of first choice to prevent and treat atony of the uterus[7].

Given its relative frequency, maternity staff should have a high index of suspicion of the possibility of postpartum haemorrhage. In clinical situations such as prolonged labour or second stage caesarean section, the likelihood of an atonic uterus should be anticipated. Syntocinon and ergometrine should be used, given slowly intravenously, or as one ampoule of syntometrine intramuscularly. Additionally it is good practice to start a syntocinon infusion immediately after delivery of the baby, with 40 units of syntocinon in 500 mls of saline to run intravenously over the next two to four hours.

The identification and management of placenta percreta

Placenta praevia with a morbidly adherent placenta caused three maternal deaths where profuse bleeding was impossible to control. Cases such as those where a woman has an anterior placenta praevia and a previous caesarean section scar require all the energies and planning of consultant obstetricians, gynaecological surgeons, anaesthetists, interventional radiologists, blood transfusion specialists and on occasion, vascular surgeons and urologists.

All women who have had a previous caesarean section must have their placental site determined. If there is any doubt, magnetic resonance imaging (MRI) can be used along with ultrasound scanning in determining if the placenta is accreta or percreta[8]. Should either be the case it may be preferable in some cases to leave the placenta in the uterus after delivery of the baby by classical caesarean section. There are reports citing successful outcomes where the placenta is left in situ[9]. It might be difficult to do this in an acute bleeding situation although it should be considered. If a placenta percreta is clearly expected in an elective procedure, then delivery of the baby through the upper part of the uterus may allow a procedure which entails little blood loss. Some would then treat the patient with methotrexate to aid disintegration of the placenta.

Interventional radiological techniques may be useful in both the elective and emergency situation. Balloon tamponade of the internal iliac arteries is helpful in reducing the severity of haemorrhage whilst surgical haemostasis is achieved. This procedure may be carried out in the operating theatre under image intensification using a portable C arm intensifier. Although the procedure has been used successfully many times, the precise place of uterine artery embolisation is not yet clearly defined, particularly if it requires transfer of a sick and bleeding woman to the radiology department.

Ruptured uterus

This is the fourth successive triennial Report to include at least one case of uterine rupture in a parous woman after induction of labour with repeated doses of vaginal prostin:

> *An older parous woman with a history of precipitate labour developed hypertension in the third trimester, which worsened despite treatment. Her labour was induced with two 3mg prostin pessaries. At full dilatation fetal bradycardia developed and the baby was delivered rapidly. Her blood pressure subsequently fell but improved after infusion of gelfusin. She complained of abdominal pain, her blood pressure fell again and a massive postpartum haemorrhage occurred. The consultant attended and treated the bleeding with a vaginal pack but she sustained a cardiac arrest. After resuscitation a laparotomy revealed a ruptured uterus but despite a hysterectomy she died shortly afterwards.*

Although 3mg is the dose recommended by the manufacturers, many obstetricians prefer lower doses in parous women. The assessors consider this dosage of prostin to be high for a woman who has had a previous precipitate labour. The classic picture of ruptured uterus – precipitate labour, fetal bradycardia and maternal shock – was not recognised until cardiac arrest occurred.

Severe morbidity

Peripartum hysterectomy for severe obstetric haemorrhage

A case-control study of peripartum hysterectomy was carried out through the United Kingdom Obstetric Surveillance System (UKOSS) from February 2005 to February 2006[10]. Peripartum hysterectomy is usually carried out in the context of life-threatening obstetric haemorrhage and may therefore be regarded as a "near-miss" event for maternal mortality from haemorrhage. All consultant-led obstetric units in the UK participate in UKOSS and the results of this study therefore provide an indication of the maternal morbidity underlying the deaths reported in this Chapter.

During the thirteen months of the study, 315 women were reported to have had a peripartum hysterectomy to control haemorrhage, a rate of 41.0 per 100,000 maternities with a 95% confidence interval from 36.6 to 45.8 oer 100,000 maternities. This suggests that more than 60 women undergo a peripartum hysterectomy for each woman who dies from haemorrhage. The underlying factors identified for the women who died of haemorrhage are also reflected in this group of women who underwent hysterectomy. Women who had undergone a previous delivery by caesarean section were at higher risk of requiring a peripartum hysterectomy, with an odds ratio of 3.52 with a 95% confidence interval from 2.35 to 5.26. This risk increased with the number of previous caesarean sections; women who had had two or more previous caesarean section deliveries had more than an eighteen times higher odds of requiring a peripartum hysterectomy than women who had not had any caesarean section deliveries. Assuming causality, an estimated 28% of hysterectomies were attributable to prior caesarean delivery.

The causes of haemorrhage reported in the UKOSS study also reflect those identified in the women who died. Of women requiring hysterectomy, 53% were reported to have uterine atony and 38% had a morbidly adherent placenta, either placenta accreta, percreta or increta. The management of these women was variable. One hundred and thirty seven women had haemorrhage due to uterine atony alone. Four of these women (3%) did not receive any uterotonic therapy in the form of syntocinon infusion, ergometrine, prostaglandin F2α or misoprostol. Eleven (8%) were not managed with a syntocinon infusion and only 84 (61%) were given ergometrine. Twenty three women with haemorrhage due solely to morbidly adherent placenta (25%) did not receive any uterotonic treatment.

Fifty women were reported to have had a hysterectomy following a B-Lynch or other brace suture, twenty-eight following the use of activated factor VII and nine following arterial embolisation. It was noted in the previous Report that no deaths occurred in women managed with arterial embolisation but the use of these newer therapies requires further analysis and review.

Conclusions

The incidence of severe bleeding in childbirth has been estimated in various surveys to range between 4 and 5 per 1000 maternities, or one in 200 to 250 deliveries. In developed countries treatment is generally effective and this gives an approximate case fatality rate between 1 in 600 and 1 in 800 cases of obstetric bleeding[1,3,11]. Nevertheless as both this Report and the UKOSS study have shown, obstetric haemorrhage remains a problem both in terms of mortality and severe morbidity.

It is clear that previous caesarean section is a risk factor for haemorrhage and the operation is not as risk free as many have thought. Whilst recognising its clinical benefits, women must be advised of the potential risks of caesarean section for their current and future pregnancies, especially for those women who have had more than one previous operative delivery. All women who have had a previous caesarean section must have their placental site determined. If there is any doubt, magnetic resonance imaging (MRI) can be used along with ultra sound scanning in determining if the placenta is accreta or percreta.

Box 4.1
Learning points: obstetric haemorrhage

Dealing with ill, bleeding women requires skilled teamwork between obstetric and anaesthetic teams with appropriate help from other specialists including haematologists, vascular surgeons and radiologists.

Senior staff should be involved as early as possible, and should have appropriate experience.

The management of placenta percreta requires a large multidisciplinary team and forward planning.

References

1 Brace V, Penney G, Hall M. *Quantifying severe maternal morbidity: a Scottish population study.* BJOG 2004 May; 111(5):481-4.

2 Waterstone M, Bewley S, Wolfe C. *Incidence and predictors of severe obstetric morbidity: case-control study.* BMJ.2001 May 5;322(7294):1089-93;discussion 1093-4.

3 Ronsmans C, Graham WJ. *Maternal Mortality: who, when, and why.* Lancet 2006 Sep 30;368 (9542):1189-200.

4 AbouZahr C. *Global burden of maternal death.* In: British Medical Bulletin. Pregnancy: Reducing maternal death and disability. British Council. Oxford University Press.2003. 1-13. www.bmb.oupjournals.org

5 Moir JC. *The action of ergot preparations on the postpartum uterus.* Br Med J. 1932; 1: 520-523

6 Winter C, Macfarlane A, Deneux-Tharaux C, Zhang W H, Alexander S, Brocklehurst P et al. *Variations in policies for management of the third stage of labour and the immediate management of postpartum haemorrhage in Europe* BJOG. 2007 Jul;114(7):845-54.

7 Moussa H, Alfirevic Z. *Treatment for Primary Postpartum Haemorrhage.* Cochrane Database Syst Rev. 2007 Jan; CD003249.

8 Warshak CR, Eskander R, Hull AD, Scioscia AL, Mattrey RF, Benirschki K, Resnik R. *Accuracy of ultrasonography and magnetic resonance imaging in the diagnosis of placenta accreta.* Obstet Gynecol. 2006 Sep;108:573-81.

9 Kayem G, Davy C, Goffinet F, Thomas C, Clement D, Cabrol D. *Conservative versus extirpative management in cases of placenta accreta.* Obstet Gynecol. 2004 Sep;104:531-6.

10 Knight M, Kurinczuk JJ, Spark P and Brocklehurst P. *United Kingdom Obstetric Surveillance System (UKOSS) Annual Report 2007.* National Perinatal Epidemiology Unit, Oxford.

11 Zhang W-H, Alexander S, Bouvier-Colle M-H, Macfarlane A, the MOMS-B Group. *Incidence of severe pre-eclampsia, postpartum haemorrhage and sepsis as a surrogate marker for severe maternal morbidity in a European population-based study: the MOMS-B survey.* BJOG. 2005;112:89-96.

5 Amniotic fluid embolism

Robin Vlies

Amniotic fluid embolism (AFE): Specific recommendations

Clinical practice and ongoing education and training

The management of amniotic fluid embolism is the same as the management of any woman who collapses before, during, or after labour. All staff require regular training for the identification and management of severe maternal illness or collapse. This is also a key recommendation of this Report.

Pathology

At autopsy fetal squames and lanugo hair should be searched for in any pregnant or recently delivered woman. All possible attempts should be made to confirm a diagnosis of amniotic fluid embolism at autopsy. Histology, and if necessary, immunocytochemistry staining should be available.

National Amniotic Fluid Embolism Study

All cases of suspected or proven amniotic fluid embolism, whether fatal or not, should be reported through the monthly card notification system to:

The United Kingdom Obstetric Surveillance System (UKOSS)
The National Perinatal Epidemiology Unit
University of Oxford
Old Road Campus
Old Road
Headington
Oxford, OX3 7LF

Summary of key findings for 2003-05

In this triennium, the deaths of 19 mothers who died of amniotic fluid embolism (AFE) were reported to this Enquiry. Of these, 17 were *Direct* deaths while a further two, although discussed here, are counted as *Late Direct* deaths in Chapter 14. This is because although both these mothers survived the initial event, it resulted in a persistent vegetative state from which they died many weeks later.

As shown in Table 5.1, compared with the five cases reported in 2000-02 and eight in 1997-99, the 17 deaths and the mortality rate of 0.80 per 100,000 maternities attributed to amniotic fluid embolism this triennium appears high. The difference between the rate for 2003-05 and that for the previous triennium, shown in Table 5.1 was 0.55, with a 95 confidence interval from 0.10 to 1.06, which was only just statistically significant. In addition, the 17 *Direct* deaths were not evenly spread throughout the three year period, with only three occurring in 2005, so this does not represent a consistent upwards trend. Thus, although AFE is the second leading cause of *Direct* maternal death for the first time since it was identified as a cause of death in these Reports, it cannot be assumed that this pattern will persist.

Table 5.1
Direct deaths attributed to amniotic fluid embolism and rates per 100,000 maternities;
United Kingdom: 1985-2005.

Triennium	Number	Rate	95 per cent CI	
1985-87	9	0.40	*0.21*	*0.75*
1985-87	11	0.47	*0.26*	*0.83*
1991-93	10	0.43	*0.23*	*0.80*
1994-96	17	0.77	*0.48*	*1.24*
1997-99	8	0.38	*0.19*	*0.74*
2000-02	5	0.25	*0.11*	*0.59*
2003-05	17	0.80	*0.50*	*1.29*

The diagnosis of amniotic fluid embolism

Since the 1991-3 Report, deaths from AFE based on firm clinical diagnoses have been accepted in this Chapter as well as those confirmed at autopsy. This is a crucial point as in many other countries where pathological services are not requested or are less widely available, it is often convenient to ascribe the deaths of all women who suddenly collapse and die to AFE. Since deaths from AFE are often unavoidable the question of possible sub-standard care is thus avoided. In the United Kingdom however, the Enquiry assessors are assiduous in determining whether or not such deaths were due to AFE or other causes. Table 5.2 shows some possible distinguishing features between AFE and pulmonary embolism. The latter is a potentially preventable cause of maternal mortality, and anecdotally, is sometimes reported as AFE in some other countries to avoid possible blame.

Table 5.2
The clinical features of amniotic fluid embolism compared with pulmonary embolism.

	Amniotic fluid embolism	Pulmonary embolism
Timing of onset:	Most likely to occur during delivery.	Any time.
Early symptoms:	Dyspnoea, restlessness, panic, feeling cold, paraesthesiae. Pain less likely.	Dyspnoea, cough, haemoptysis, pleuritic pain.
Collapse:	Highly likely.	May occur.
DIC:	Highly likely.	Absent.
ECG:	Non-discriminatory.	Non-discriminatory.
Chest x-ray:	Pulmonary oedema, ARDS, right atrial enlargement, prominent pulmonary artery.	Segmental collapse, raised hemidiaphragm, unilateral effusion.
Arterial blood gases:	Non-discriminatory.	Non-discriminatory.
CT pulmonary artery:	Negative.	Positive.

In this triennium there was complete clinical and pathological correlation in 11 of the 19 cases. In two cases where the clinical diagnosis was in doubt, histological evidence of amniotic fluid embolism was proven at autopsy. Of the remaining cases the clinical diagnosis was not confirmed at autopsy, either because it was not performed (one case), was inadequately investigated (three cases) or because death occurred many weeks after the initial collapse (two cases). Strict correlation is made more difficult as it is known that fetal squames can be found in the maternal circulation in living patients without symptoms of amniotic fluid embolism[1]. Future clarity may be found in the measurement of complement, which may be activated following AFE, or the fetal antigen sialyl Tn[2]. The latter can be measured serologically or by immunocytochemistry on lung tissue but, as yet, is not widely available.

The reasons for the large increase in deaths from AFE for this triennium are not immediately obvious. The main criterion for diagnosis is the finding of fetal squames in the pulmonary vasculature at autopsy. The improved quality of examination and reporting at autopsy may have resulted in some increase in diagnosis, providing there is clinicopathological correlation. Such increased ascertainment therefore could account for some, though not all, of this increase. Excluding the two *Late* deaths, which had to be classified on clinical features alone, there were three other deaths in which the diagnosis was made clinically, supported by the Enquiry assessors, but not confirmed at autopsy. For example:

> *A multigravid woman who had a normal pregnancy was admitted in late pregnancy because of pre-eclampsia. She had labour induced with 3mg of oral prostaglandin followed a few hours later by a further 3 mg. A rapid labour ensued which resulted in a vaginal delivery with an incomplete placenta. She was transferred to theatre for manual removal of the placental remains at which stage her observations were stable. She collapsed an hour or so later and developed disseminated intravascular coagulation (DIC). She sustained another cardiac arrest shortly afterwards from which she could not be resuscitated.*

At autopsy there were numerous petechial haemorrhages on her serosal surfaces. Extensive histology demonstrated the features of severe pre-eclampsia but found no retention of products in the uterus and no evidence of amniotic fluid embolism was identified within the pulmonary capillaries.

There were another three maternal deaths where the fetal squames were scanty and only detected after prolonged searching. It is therefore conceivable that these six cases may not have been categorised as amniotic fluid embolism in previous Reports. Some of these cases also had an atypical clinical presentation. For example:

> *A primigravid woman presented at term in spontaneous labour. She collapsed a few hours later, just as arrangements were being made for an emergency caesarean section for fetal distress. She was successfully resuscitated but at operation an excess of blood was found in her abdomen and an exploratory laparotomy revealed a two centimetre tear on the inferior aspect of the left lobe of the liver. Despite transfusion and blood products she continued to bleed and, even though she was transferred to a liver unit, she eventually died.*

Her autopsy confirmed the liver rupture but there was no underlying liver pathology on histology. Cytokeratin positive squames were found in her lung capillaries as well as in a medium-sized artery on immunochemistry. Her cause of death was attributed to spontaneous rupture of the liver but it is also conceivable that vigorous resuscitation caused rupture of the liver in a patient with a bleeding diathesis from amniotic fluid embolus.

The women who died

The classical scenario of amniotic fluid embolism usually involves an older, multiparous woman in advanced labour who suddenly collapses, develops DIC and dies rapidly thereafter:

> *A woman with a history of previous normal deliveries had labour induced with 3mg of vaginal prostaglandin which was repeated a few hours later and labour then rapidly commenced. She collapsed at the start of the second stage and, following successful cardiopulmonary resuscitation, an emergency caesarean section was performed. She developed DIC with an estimated blood loss*

of over ten litres. Despite a hysterectomy, and excellent Critical Care, she died shortly afterwards. Autopsy confirmed the presence of fetal squamous cells in her pulmonary vasculature.

The ages of the women who died this triennium ranged from 17 to 39 years with a median age of 33 years. Thirteen were multiparous. All but one had reached their estimated due delivery date of between 38-41 weeks' gestation with the other woman having a slightly premature delivery. Fifteen women died within 24 hours of collapse.

All the women were in stable relationships and only one family was unemployed. Five were from Black and Minority Ethnic groups, four of whom did not speak English. All but three sought and received appropriate and timely antenatal care. The other women, all Black African mothers with previous children, had booked for maternity care at around six months of pregnancy.

The clinical circumstances

Only one of the women whose deaths are discussed in this Chapter died undelivered. Four women who collapsed before the onset of labour were delivered by emergency caesarean section. Of the others, five had a spontaneous vaginal delivery, two required low cavity forceps and the remaining women were delivered by caesarean section, ten of which were peri or post mortem sections carried out during active maternal resuscitation. Four women collapsed after delivery, two within minutes and the others between one and four hours. Hysterectomy was also performed in four cases.

Ten babies survived including one set of twins and the three babies who were delivered before their mothers collapsed. Unusually, a third of the babies who were delivered by peri or post mortem caesarean section also survived, probably because their mothers collapsed in a delivery suite or maternity ward fully equipped for rapid emergency caesarean sections and neonatal resuscitation.

Eight women had received uterine stimulation, five with prostaglandins and three with oxytocin. Nine had ruptured membranes, two artificially. In 11 cases, premonitory symptoms were recorded which included breathlessness, chest pain, feeling cold, light headedness, restlessness, distress, panic, a feeling of pins and needles in the fingers and nausea and vomiting. The interval between the onset of these symptoms and delivery varied from almost immediately to over four hours later.

All the cases described here involved resuscitation and advanced life support. In many cases there were excellent examples of multidisciplinary team working and excellent support was provided for both staff and relatives.

Box 5.1
Learning points: AFE

In many cases, women who suffer an amniotic fluid embolism report some or all of the following premonitory symptoms:

Breathlessness, chest pain, feeling cold, light headedness, restlessness, distress, panic, a feeling of pins and needles in the fingers, nausea and vomiting.

In several cases the severity of the mother's condition was not recognised until too late which compromised the delivery of timely and effective resuscitation.

Sub-standard care

Care was judged to be sub-standard in seven (36%) cases. Even though many of these deaths would probably have been inevitable, the defining feature of most of them was a delay in instituting resuscitation although there were other contributory features, as discussed later. In three cases there was a failure to recognise the severity of the acutely ill women and in two further cases resuscitation was delayed because women were sent for unnecessary diagnostic scans. For two other women more resuscitation was delayed because either the relevant drugs and equipment were not readily to hand or the cardiac arrest team were unable to gain access to the labour ward.

Care for these women could also be judged sub-standard for other reasons. One woman who collapsed just after delivery had had a seven to eight hour second stage before eventual delivery. For three women who were delivered by emergency caesarean section there was a delay in delivery, in one case for more than five hours. The Managing Obstetric Emergencies and Trauma (MOET) course recommends caesarean section delivery of the infant within five minutes of cardiac arrest to facilitate resuscitation[3].

One woman's care was compromised by having to be transferred from an isolated maternity unit in a haemodynamically unstable condition and in a further case the mother was left unattended in labour for half an hour after being given pethidine and then found collapsed. One woman, who due to her beliefs refused to accept blood transfusion, had no advanced care plan regarding the management of any obstetric emergency.

Pathology

At post mortem the initial features of AFE are of congested, relatively airless lungs with petechial haemorrhages on mesothelial, particularly pleural surfaces. Often other organ systems are normal and the diagnosis can only be confirmed on histology. Fetal squames can often be identified within the maternal lung capillaries on routine H&E staining and amniotic fluid mucins and lanugo hairs may also be present. Sometimes the material may be so scanty, as with three cases this triennium, that immunochemistry is required for identification.

In this triennium an autopsy was performed for all but one of the women. In one case the report was not available to the assessors and histology was not performed, or not available, in another. The one woman who did not have an autopsy collapsed a few minutes after delivery. This woman was a *Late* death, dying two months later, and the diagnosis in her case was made clinically. In three other cases AFE was not confirmed and the diagnosis was also made clinically and, for a further three, the diagnosis was difficult and only confirmed by immunocytochemistry. In the remaining cases fetal squames were either so obvious on routine staining that no special stains were required or were confirmed by immunochemistry.

The incidence of amniotic fluid embolism

A prospective, national study of amniotic fluid embolism is currently being undertaken by UKOSS[4]. Over the first eighteen months of the study from February 2005 to July 2006, 19 confirmed cases of amniotic fluid embolism were reported in an estimated 1,080,000 total births. This gives an estimated incidence in the UK of 1.8 cases per 100,000 maternities with a 95% confidence interval from 1.1 to 2.8.

Acknowledgements

This Chapter has been seen and commented on by Derek Tuffnell FRCOG.

References

1 Clark SL, Pavlova Z, Greenspoon J, Horenstein J, Phelan JP. *Squamous cells in the maternal pulmonary circulation.* Am J Obstet Gynecol 1986; 154:104-6.

2 Benson MD, Kobayashi H, Silver RK, Oi H, Greenberger PA, Terao T. *Immunologic studies in presumed amniotic fluid embolism.* Obstet Gynecol 2001; 97(4):510-4.

3 Grady K, Prasad BGR, Howell C. *Cardiopulmonary resuscitation in the non-pregnant and pregnant patient.* In: Johanson R, Cox C, Grady K, Howell C, editors. Managing Obstetric Emergencies and Trauma. London: RCOG Press; 2003. p 24.

4 Knight M, Kurinczuk JJ, Spark P and Brocklehurst P. *United Kingdom Obstetric Surveillance System (UKOSS) Annual Report 2007.* National Perinatal Epidemiology Unit, Oxford.

6 Early pregnancy deaths

James Neilson

Early pregnancy deaths: Specific recommendations

In women of reproductive age who present to practitioners with diarrhoea and vomiting and/or fainting, the possibility of ectopic pregnancy should be considered.

Medical treatment of ectopic pregnancy should be based on strict adherence to protocols, with women having immediate access to in-patient facilities if complications occur.

Women admitted to hospital with ovarian hyperstimulation syndrome should receive thromboprophylaxis.

Summary of key findings for 2003-2005

The deaths of fourteen women who died of causes directly attributed to complications arising in early pregnancy, before 24 completed weeks of gestation, who were reported to the Enquiry during this triennium are counted and discussed in this Chapter. These are shown in Table 6.1. These include ten deaths from ruptured ectopic pregnancies, one following a miscarriage, two deaths after termination of pregnancy, one illegal, and a death from ovarian hyperstimulation syndrome (OHSS).

An additional 18 women died from thromboembolism occurring before 24 weeks' completed gestation whose deaths are counted and discussed in Chapter 2 - Thrombosis and thromboembolism. Apart from the death following miscarriage attributable to anaphylaxis to analgesia which is counted in this Chapter, there were another five *Direct* deaths from sepsis associated with miscarriage which are counted and discussed in Chapter 7 - Genital tract sepsis. The case of a woman who died from anaesthesia following surgery for an ectopic pregnancy is counted and discussed in Chapter 8.

Table 6.1
Numbers of *Direct* deaths in early pregnancy counted in this Chapter by cause; United Kingdom: 1988-2005.

Triennium	Ectopic pregnancy	Miscarriage	Termination of pregnancy	Other	All deaths counted in Chapter 6	Counted as deaths from sepsis in chapter 7
1985-87	11	4	1	0	16	0
1988-90	15	6	3	0	24	0
1991-93	9	3	5	0	17	0
1994-96	12	2	1	0	15	0
1997-99	13	2	2	0	17	5
2000-02	11	1	3	0	15	2
2003-05	10*	1	2	1	14	5

Note: Up to 1994-96, early pregnancy deaths were defined as occurring before 20 weeks of pregnancy. Since 1997-99, 24 completed weeks of gestation has been used as the upper limit. Thus, direct comparisons with data from previous triennia may be misleading.
* A further woman who died from anaesthesia for an ectopic pregnancy is counted among the anaesthetic deaths.

The women who died

The ages of the women who died ranged between 18-40 years with a median age of 31. In contrast to the last Report, all but two mothers were White. Most women were in long term stable relationships and a few were health care workers.

Sub-standard care

As in previous years, the major challenge is to reduce the number of deaths from ectopic pregnancy, especially those associated with sub-standard care. Overall, 11 of the 14 deaths counted in this Chapter were assessed as having sub-standard care. Seven of the ten deaths from ectopic pregnancy were associated with sub-standard care, as were all the deaths from other causes counted in this Chapter.

Ectopic pregnancy

The maternal death rates from ectopic pregnancy for this and previous triennia are shown in Table 6.2.

Table 6.2
Numbers of deaths from ectopic pregnancies and rates per 100,000 estimated ectopic pregnancies; England and Wales 1988-1990 and United Kingdom: 1991-2005.

Triennium	Total estimated pregnancies	Total estimated ectopic pregnancies	Ectopic pregnancies per 1,000 pregnancies			Deaths from ectopic pregnancies	Death rate per 100,000 estimated ectopic pregnancies		
	Number	Number	Rate	*95 per cent CI*		Number	Rate	*95 per cent CI*	
England and Wales									
1988-90	2,880,814	24,775	8.6	*8.5*	*8.7*	15	0.52	*0.31*	*0.86*
United Kingdom									
1991-93	3,141,667	30,160	9.6	*9.5*	*9.7*	9	0.29	*0.15*	*0.55*
1994-96	2,917,391	33,550	11.5	*11.4*	*11.6*	12	0.41	*0.24*	*0.72*
1997-99	2,878,018	31,946	11.1	*11.0*	*11.2*	13	0.45	*0.26*	*0.77*
2000-02	2,736,364	30,100	11.0	*10.9*	*11.1*	11	0.40	*0.22*	*0.72*
2003-05	2,891,892	32,100	11.1	*10.9*	*11.1*	10	0.35	*0.19*	*0.64*

Ten women died from ruptured ectopic pregnancies during the period of this Report. Another woman, whose death is counted in the anaesthetic Chapter (Chapter 8), died of the consequences of the anaesthetic she received for treatment of an ectopic pregnancy. Among the ten deaths counted in this Chapter was one corneal (interstitial) pregnancy. Another woman had a heterotopic pregnancy (combined intra- and extra-uterine pregnancies). She presented with diarrhoea and vomiting, as did three other women with (non-heterotopic) ectopic pregnancies in whom misdiagnosis occurred. Recent Reports have repeatedly emphasised the importance of diarrhoea and vomiting as a possible, atypical clinical presentation of ectopic pregnancy:

> *A woman who had diarrhoea and vomiting also had vaginal bleeding, fainting and severe abdominal pain. She was known to be pregnant and was diagnosed as having gastroenteritis by a very junior gynaecologist in an Emergency Department (ED), and discharged. She returned to the ED the following day with increased pain, having collapsed at home. She was found to be hypotensive and tachycardic by the nursing staff, given a very large amount of intravenous*

fluid for what was thought to be dehydration from 'gastroenteritis' and again discharged. Her haemoglobin was not checked. She was tachycardic throughout. She returned a few hours later in extremis. Autopsy revealed a large haemoperitoneum from a ruptured tubal pregnancy.

It is important to re-emphasise that early pregnancy plus fainting points to ectopic pregnancy until proven otherwise. The importance of observation of vital signs also needs to be remembered. There is a recurring theme in this Report of junior medical staff disregarding important, basic clinical signs – tachycardia, hypotension, rapid respiration – this is one such case.

There were also potentially avoidable deaths in women who were under the care of specialist gynaecological services:

One woman had a modestly raised ßhCG level, no evidence of an intrauterine pregnancy and a pelvic mass on ultrasound compatible with ectopic pregnancy. While in hospital and awaiting a repeat ßhCG assay she collapsed with a ruptured tubal pregnancy from which she could not be resuscitated.

Another woman was having medical treatment with methotrexate for a known ectopic pregnancy. Her ßhCG levels rose rather than fell after one week of treatment, but it was not clear who saw these results. She became unwell, with diarrhoea and vomiting, and subsequently collapsed, but phone calls to the early pregnancy unit in the local hospital did not elicit the appropriate responses. Her GP found her shocked at home and she had a fatal cardio-respiratory arrest in the ambulance en route to hospital.

Many ectopic pregnancies in modern practice follow a benign clinical course which allows a more conservative approach to management. However, ectopic pregnancy remains a dangerous condition and these two cases are tragic reminders that deaths still occur. Medical treatment, in particular, must be based on strict adherence to protocols and immediate access to hospital services[1].

Another woman underwent salpingectomy at laparotomy. Although she had a large haemoperitoneum, her vital signs were stable during the procedure. She had been extubated and was breathing, when she had a cardiac arrest. The cause of death is not certain but the possibility of a cardiac arrythmia resulting from (relatively) cold intravenous fluids needs consideration.

Miscarriage

One woman had an anaphylactic reaction to an opioid analgesic administered by a paramedic. She was known to have a probable anembryonic pregnancy and was, appropriately, awaiting a further ultrasound, one week after the first, for definitive diagnosis. She was given the opioid for severe pain associated with spontaneous miscarriage.

One of the women whose death is counted in Chapter 7 - Sepsis, was initially and correctly thought to have had a septic miscarriage when seen in the Emergency Department, but the diagnosis was revised to probable ectopic pregnancy, despite a temperature of over 40°C.

Termination of pregnancy

The 50-year review of Confidential Enquiries in the last Report noted that 'the most striking change during the past 50 years has been the disappearance of unsafe, illegal abortion as a cause of early pregnancy Direct deaths in this country. The first full working year of the Abortion Act was 1969, but it was not until 1982-4 that no deaths from illegal abortion were recorded'. There have been no further such deaths until now:

A woman who had not been long in the UK, but who spoke English well, requested termination of an early pregnancy because of her social circumstances. She was referred from a community clinic to a hospital clinic for a surgical termination. In the meantime, she attended an Emergency Department with rigors and severe low abdominal pain, where she was found to be markedly pyrexial and tachycardic. She declined admission and was discharged by a junior gynaecologist on a broad spectrum antibiotic for what was thought to be a urinary tract infection. She returned to the hospital the next day, still very pyrexial, and intravenous fluids and antibiotics were given after significant delay. Shortly after a pelvic ultrasound examination, which showed free fluid in her pelvis, she suffered a cardiac arrest from which she could not be resuscitated. A laparotomy was done in case she had an ectopic pregnancy. Although there was blood in the pelvis there was no ectopic pregnancy. Microbiological cultures grew an unusual organism, usually found in water, from several tissues, and careful inspection at autopsy showed evidence of unusual trauma in her genital tract.

It is not known why this woman opted for an unsafe abortion, having already engaged with NHS services. One can only speculate if there may have been cultural issues, or coercion. Globally, unsafe, illegal abortion is very common and is one of the leading causes of maternal death. With increasing migration, this sad case is an important reminder to clinicians that this can happen in the UK too. Another woman died following a legal termination of pregnancy:

A young woman who underwent a medical termination of pregnancy was subsequently readmitted to hospital with vaginal bleeding. Because the bleeding settled and because ultrasound examination showed no evidence of retained tissues, she was discharged without further treatment. She re-presented again with a pounding headache and breathlessness on exertion, and was found to be pale and tachycardic. She was given a large amount of intravenous crystalloid and colloid while a blood count was analysed and re-analysed. The haemoglobin concentration indicated severe anaemia. She had a cardio-respiratory arrest before a blood transfusion was started. Although she was resuscitated, she developed overwhelming pulmonary oedema. Profound cerebral damage became evident. Her death was attributed to severe anaemia from haemorrhage from retained products (found at autopsy), exacerbated by intravenous fluid infusion.

This case again illustrates a failure to recognise basic clinical signs and symptoms. The initial extremely low haemoglobin result should have prompted a re-inspection of the conjunctivae, urgent blood transfusion, and senior review rather than additional venepuncture and further delay whilst awaiting re-analysis in the haematology laboratory.

Ovarian hyperstimulation

There has been debate as to whether deaths from ovarian hyperstimulation should be included in this Report. As discussed in Chapter 1, in the view of the assessors these deaths should be reported to, and assessed by this Enquiry, as they occurred as a direct consequence of a woman trying to become pregnant. Further, they contain important lessons for the provision of infertility treatment, a growing area of medical intervention which is not currently subject to such critical review.

One death reported to the Enquiry was of a woman who had undergone ovarian hyperstimulation and intrauterine insemination. There are conflicting reports about whether a pregnancy test was positive, or not, at the time of her death. She was admitted with ovarian hyperstimulation syndrome and deteriorated over three days in the gynaecology ward before being transferred to Critical Care Unit, extremely ill. She did not receive thromboprophylaxis. Autopsy showed fluid in body cavities and patchy infarction throughout the body, including bowel. Women admitted to hospital with severe ovarian hyperstimulation syndrome should receive thromboprophylaxis.[2]

Box 6.1
Learning points: early pregnancy deaths

Clinicians in primary care and Emergency Departments, in particular, need to be aware of atypical clinical presentations of ectopic pregnancy and especially of the way in which it may mimic gastrointestinal disease. This needs to be taught to undergraduate medical and nursing students and highlighted in textbooks.

Fainting in early pregnancy suggests the possibility of ectopic pregnancy.

More conservative approaches to the treatment of ectopic pregnancy should not blind clinicians to the dangers of this condition. Laparoscopy or laparotomy should be undertaken without delay if there are clinical signs suggestive of tubal rupture. Medical treatment of ectopic pregnancy should be based on strict adherence to protocols, with women having immediate access to in-patient facilities if complications occur.

Illegal, unsafe abortion is common globally; it can occur in the UK.

Acknowledgements

This Chapter was seen and discussed with Dr Davor Jurkovic (London).

References

1   RCOG Guideline No. 21. *The Management of Tubal Pregnancy.* London: Royal College of Obstetricians & Gynaecologists; May 2004. www.rcog.org.uk

2   *RCOG Green-top Guideline no. 5. The Management of Ovarian Hyperstimulation Syndrome.* London: Royal College of Obstetricians & Gynaecologists: September 2006. www.rcog.org.uk

7 Genital tract sepsis

Ann Harper

Summary of key findings for 2003-05

Twenty-two women died in this triennium from genital tract sepsis. Of these, 18 *Direct* deaths are counted in this Chapter. A further *Direct* death from sepsis following an illegal abortion, is counted in Chapter 6 - Early pregnancy deaths. The remaining three were *Late* deaths which occurred more than six weeks after delivery, outside the international definition for maternal deaths. These *Late Direct* deaths are counted in Chapter 14 but are discussed here. Genital tract infection was also a leading co-factor in a further *Late Direct* death which was attributed to thromboembolism associated with an infected retained vaginal tampon.

Table 7.1
Direct deaths associated with genital tract sepsis and rate per 100,000 maternities; United Kingdom: 1985-2005.

Triennium	Sepsis in early pregnancy*	Puerperal sepsis	Sepsis after surgical procedures	Sepsis before or during labour	All *Direct* deaths from sepsis counted in this chapter				*Direct* deaths from sepsis counted as early pregnancy deaths	*Late* deaths** from sepsis
					Number	Rate	95 per cent CI		Number	Number
1985-87	3	2	2	2	**9**	0.40	0.21	0.75	0	0
1988-90	8	4	5	0	**17**	0.72	0.45	1.15	0	0
1991-93	4	4	5	2	**15**	0.65	0.39	1.07	0	0
1994-96	0	11	3	1	**16**	0.73	0.45	1.18	2	0
1997-99	6	2	1	7	**18**	0.85	0.54	1.34	0	2
2000-02	2	5	3	1	**13**	0.65	0.38	1.11	2	0
2003-05	5	3	2	8	**18**	0.85	0.54	1.35	1	3

* Early pregnancy includes deaths following miscarriage, ectopic pregnancyand other causes.
** *Late* deaths are not counted in this Chapter or included in the numerator.

The women who died

The ages of the women ranged from 18 to 40 years with a median age of 32. All but four were White, three were Black African and one was Black Caribbean. The majority were overweight and only four had a Body Mass Index (BMI) of less than 25 at booking. Seven women had a BMI greater than 30, three of whom were morbidly obese with a BMI exceeding 35. For two women their BMI was not recorded.

Twelve of the women whose cases are discussed in this Chapter were primigravidae. Five women died before 24 weeks' gestation. Six women had a vaginal delivery and seven had a caesarean section after 24 weeks' gestation, as did the three *Late Direct* deaths. There were four twin pregnancies. Eleven babies survived, including two sets of twins. There were five miscarriages and nine stillbirths, including the other two sets of twins.

Two women had concealed their pregnancies, a further two had not booked by the time they died around 18 weeks' gestation and one woman booked very late despite having a known underlying and serious medical condition. Two women had learning disabilities.

The organisms that killed them

The most common pathogens identified among the cases discussed in this Chapter were the beta-haemolytic streptococcus - Lancefield Group A (8 cases), *E. coli* (7 cases) and *pseudomonas* (three cases). There were two cases each from *staphylococcus aureus and proteus*, and one case each of beta-haemolytic *streptococcus* - Lancefield Group B, *streptococcus pneumoniae, citrobacter koserii, actinobacter* and *listeria*. Some women had mixed infection with two or more organisms. For one obviously septic woman no pathogen was identified because the tests were not done. Methicillin resistant staphylococcus aureus (MRSA) infection developed in three women who had prolonged stays in Critical Care Units, but this was not the eventual cause of their death.

Sub-standard care

The assessors considered care to have been less than optimal in 15 of the 21 cases discussed in this Chapter although different management would not necessarily have altered the outcome. All of the women died in hospital but many were already seriously ill or moribund on arrival and deteriorated rapidly with little opportunity for altering the course of events. Nine women died within 24 hours of admission and only seven survived for more than three days. However, in some cases opportunities for early intervention were missed.

As in previous Reports there was failure or delay in diagnosing sepsis, failure to appreciate the severity of the woman's condition with resultant delays in referral to hospital, delays in administration of appropriate antibiotic treatment and late or no involvement of senior medical staff. There were some cases where doctors said they were already so busy dealing with other urgent problems that they were unable to see women for some time after admission. It was also clear that many doctors, midwives and community midwives were unfamiliar with the signs and symptoms of sepsis, did not realise when a woman was deteriorating or critically ill and failed to appreciate how quickly the clinical condition of a septic woman can deteriorate. There were also failures to take routine basic observations, to recognise abnormal fetal cardiotocograph (CTG) patterns and to ask for senior advice at an early stage.

In general, once consultants became involved the standard of care provided was of very high quality, particularly in relation to Critical Care, but there were also situations where seriously ill women were managed in units that were not equipped to deal with them. There were also a very few occasions where women declined treatment or delayed seeking help as they did not realise how ill they were.

Sepsis in early pregnancy

Six women died of genital tract sepsis occurring before 24 weeks' completed gestation. One death from sepsis following illegal abortion is counted and discussed in Chapter 6 - Early pregnancy deaths. Of the five cases counted here, four were associated with septic miscarriage and one woman died following an evacuation of her uterus for retained products following a miscarriage. Care was sub-standard in most cases and the lessons to be learnt from these are summarised in Box 7.1 .

Box 7.1
Learning points: sepsis in early pregnancy

Care should be taken to ensure that the uterus is empty following a surgical evacuation of the uterus. An ultrasound scan should be performed if there is any doubt.

Screening for infection and antibiotic prophylaxis is recommended in women undergoing surgical evacuation if there is an increased risk of infection.

Three women had septic miscarriages at around 16 weeks' gestation. Two of these women were unbooked. For one of these women this was despite several hospital attendances and two previous admissions with lower abdominal pain, dysuria and vaginal discharge. No consultant was ever involved in this woman's care and the seriousness of her condition was unrecognised until she collapsed, when inadequate venous access hindered resuscitation. In another case:

> A woman attended an Emergency Department (ED) with a four day history of vaginal bleeding, backache, feeling shivery, vomiting and having fainted twice. She was hypotensive, had a pulse rate of 146bpm and temperature of 400C. She had not sought antenatal care but thought that she was about four months pregnant. She was correctly started on intravenous fluids and antibiotics, however, her initial, correct, diagnosis of a septic miscarriage was then revised to a probable ectopic pregnancy despite her pyrexia. As the gynaecologists were occupied in theatres and could not attend immediately she was transferred to another hospital ill-equipped to treat such severe sepsis. She died shortly after. All in all she died within three hours of first walking into the ED. Autopsy showed suppurative chorio-amnionitis from Group A streptococcal infection.

This woman was already critically ill by the time she arrived at hospital and it is extremely unlikely that different management would have saved her, but the case does illustrate how inappropriate decisions are sometimes made when hospitals are very busy. Such an ill woman would have been more appropriately managed in the resuscitation room or critical care unit. An ultrasound scan in the ED would have excluded ectopic pregnancy. The consultant gynaecologist was available, but not called, until just before she died.

Sepsis before delivery

Eight women died from genital tract sepsis present before delivery. A cervical suture was the probable portal of entry for infection in two women. The following describes a classical presentation:

> *A woman who had a cervical suture inserted in early pregnancy with antibiotic prophylaxis was readmitted on several occasions feeling unwell with vaginal discharge, for which antibiotics were prescribed. In mid pregnancy she attended another hospital with a short history of intermittent severe suprapubic pain and tachycardia of 130-152 bpm; intravenous antibiotics were commenced. A few hours later she suffered an intrauterine fetal death, her suture was removed and she started to labour. She had an epidural for severe abdominal pain unresponsive to opiate analgesia after which she suddenly delivered the baby and suffered a terminal cardiac arrest. Autopsy showed marked acute inflammation of the cervix and placenta. Mixed coliforms and enterococci were cultured from the cervical suture and coliforms and proteus from the baby.*

The only outward clinical signs of this woman's overwhelming sepsis were tachycardia, fetal death and the severity of her abdominal pain; she was apyrexic throughout. The epidural given against a background of fulminating septicaemia may have precipitated her inevitable demise.

Box 7.2
Learning points: Cervical sutures

Although cervical cerclage may be justified in certain situations, it is a potential source or portal of infection.

It is important to monitor such women for signs of infection and to carry out appropriate investigations including vaginal/cervical swabs if any symptoms develop.

Care should be taken to ensure that the uterus is empty following a surgical evacuation of the uterus. An ultrasound scan should be performed if there is any doubt.

Screening for infection and antibiotic prophylaxis is recommended in women undergoing surgical evacuation if there is an increased risk of infection. One woman had listeriosis. She had received appropriate advice about which foods to avoid during pregnancy, but it is unknown whether she had any contact with animals. Listeria infection in pregnancy is well known to cause preterm labour and intrauterine fetal death, and is sometimes associated with maternal hepatitis, liver abscess, septicaemia, meningo-encephalitis and ARDS. Maternal death due to listeriosis is extremely rare and apart from this death, only two other cases, both in association with immuno-compromise, have been reported[1].

Five other women were admitted with abdominal pain and fetal death either before or shortly after admission. In some cases there were delays in diagnosing sepsis and starting antibiotics and in one case an abnormal CTG was not recognised. Four of the women were initially thought to have placental abruption, two of whom had a history of recent abdominal trauma, which may have misled staff. One woman with a concealed pregnancy was admitted in labour with a subsequent intrauterine fetal death. Apart from her severe abdominal pain there were no signs or symptoms of sepsis until delivery of very offensive smelling placenta and membranes.

> **Box 7.3**
> **Learning points:** Sepsis in later pregnancy
>
> Genital tract sepsis must be considered in the differential diagnosis when a woman presents with symptoms suggestive of placental abruption.
>
> Disseminated intravascular coagulation and uterine atony are common in genital tract sepsis and often cause life-threatening postpartum haemorrhage.
>
> Treatment, including delivery, should not be delayed once septicaemia has developed because deterioration can be extremely rapid. Women should be fully informed of the dangers of conservative management.

Sepsis after vaginal delivery; puerperal sepsis

Three women died from puerperal sepsis after uneventful pregnancies and a normal vaginal delivery at term. One mother developed sepsis whilst still in hospital and, once the severity of her condition was recognised, was transferred quickly to intensive care where she died a few days later from multi-organ failure and disseminated intravascular coagulation. Two women became ill in the community after postnatal discharge but the warning signs were initially overlooked. Although they were eventually admitted, both died within 24 hours despite excellent critical care. In one case both the midwife and General Practitioner (GP) failed to recognise the severity of the illness, in the other the midwife did not visit when the partner called with concerns but gave advice over the phone.

These cases of classical puerperal sepsis due to Group A haemolytic streptococcal infection demonstrate that by the time sepsis is clinically obvious, infection is already well established and deterioration into widespread septicaemia, metabolic acidosis, coagulopathy and multi-organ failure is very rapid and often irreversible. The best defence against this situation is awareness of the early signs of sepsis and early recognition by routine regular basic clinical observations. Earlier detection of pyrexia might have made a difference in these three cases. Postnatal observations of pulse, temperature, BP, respiration, and lochia should be done regularly while the woman is still in hospital and for several days after discharge by her community carers. This is particularly important in women who leave hospital a few hours after birth, 'early discharge', or if a woman complains of feeling feverish or unwell.

Good communication is essential between hospital and community carers. Early discharge after delivery is common and GPs and community midwives must be reliably informed at the time of the woman's discharge if there have been any problems during her hospital stay. Recently delivered mothers should be visited regularly after discharge from hospital and basic maternal observations of pulse, BP, temperature, respiratory rate, and lochia made. Community carers should be aware of the importance of early referral to hospital of recently delivered women who feel unwell and have pyrexia.

> **Box 7.4**
> **Learning points:** Puerperal sepsis
>
> Any problems noted during a woman's hospital stay should be reported directly to her community carers (GP, midwives and health visitors) when she is discharged in order that appropriate follow up visits may be arranged and the significance of developing symptoms recognised.
>
> Early discharge means that some women will develop complications after they return home.
>
> Routine observations of pulse, BP, temperature, respiratory rate, and lochia should be made in all recently delivered women for several days postpartum.
>
> Sepsis is often insidious in onset with a fulminating course. The severity of illness should not be underestimated. Community midwives and GPs need to be vigilant and visit regularly. Early referral to hospital may be life saving.
>
> Sepsis should be considered in all recently delivered women who feel unwell and have pyrexia.

Sepsis after surgery

Ten women died from genital tract sepsis following a caesarean section. Five of the women were already very ill from sepsis before an emergency caesarean section was performed. The remaining five women died following caesarean wound infection. All were overweight, two were morbidly obese and one was a gestational diabetic. All were given antibiotic prophylaxis at operation. All had obstetric indications for the operation, one was an elective procedure and the others were undertaken for breech presentation or fetal distress. Three of the women had pre-labour spontaneous rupture of their membranes (SROM), one prolonged.

None of the other women had any evidence of infection until two to seven days after birth when they all rapidly developed pyrexia, rigors and abdominal pain. Three required further surgery including exploratory laparotomy and one woman with necrotising fasciitis required wound debridement. All had a relapsing course despite multidisciplinary consultant involvement and intensive multiple antibiotic therapy.

Risk factors for, and the identification and management of, genital tract sepsis

Successive Reports have identified women who appear to be at increased risk of, or have predisposing factors for, pelvic sepsis as shown in Box 7.5.

Box 7.5
Risk factors for maternal sepsis as identified from the Confidential Enquiries into Maternal Deaths

- Obesity
- Impaired glucose tolerance / diabetes
- Impaired immunity
- Anaemia
- Vaginal discharge
- History of pelvic infection
- History of Group B streptococcal infection
- Amniocentesis, and other invasive intrauterine procedures
- Cervical cerclage
- Prolonged SROM
- Vaginal trauma
- Caesarean section
- Wound haematoma
- Retained products of conception post miscarriage or post delivery.

Many of the women had one or more of these risk factors for sepsis, including cervical cerclage, gestational diabetes, wound haematoma, retained products, and impaired immunity. Obesity is a risk factor for infection and can also lead to practical difficulties in managing care:

A woman collapsed and died due to a pulmonary embolism. She had several risk factors for this including obesity, laparotomy for primary PPH, suboptimal thromboprophylaxis and vaginal sepsis due to inadvertent retention of a tampon inserted during repair of vaginal tear. Vaginal examination was extremely difficult because of her high BMI which was over 35. She had offensive lochia but the tampon remained undiscovered despite several vaginal examinations until it was extruded a month later. This case highlights some of the problems encountered in obese women and emphasises the importance of accurate swab counts on all occasions.

Signs and symptoms

The signs and symptoms of genital tract sepsis are listed in Box 7.6. Most are non-specific and unless genital tract sepsis is specifically considered in the differential diagnosis it may be missed until too late. Severe sepsis with acute organ dysfunction has a 20-40% mortality rate. It can be insidious in onset and patients often appear deceptively well until they suddenly deteriorate and collapse. If septicaemic shock (sepsis with hypotension refractory to fluid resuscitation) develops, the mortality rate rises to around 60%.

Tachycardia, over 100 bpm, and unusually severe abdominal pain are important and common signs and symptoms requiring urgent review by a doctor. Gastro-intestinal symptoms, especially diarrhoea, are common in pelvic sepsis. Pyrexia is not always present although a temperature of 38°C or higher should always prompt a thorough investigation for infection including vaginal, cervical, wound and throat swabs and blood and urine cultures. The white cell count is not always elevated and may be low. C-reactive protein (CRP) is a useful indicator of infection.

Box 7.6
Common symptoms and signs of genital tract sepsis

Symptoms	Signs
• Fever	• Tachycardia
• Diarrhoea	• Tachypnoea
• Vomiting	• Pyrexia
• Abdominal pain	• Possible elevated white cell count
• Rash (generalised streptococcal maculopapular rash)	• Elevated C-Reactive Protein
• Vaginal discharge, wound infection	

In some cases routine observations were often not taken or their significance was not appreciated. One woman did not have her temperature taken for over 24 hours after delivery, when she collapsed. Routine observation of vital signs is essential for the early detection of severe illness. In hospital practice, a Modified Obstetric Early Warning Scoring (MEOWS) system such as one recommended and discussed in Chapter 19 - Critical Care, should help to reduce deaths due to the late recognition of serious illness.

Once septicaemia develops the woman's clinical condition may deteriorate very rapidly over the course of a few hours, particularly when endotoxin-producing organisms are responsible. The features of septicaemic shock are shown in Box 7.7. Increased respiratory rate and severe tachycardia are important symptoms. Hypotension results in inadequate organ perfusion and lactic acidosis. Rapid development of disseminated intravascular coagulation (DIC) is a common complication. Several of the women who developed septic shock around the time of delivery had massive haemorrhage due to a combination of unresponsive uterine atony and DIC. Cardiac arrest in septic women often occurs with little warning and resuscitation is often unsuccessful.

Box 7.7

Features of septicaemic shock

- Tachycardia   over 90 beats per min
- Tachypnoea   over 20 breaths per min
- Pyrexia   over 380C
- Hypothermia   below 350C
- Hypotension   Systolic BP 90mm/Hg or below in absence of other causes e.g. bleeding
- Hypoxemia
- Poor peripheral perfusion, mottled skin
- Oliguria
- Metabolic acidosis
- Elevated lactate
- Positive blood cultures
- Abnormal coagulation and bleeding
- Abnormal liver and renal function tests

Treatment

A recurring feature in the cases described here and in previous Reports is a delay in starting intravenous antibiotics. In some cases no antibiotic was ever given. In one case antibiotics were stopped because a streptococcal rash was mistaken for a drug allergy. The guiding principles are given in Box 7.8.

Box 7.8

Guiding principles for antibiotic therapy in genital tract sepsis

If pelvic sepsis is suspected prompt early treatment with a combination of high-dose broad-spectrum intravenous antibiotics, such as cefuroxime and metronidazole, may be lifesaving. Do not wait for microbiology results.

Ensure that serum levels of antibiotics are within the therapeutic range.

The expert advice of a consultant microbiologist should be sought at an early stage.

Microbiology results should be obtained as soon as possible.

If there is no response within 24-48 hours or the woman's condition is deteriorating, the antibiotics should be changed and gentamicin or alternative antibiotics added, guided by microbiological advice.

The source of sepsis should be sought and dealt with if possible and appropriate, for example - by delivery or ultrasound scans to detect retained intrauterine products and evacuation of products if present.

Multidisciplinary care, staffing and facilities

Consultants should be involved in the patient's care as early as possible. A multidisciplinary team approach is required including haematologists, microbiologists, anaesthetists and intensive care specialists. Critically ill patients should be cared for in a critical care or high dependency unit with adequate staff and facilities.

Conclusion

In the past, puerperal sepsis or 'childbed fever' was a leading cause of maternal death and its signs and symptoms were widely known. Antisepsis, antibiotics and changing practice over the years mean that genital tract sepsis has become much less common and death is rare. The fear and respect with which it was held in the past by obstetricians, midwives and patients has disappeared from our collective memory. Action is now required to raise awareness of the signs and symptoms of sepsis and recognition of critical illness among staff in maternity units or in the community, Emergency Departments, and among GPs and health visitors.

The cases in this Report clearly demonstrate that genital tract sepsis is still a problem, that is repeatedly missed and there is often failure to treat women early and aggressively enough. Some of these maternal deaths may have been prevented if the signs and symptoms of sepsis and developing septicaemic shock had been recognised and treated earlier. Nevertheless the clinical picture of life-threatening sepsis often develops very rapidly and in many of the cases the outcome could not have been prevented.

References

1   Mylonakis E, Paliou M, Hohmann EL, Calderwood SB, Wing EJ. *Listeriosis during pregnancy. A Case Series and Review of 222 Cases.* Medicine 2002: 81(4); 260-269.

8 Anaesthesia

Griselda Cooper and John McClure

Anaesthesia: Specific recommendations

All patients, including women in early pregnancy whose treatment is generally managed by gynaecological services, require the same high standard of anaesthetic care. This includes early recovery from anaesthesia for which anaesthetic services have full responsibility. Recovery staff must be able to receive immediate effective assistance from an anaesthetist until the woman is fully conscious and has stable vital signs.

Trainee anaesthetists must be able to obtain prompt advice and help from a designated consultant anaesthetist at all times. They and their consultants must know the limits of their competence and when close supervision and help are needed. Morbidly obese women should not be anaesthetised by trainees without direct supervision.

Trainees across all specialties may not have the experience or skill to recognise a seriously ill woman. Referral to a consultant or senior trainee should occur if there is any doubt about a woman's condition. Early warning scores may help identify the mother who is seriously ill. Bedside estimation of haemoglobin concentration is valuable. Many of these points are reiterated in the "top-ten" Recommendations of this Report.

Summary of key findings for 2003-05

The central assessors in anesthesia reviewed 150 cases where a woman who died from either a *Direct* or *Indirect* cause of maternal death was also known to have had an anaesthetic. These comprise around half of the maternal deaths this triennium. From these cases the assessors identified six women who died from problems directly associated with anaesthesia and whose deaths are counted in this Chapter. This is the same number and a similar rate to 2000-02. The overall mortality rates from deaths from anaesthesia over the past seven triennia are shown in Table 8.1.

Table 8.1
Direct deaths attributed to anaesthesia and rate per 100,000 maternities; United Kingdom: 1985-2005.

Triennium	Direct deaths attributable to anaesthesia n (%)	Total number of *Direct* deaths	Rate per 100,000 maternities	95 per cent CI	
1985-87	6 (4.3)	139	0.26	0.12	0.58
1988-90	4 (2.8)	145	0.17	0.07	0.44
1991-93	8 (6.3)	128	0.35	0.18	0.68
1994-96	1 (0.7)	134	0.05	0.01	0.26
1997-99	3 (2.8)	106	0.14	0.05	0.42
2000-02	6 (5.7)	106	0.30	0.14	0.66
2003-05	6 (4.5)	132	0.28	0.13	0.62

In addition to the six women who died from *Direct* anaesthetic causes, the assessors considered that in a further thirty-one cases poor perioperative anaesthetic management may have contributed to the outcome. These deaths are counted in the relevant Chapters of this Report, but the lessons for anaesthetists to be learnt from them are included here.

It is clear that the workload and challenges presented to the obstetric anaesthetist are increasing in number, complexity and severity because of increasing interventions, maternal age, obesity and other co-morbidities.

Deaths directly due to anaesthesia

The women who died

The ages of the women who died ranged between 23 and 33 years, with a median age of 30. All but one were White and, where relevant, all attended for regular antenatal care. Four were obese, two morbidly so with a Body Mass Index (BMI) greater than 35. Two, whose care was managed by the gynaecological services, died in early pregnancy.

Postoperative respiratory failure

> *An obese asthmatic woman died as a result of failed re-intubation during the recovery phase after anaesthesia for laparoscopic surgery for an ectopic pregnancy. She developed acute respiratory distress due to severe bronchospasm on extubation. A senior anaesthetist was called but by then she had suffered an irreversible cardiac arrest.*

As highlighted in the previous Report there is great concern that trainees in anaesthesia now take longer to become experienced in laryngoscopy, intubation and other advanced airway techniques. Fortunately there have been no deaths this triennium from unrecognised oesophageal intubation at caesarean section but this case reiterates the need for intubation skills throughout anaesthetic practice. Better training in tracheal intubation and dealing with consequent problems is still required. Undoubtedly this can only be gained outside obstetric practice and is a departmental responsibility. Tracheal extubation has been added as a specific skill to the Initial Test of Competence in the CCT syllabus[1].

> *Another obese woman, also in early pregnancy, was anaesthetised by a trainee. A second, relatively large dose of fentanyl was given at the end of the procedure and the woman was then transferred to recovery and left with the recovery nurse. Within five minutes she developed breathing difficulties and the anaesthetist was called back after having left the unit. The immediate efforts of the nursing staff to support ventilation were not adequate and the woman became bradycardic and then suffered a fatal cardiac arrest.*

The anaesthetist did not appreciate the profound ventilatory depression caused by the opioid. Anaesthetists are fully responsible for their patients until full consciousness has returned, with stable cardiovascular and respiratory systems. They may delegate immediate supervision to a trained recovery nurse but must stay close by and be able to attend immediately in case problems arise.

In these two cases, trainees without immediate senior backup, administered the anaesthetics. Their relative inexperience was relevant because, in both cases, the problems were avoidable and once they had happened should have been retrievable. The close proximity of additional skilled help may have been able to avert these deaths.

The third case also highlights the problems in caring for a morbidly obese woman with asthma where her compromised breathing should have received attention and treatment:

A morbidly obese asthmatic woman had an elective caesarean section for which a consultant anaesthetist administered spinal anaesthesia. She became agitated and short of breath after surgery but she was sent to the postnatal ward a few hours later. She received oxygen but remained agitated and short of breath. She was reviewed by an anaesthetist but had a fatal cardiac arrest a few hours later. There were additional problems with the ready availability of resuscitation equipment on the postnatal ward.

The anaesthetist failed to recognise postoperative respiratory failure and did not monitor her appropriately, which should have included arterial blood gases. Appropriate treatment (bronchodilators, optimal positioning, early assisted ventilation) was not given. Asthma which does not respond to bronchodilators constitutes a medical emergency, particularly if associated with obesity, agitation and tachycardia.

Drug administration error

A woman of slight build had a low dose infusion epidural during labour and was delivered by forceps. She had some bleeding and intravenous fluid and syntocinon infusions were started. Shortly after she had a grand mal convulsion followed by ventricular fibrillation from which she could not be resuscitated. She had received 150ml of a 500ml bag of 0.1% bupivacaine in saline intravenously in error. Blood samples taken after the arrest showed serum bupivacaine concentrations of 2.1 and 4.2 mg/l.

It is unclear why 500 ml bags of plain 0.1% bupivacaine were in use and why they were stored in an area where the bags could be confused with conventional IV fluids. Epidural infusion analgesia has been in common use for 30 years but, in spite of great advances in pump technology, the disposable equipment is basically the same as that used for intravenous infusion. This was a systems error and until such time as specific equipment and connectors are used for central neural drug administration these errors will recur. Strategies to avoid such errors have now been described in a National Patient Safety Agency (NPSA) patient safety alert[2].

Lipid emulsion has been used to end otherwise refractory cardiac arrest in patients apparently intoxicated with local anaesthetics, including bupivacaine. As a result of these successes many departments have decided to stock a 'lipid rescue' pack in their theatres and labour wards[3]. Although the cases are anecdotal the authors have volunteered to establish an educational website, www.lipidrescue.org, in order to collect and disseminate information that can only be assimilated through such case reports as clinical trials would clearly be unethical. We encourage anaesthetists to contribute to this.

Anatomical compromise

A woman with pectus excavatum presented in mid pregnancy with reduced fetal movements, fulminant pre-eclampsia and HELLP syndrome. She was severely hypertensive, hyperreflexic with clonus, oliguric and had abnormal liver function tests. She was given oral labetalol, magnesium and hydralazine to little effect. An urgent caesarean section was planned with prior insertion of arterial and central venous pressure monitoring. Right internal jugular cannulation was unsuccessful but the consultant anaesthetist was able to cannulate the subclavian vein at the second attempt. Shortly after she had a cardiac arrest from which she could not be resuscitated. At autopsy a large right haemothorax was found.

There were good indications for invasive monitoring techniques in this woman with severe hypertension and oliguria. The difficulties with central venous placement were probably caused by abnormal great vessel anatomy because of her pectus excavatum. The haemothorax was secondary to trauma of the proximal part of the intrathoracic internal jugular vein. Such trauma may have been caused by a rigid vein dilator. Care should be taken not to advance a rigid dilator too far into the vein. It is unlikely that ultrasound guidance would have avoided this complication.

In the final *Direct* death from anaesthesia the cause of death was difficult to ascertain:

> *Another obese woman had longstanding renal problems necessitating nephrectomy. She became pregnant and had a premature labour and delivery. A few weeks later she was admitted with fever, loin pain and an ileofemoral venous thrombosis. It was planned to drain a suspected septic focus from her remaining kidney under ultrasound guidance. The woman did not want local anaesthesia and during the subsequent general anaesthesia she suffered a cardiac arrest from which she could not be resuscitated.*

The cause of her death was unascertained but pulmonary embolus and anaphylaxis were excluded. Although the details are incomplete the assessors consider her death was likely to be due to a cardiac arrhythmia, presumed to be secondary to an electrolyte disturbance.

Deaths to which anaesthesia contributed

There were 31 further *Direct* or *Indirect* maternal deaths in which perioperative/ anaesthesia management contributed and from which lessons can be learned. These deaths are counted in the relevant Chapters in this Report and discussed here in the following categories:

- Failure to recognise serious illness
- Poor management of
    - haemorrhage (including the use of syntocinon),
    - sepsis and
    - pre-eclampsia/eclampsia.
- The management of obese pregnant women
- The quality of in-house hospital Trust enquiries into serious untoward incidents including maternal deaths.

Failure to recognise serious illness

As highlighted in almost every Chapter of this Report, and one of its "top ten" key recommendations, the early recognition and management of severe illness in pregnant or recently delivered women remains a challenge for everyone involved in their care. The relative rarity of such events, combined with the normal changes in physiology associated with pregnancy and childbirth, compounds the problem. As discussed in Chapter 19 - Critical Care, modified early warning scoring systems have been successfully introduced into hospital practice which could be adapted and introduced for use in maternity units.

Haemorrhage

Less than optimal anaesthetic management was considered to have contributed to many of the 17 maternal deaths from haemorrhage or ruptured uterus counted in Chapter 4. Twelve of these women died from postpartum haemorrhage. Although some women with obstetric haemorrhage were clearly managed very well with excellent team debriefing afterwards there are still areas of concern which have also been highlighted in Chapter 4. The following is representative of a typical case:

A woman suffered a concealed haemorrhage after a caesarean section for pre-eclampsia. The team of obstetrician, anaesthetist and midwives failed to interpret the classical signs of peripheral shutdown and tachycardia and misdiagnosed her abnormal twitching movements as incipient eclampsia. Ischaemic findings on an electrocardiograph (ECG) were interpreted as primary cardiac disease, rather than being due to severe anaemia. Once the correct diagnosis was made further delays occurred in obtaining her blood results and cross-matched blood. She died shortly afterwards, just as consultant help arrived.

Here there was a failure to interpret the vital signs and to consider concealed haemorrhage as a possibility. There was also failure to realise that cardiac ischaemia may be caused by severe anaemia and a further failure to estimate her haemoglobin level either urgently in the laboratory or at the bedside.

The remediable factors also illustrated in the other cases of obstetric haemorrhage include:

- Poor recognition of concealed intra-abdominal bleeding.

- The classical signs related to intra-abdominal haemorrhage of peripheral shutdown, tachycardia and tachypnoea, are still being ignored. Hypotension is often a late sign in young fit adults.

- A reluctance to believe low blood pressure recordings recorded by non-invasive devices.

- Inconsistent use of invasive monitoring.

- The wrong administration of large volumes of cold clear fluid and unwarmed blood products.

- Poor postoperative care and observations in recovery, postnatal or gynaecological wards where continuing haemorrhage may go unnoticed.

- Poor management of women with placenta accreta, as also discussed in Chapter 4.

- Recognising that women who decline blood and blood products require consultant anaesthetic and obstetric care and, where possible, access to cell salvage facilities.

Box 8.1
Management of obstetric haemorrhage: anaesthetic and other learning points

Women with placenta praevia who have had a previous caesarean section are at risk of massive haemorrhage and should be managed in units with direct access to blood transfusion and Critical Care. These cases require consultant obstetrician and consultant anaesthetist involvement with additional obstetric and anaesthetic help. Balloon tamponade by iliac artery catheters may be helpful in the planned and emergency management of these patients.

The earlier recognition of hypovolaemia would be helped by the routine use of an early warning score system as advocated in the key recommendations.

Blood pressure parameters may need adjusting in patients with pregnancy induced hypertension.

Where there is a possibility of bleeding, a near-patient method of haemoglobin estimation may be life-saving. Such a device should be available in all obstetric units.

High volume infusions of intravenous fluid must be warmed beforehand. Women who are being resuscitated should be insulated and actively warmed. Hypothermia at temperatures below 33 o C produces a coagulopathy that is functionally equivalent to significant (< 50% of normal activity) factor-deficiency states under normothermic conditions, despite the presence of normal clotting factor levels[4]. In the situation of hypothermia and dilutional coagulopathy, both rewarming and administration of coagulation factors are required[5].

Where tachycardia persists after intraoperative haemorrhage, the woman must remain in theatre until both surgeon and anaesthetist are satisfied that her condition is stable.

Invasive monitoring via appropriate routes should be used particularly when the cardiovascular system is compromised by haemorrhage or disease.

Hands on help from other anaesthetists, and, in particular the consultant anaesthetist, should be present for these cases.

Syntocinon

The majority of anaesthetists have changed from using a single intravenous bolus injection of 10 units of syntocinon to using the recommended dose of 5 units[6] after the 1997-1999 Confidential Enquiry Report. It was disappointing to see in a number of cases that the larger bolus dose was still being given. It may be that a perceived conflict of interest arises between obstetricians and anaesthetists, the former wishing to maintain tone in the uterus and the latter trying to maintain cardiovascular stability. These two aims are not incompatible. Uterine tone should initially be stimulated by slow administration of intravenous syntocinon five units, maintaining cardiovascular stability[7] and thereafter maintained by an infusion of syntocinon, intramuscular or slow intravenous administration of ergometrine and intramuscular carboprost as recommended in Chapter 4.

Box 8.2
Learning point: uterine atony

Uterine atony may be prevented by slow intravenous administration of syntocinon. Syntocinon causes hypotension when given intravenously by bolus dose in the hypovalaemnic woman. It may be given slowly in the presence of hypovolaemia. Uterine atony should be treated by giving a continuous infusion of syntocinon as a first measure.

Sepsis

Poor anaesthetic or resuscitation management were considered to have contributed to ten maternal deaths from sepsis. Regardless of the woman's gestation, early or late in pregnancy, there were common themes in the cases reviewed. The failure of trainee medical staff to appreciate the seriousness of the woman's condition was frequent, yet again suggesting that an early warning score system would be valuable. When cardiac arrest occurred there were some problems with the availability of resuscitation equipment and suction and difficulty in resuscitating obese women.

One woman, septic and tachycardic after a midtrimester fetal loss, collapsed immediately after an epidural test dose. There was no evidence that the local anaesthetic was given intrathecally or intravenously or that an incorrect drug was given. It is unlikely that a small dose of epidural local anaesthetic precipitated her collapse. However epidural anaesthesia is contraindicated in patients who have obvious septicaemia or those who are tachycardic secondary to the cardiovascular response to systemic infection.

Another woman who had a medical termination of pregnancy delayed seeking care afterwards when she was continuing to bleed and developing an infection secondary to retained products of conception. Having finally sought medical care her condition rapidly deteriorated in a gynaecology ward under the care of trainee medical staff. She was both severely anaemic and septic and the rapid resuscitation with intravenous fluid she was eventually given suddenly resulted in pulmonary oedema. Here early diagnosis and careful resuscitation with blood and inotropes guided by invasive monitoring in a Critical Care Unit was indicated.

Box 8.3
Learning point: anaesthesia and sepsis

Cardiovascular collapse can happen suddenly in sepsis. Circulatory support requires invasive monitoring and careful fluid resuscitation in a Critical Care unit or operating theatre environment.

Pre-eclampsia/eclampsia

Four women died from pre-eclampsia/eclampsia to which poor anaesthetic management contributed. In all cases there was inadequate control of their high systolic blood pressure either at the time of caesarean section or in the postoperative period. The importance of ameliorating the hypertensive response to laryngoscopy should be remembered. The immediate postoperative management of women with preeclampsia/eclampsia is the responsibility of both the consultant obstetrician and the consultant anaesthetist. It should be a joint decision whether care, treatment and monitoring are provided in a Critical Care Unit, high dependency unit or the postnatal ward.

Obesity

The problems that morbid obesity pose for pregnant women are numerous and have been mentioned throughout this Report. They have also been recently reviewed in relation to anaesthetic practice[8]. It was pleasing to note that there were many good aspects of both anaesthetic and surgical management of women with morbid obesity even up to a Body Mass Index (BMI) of 66. However these women present many challenges and this Report makes a recommendation that the management of obese pregnant women, especially the morbidly obese, is an important area requiring a evidence based clinical guideline.

Box 8.4
Learning points: anaesthesia and obesity

All obstetric units should develop protocols for the management of morbidly obese women. These should include pre-assessment procedures, special community, ward and theatre equipment such as large sphygmomanometer cuffs, hoists, beds and operating tables and long regional block needles.

Morbidly obese women should be referred for anaesthetic assessment and advice as part of their antenatal care.

Management by consultant anaesthetists is essential and difficulties with airway management and intubation should be anticipated.

Positioning the women requires skill and sufficient manpower in the event of a requirement for induction of general anaesthesia.

Direct arterial pressure measurement may be useful in the morbidly obese women where sphygmomanometry is often inaccurate.

All morbidly obese women in childbirth should be given prophylactic low molecular weight heparin and the duration of therapy needs to be determined in view of likely immobility. Thromboembolic stockings of appropriate size need to be available.

Hospital enquiries

A new but recurring feature in many of the cases reviewed in this Report, is that it is the first triennium where there have been a substantial number of reports of internal hospital enquiries related to the maternal death included in the documentation sent to CEMACH. These have been welcome in that that they reveal clinical reflections and also aspects of the culture of working in specific institutions. Whilst some of these reports have been insightful, it is fair to say that others have not been. In some cases the hospital enquiries were improperly conducted: investigatory panels did not include clinicians from relevant disciplines (including anaesthesia) and therefore lacked clinical insight and relevance, or included clinicians who were directly involved in the death and were therefore potentially biased in their assessments. Hospital managers should consider for each case whether unbiased external input would assist real learning from individual deaths: it is often after this has been received that the benefit is realised.

What the practitioners learnt

A new feature of completing the case details on the CEMACH form is an invitation for the practitioner to reflect on the case. Some of the comments are poignant and insightful whereas others are disappointing.

> ## What did you learn from this case and how has it changed your practice?
>
> *"After the death of a woman who refused blood transfusion I no longer treat such patients for elective surgery and have reservations about continuing on-call because of the ethical concerns about being forced to accept treating those who refuse blood transfusion."* (Consultant anaesthetist)
>
> *"The relatives want Dr X to know that they bear no grudge, and hope that Dr X will not give up anaesthesia as a result of this case."*
>
> *"No lessons to be learned."* (Consultant anaesthetist, although in the opinion of the assessors there clearly were)
>
> *"Should I have done a pre-op ECG? Would there have been a case for an echo? In future I would not rely on non-invasive blood pressure monitoring but would insert an arterial line, or at least try."* (Reflections from a consultant anaesthetist who had realised the problems of an obese hypertensive woman with pre-eclampsia)
>
> *"I am even more keen to obtain consultant advice and participation early with such patients."* (Lesson from staff grade about a woman with HELLP syndrome and bleeding)
>
> *"There was an emphasis on urgency because of possible abruption, such that the warning bells about pre-eclampsia may not have registered. It is disappointing that the anaesthetist did not reflect on the need for ameliorating the pressor response to intubation when writing his/her report."* (Central assessor)

Acknowledgements

This Chapter has been seen and discussed with the National and Regional Assessors in Anaesthesia.

References

1 Royal College of Anaesthetists. *Initial Assessment of Competence. The CCT in Anaesthesia II Competency based Basic level.* 2006.

2 National Patient Safety Agency (2007): *Patient safety alert 21: Safer practice with epidural injections and infusions.* www.npsa.nhs.org.uk

3 Picard J, Meek T, Weinberg G and Hertz P. *Lipid emulsion for local anaesthetic toxicity.* Anaesthesia 2006; 61: 1116-7.

4 Johnston TD, Chen Y, Reed RL. *Functional equivalence of hypothermia to specific clotting factor deficiencies.* J Trauma 1994; 37: 413-7.

5 Gubler KD, Gentilello LM, Hassantash SA and Maier RV. *The impact of hypothermia on dilutional coagulopathy.* J Trauma 1994; 36: 847-51.

6 Bolton TJ, Randall K, Yentis SM. *Effect of the Confidential Enquiries into Maternal Deaths on the use of Syntocinon® at caesarean section in the UK.* Anaesthesia 2003; 58: 277-9.

7 Thomas JS, Koh SH, Copper GM. *Haemodynamic effects of oxytocin given as i.v. bolus or infusion on women undergoing Caesarean section.* British Journal of Anaesthesia, 2007; 98: 116-9.

8 Saravanakumar K, Rao SG, Cooper GM. *Obesity and obstetric anaesthesia.* Anaesthesia, 2006; 61: 36-48.

9 Cardiac disease

Catherine Nelson-Piercy

Cardiac disease: Specific recommendations

As recommended in other Chapters of this Report, pregnant immigrant women require a complete medical examination, including cardiovascular examination, by an appropriately trained doctor at booking.

Maternity health care professionals must remember the possibility of rheumatic heart disease in immigrant women and there should be a low threshold for investigation if any symptoms develop.

Women at higher risk of developing cardiac disease in pregnancy, i.e. the obese, those who smoke or who have existing hypertension and/or diabetes, a family history of heart disease and those over the age of 35, should be appropriately counselled of these risks pre-conception and particularly prior to receiving assisted reproductive technology (ART) or other infertility treatment.

Clinicians should have a low threshold for further investigating pregnant or recently delivered women, especially those with any of the above risk factors, with severe chest pain, chest pain that radiates to the neck, jaw or back, chest pain associated with other features such as agitation, vomiting or breathlessness, tachycardia, tachypnoea or orthopnea. Appropriate investigations include an electro-cardiogram (ECG), a chest x-ray (CXR), cardiac enzymes (Troponin), echocardiogram and CT pulmonary angiography.

If a clinician is not confident or competent to interpret an ECG, he/she should discuss the woman's case and show her ECG to someone who is.

Summary of key findings for 2003-05

In this triennium cardiac disease was the commonest cause of maternal death overall. A total of 48 women who died from heart disease associated with, or aggravated by, pregnancy were reported to the Enquiry in 2003–05. All but one of these cases were fully assessed and these deaths are discussed further in this Chapter. These are classified as *Indirect* maternal deaths. This compares with 44 deaths in 2000-2002 and 35 deaths in 1997–99, as shown in Table 9.1. This Table shows a clear rise in mortality from cardiac causes since the late 1980s, but no further rise in 2003-05. The maternal mortality rate for cardiac disease was 2.27 per 100,000 maternities in 2003-05.

In addition, lessons arising from 34 other women known to the Enquiry who died from cardiac disease later after delivery are discussed and considered here although they are counted as *Late* deaths in Chapter 14. Future Reports will continue to consider all maternal deaths from cardiac disease which occur during pregnancy or within six weeks of birth, as well as those *Late* cardiac deaths which arise directly or indirectly from the woman having been pregnant, such as deaths attributed to peripartum cardiomyopathy.

Three other maternal deaths to which cardiac disease contributed are counted and considered in other Chapters. One woman died from pulmonary embolus although aortic dissection was a contributing feature, another from liver disease with pulmonary hypertension and the third from amniotic fluid embolism.

Table 9.1
Indirect maternal deaths from congenital and acquired cardiac disease and rates per 100,000 maternities; United Kingdom: 1985-2005.

Triennium	Congenital	Acquired		Total	Rate	95 per cent CI	
		Ischaemic	Other				
	n (%)	n (%)	n (%)	n (%)			
1985-1987	10 (43)	9 (39)	4 (17)	23 (100)	1.01	0.68	1.52
1988-1990	9 (50)	5 (28)	4 (22)	18 (100)	0.76	0.48	1.21
1991-1993	9 (24)	8 (22)	20 (54)	37 (100)	1.60	1.16	2.20
1994-1996	10 (26)	6 (15)	23 (59)	39 (100)	1.77	1.30	2.43
1997-1999	10 (29)	5 (14)	20 (57)	35 (100)	1.65	1.19	2.29
2000-2002	9 (20)	8 (18)	27 (61)	44 (100)	2.20	1.64	2.96
2003-2005	4 (8)	16 (33)	28* (58)	48 (100)	2.27	1.67	2.96

* Includes one case which was not assessed.

The leading cardiac causes of maternal death are now myocardial infarction, mostly related to ischaemic heart disease, and dissection of the thoracic aorta. Maternal deaths from pulmonary hypertension and from congenital heart disease were less common than in previous triennia. Rheumatic mitral stenosis has re-emerged as a cause of maternal death.

Both the relative and absolute numbers of deaths from myocardial infarction in pregnant or recently delivered women are increasing. Although not directly or indirectly related to pregnancy, these *Coincidental* cardiac deaths nevertheless contain important public health lessons by demonstrating that the large increase in the proportion of women dying of myocardial infarction is due to ischaemic heart disease which tends to be associated with avoidable or remediable lifestyle factors. For example, 29 of the 45 maternal deaths from cardiac disease and for whom a Body Mass Index (BMI) was available, occurred in women who were overweight or obese. Of these women, 14 were overweight with BMI over 25 and 15 were obese with a BMI over 30. Nine of these 15 women were morbidly obese with a BMI over 35, including five with a BMI greater than 40.

All the women who died from peripartum cardiomyopathy in this triennium are counted as *Late* deaths as they died some time after delivery, although most presented sooner than this. These deaths will continue to be assessed by this Enquiry. Indeed, in the opinion of the assessors, deaths from peripartum cardiomyopathy would not have occurred if the women had not been pregnant and should, in international and national terms, be classified as *Direct* deaths in future.

The assessors considered that some degree of sub-standard care was present in 23 or nearly half of the 47 cases. As with preceding Reports, a lower proportion, 36%, of women who died from *Late* cardiac causes had any degree of sub-standard care.

Table 9.2 shows the overall numbers of cardiac maternal deaths in 2003-05 which were assessed, subdivided by major cause of death.

Table 9.2
Causes of maternal death from cardiac disease; United Kingdom: 2003-2005.

Type and cause of death	*Indirect*	*Late**
Acquired		
Aortic dissection	9	0
Myocardial infarction	12	4
Ischaemic heart disease	4	0
Sudden Adult Death Syndrome (SADS)	3	9
Peripartum cardiomyopathy	0	12
Cardiomyopathy	1	4
Myocarditis or myocardial fibrosis	5	0
Mitral stenosis or valve disease	3	0
Infectious endocarditis	2	2
Right or left ventricular hypertrophy or hypertensive heart failure	2	1
Congenital		
Pulmonary hypertension	3	0
Congenital heart disease	3	2
Total	**47**	**34**

*Women who died from 42 days to one year after delivery and whose deaths were reported to and assessed by the Enquiry. They are not representative of the totality of *Late* deaths for cardiac disease as some cases were not assessed.

Congenital heart disease

As Table 9.1 shows, fewer women died from congenital cardiac disease in this triennium than in previous Reports. Of the four women counted here, two died from complications of surgery, either for tetralogy of Fallot or a Mustard procedure for transposition of the great arteries, another from pulmonary vascular disease and the last from severe aortic stenosis in association with a bicuspid aortic valve and severe left ventricular hypertrophy. In addition there were two Late deaths in women with severe congenital aortic stenosis, one of which was associated with coarctation of the aorta and who died after aortic valve replacement several months after delivery.

Care was considered sub-standard in only one of these cases where, although the woman was seen by a cardiologist early in her pregnancy, there was no subsequent specialist cardiological follow up. The severity of her residual problems after earlier surgery was underestimated and she died suddenly, probably from an arrhythmia, in her third trimester.

For two women who died whilst still pregnant, the pregnancy was unplanned and there was no documentation of either pre-pregnancy counselling or contraceptive advice. For example:

A young pregnant woman who had had a repair for a congenital heart condition had the midwifery aspects of her care provided by specialist teenage midwives. She was under paediatric cardiac follow up every two years and due for transfer to adult congenital heart disease services. She had moderate to severe pulmonary regurgitation and right ventricular dilation, but was well and asymptomatic. She collapsed and died suddenly in mid-pregnancy. An inadequate autopsy failed to ascertain the precise cause of her death although a specialist cardiac pathologist considered it to be most probably due to a cardiac arrhythmia. There are no details regarding her health in pregnancy.

There are some key lessons to be drawn from this case about the management of women with congenital heart disease. Firstly, because of her significant heart disease, her care should have been arranged under a specialist high-risk obstetric team[1]. As she was a teenager the team could still have put her in touch with her local teenage pregnancy midwife. Secondly, although the importance of seamless transfer from paediatric to adult congenital heart disease services is vital, so too is timely advice regarding pregnancy and contraception[1]. One of the consensus views from the RCOG Study Group on heart disease and pregnancy states[2]:

"A proactive approach to preconception counselling should be started in adolescence and this should include advice on safe and effective contraception. Proper advice should be given at the appropriate age and not delayed until transfer to the adult cardiological services".

This is the second consecutive triennium in which a death, probably arrhythmic related to right ventricular failure, has been reported in women with a surgically repaired tetralogy of Fallot, traditionally believed to be one of the less risky conditions with regard to pregnancy. However it is important to note that it is the commonest form of cyanotic heart disease, which occurs once in every 3,600 live births, and that even in historical series, survival rates into the fifth decade are similar to that of the general population[3]. Surgically repaired tetralogy of Fallot is probably the commonest condition seen in adult congenital heart disease clinics, thus its repeated appearance as a cause of maternal cardiac death may simply be a reflection of the numbers of these women now becoming pregnant. However, the fact that some may die means there is no room for complacency and those caring for these women in pregnancy should be aware that assessment of right ventricular function is vital. A recent study of pregnancy outcomes in women with congenital heart disease confirms that the presence of impaired sub-pulmonary ventricular systolic function and/or severe pulmonary regurgitation increases the risk of an adverse outcome[4].

Three women died from pulmonary hypertension, one less than reported in the last triennium. One mother, who had Eisenmenger's syndrome secondary to a ventricular septal defect (VSD), and who had been advised about the risks of becoming pregnant and continuing with her pregnancy had excellent antenatal care managed by a multidisciplinary team in a tertiary centre. Despite this she collapsed and died shortly after an elective caesarean section. The other two women died between one and four weeks after delivery; both had undiagnosed primary pulmonary hypertension with no symptoms antenatally, and these deaths, too, were probably unavoidable.

Another woman, whose death is counted in Chapter 10, died from pulmonary hypertension secondary to recurrent pulmonary emboli from antithrombin deficiency secondary to chronic liver disease.

It is encouraging that maternal deaths from pulmonary hypertension seem to be falling and this may reflect better pre-pregnancy counselling and acceptance of contraception, or, alternatively, improved care.

Incidence of pulmonary vascular disease

Over the nine month period between March and November 2006, the United Kingdom Obstetric Surveillance System (UKOSS) reported six confirmed cases of pulmonary vascular disease. This gives an estimated incidence of 1.1 per 100,000 maternities with a 95% confidence interval of 0.4 to 2.4 and with no case fatalities.[5] Three of the cases were attributed to congenital heart disease, one to chronic thromboembolism, one to sleep apnoea and one to primary pulmonary hypertension. Five cases were known prior to pregnancy and only one diagnosed during pregnancy.

Acquired heart disease

Myocardial infarction and ischaemic heart disease

Sixteen women died from either myocardial infarction and/or ischaemic heart disease. Of the twelve who died from myocardial infarction, eight deaths were due to ischaemic heart disease, in two the underlying cause was undetermined, one was due to coronary artery dissection, a recognised complication of pregnancy, and one due to a coronary embolism. Where the site of the coronary atheroma was identified at autopsy, it involved the left anterior descending coronary artery in four cases, the right coronary artery in one further case and triple vessel disease in another.

For three of the four other women whose deaths were attributed to ischaemic heart disease no myocardial infarction was seen at autopsy. The other woman died of left ventricular failure due to ischaemic heart disease. In all, ischaemic heart disease was responsible for the deaths of twelve women. This represents a four fold increase in deaths from ischaemic heart disease compared to the last triennium, probably reflecting the impact life style factors such as increasing maternal age, obesity and smoking have on the health of women of childbearing age.

The women who died

All of the women who died from ischaemic heart disease had identifiable risk factors. Six were aged 35 or over and the age range was 27 to 40 with a median of 35 years. Six were morbidly obese with a BMI of 35 or more, of whom four had a BMI over 40. All but one were parous, two had known hypertension, seven were smokers, one had a family history and two had type 2 diabetes. Three women were Asian and the others were White. Three of these women were poor attenders for antenatal care.

The *Late* deaths of four further women who died after childbirth from myocardial infarction were also considered by the assessors, three were due to coronary artery dissection and one was due to ischaemic heart disease, although there were undoubtedly more cases which remained unreported as the women will have died many months after ceasing contact with the maternity services. The one woman whose death was assessed and classified as a *Late* death from an myocardial infarction due to ischaemic heart disease fitted the classic picture of women at risk in that she was parous, obese, aged over 40 and had type 2 diabetes.

There were four postpartum deaths from myocardial infarction due to coronary artery dissection although three of these are counted as *Late*. Two involved the left anterior descending coronary artery, one the right coronary artery, and one both arteries. Although rare in general, coronary artery dissection is a not uncommon cause of coronary artery occlusion related to pregnancy.

The UKOSS study of acute myocardial infarction in pregnancy, undertaken from August 2005 to July 2006, identified four confirmed non-fatal cases, giving an estimated incidence of 0.6 cases per 100,000 maternities (95% confidence interval 0.02, 1.4)[5].

Interpreting trends in deaths from myocardial infarction

There appears to have been an increase over the past three triennia in rates of death from ischaemic heart disease. In 2003-5 eight women died from myocardial infarction due to ischaemic heart disease and another four from ischaemic heart disease without demonstrable myocardial infarction. From the table it appears that increasing deaths from ischaemic heart disease have contributed to this, although numbers are small.

Table 9.3
Deaths from myocardial infarction, numbers and rates per 100,000 maternities; United Kingdom: 1985-2005.

Triennium	Ischaemic	Dissection	Embolism	Undetermined	Total	Rate	*95 per cent CI*	
1997-1999	5	0	0	0	**5**	0.24	*0.10*	*0.55*
2000-2002	3	5	0	0	**8**	0.40	*0.20*	*0.79*
2003-2005	8	1	1	2	**12**	0.57	*0.32*	*0.99*

In considering factors which may have contributed to this rise, it is relevant to consider death rates among women in the general population, shown in Table 9.4.

Table 9.4
Death rates per 100,000 population from myocardial infarction among women of childbearing age; United Kingdom: 2000-05.

	Age, years		
	15-24	25-34	35-44
2000-02	0.11	0.44	2.42
2003-05	0.05	0.38	1.98

Source: ONS, General Register Office Scotland, General Register Office Northern Ireland.

Although age specific rates have declined slightly between the past two triennia, the most striking feature is the higher mortality among older women of childbearing age. As shown in Chapter 1, the percentage of maternities in the United Kingdom which were women aged 35-39, rose from 12.3 per cent in 1997-1999 to 15.9 per cent in 2003-05 and the percentages of maternities to women aged 40 and over rose from 2.1 per cent to 3.2 per cent. The mean age of the women dying from ischaemic heart disease associated with pregnancy in 2003-5 in the UK was 35. Similar patterns were shown in two studies of myocardial infarction in pregnancy in the United States.

A study of 151 women with acute myocardial infarction in association with pregnancy from California has demonstrated an overall incidence rate of 1 in 35,700 but the incidence of myocardial infarction in pregnancy increased throughout the 1990s[6]. The maternal mortality rate was 7.3% in this group of women. This study also demonstrated an increased risk related to maternal age. Women with an acute myocardial infarction associated with pregnancy were more likely to be older compared with women who did not have an acute myocardial infarction. Thirty per cent of those with an acute myocardial infarction were older than 35 years compared to ten per cent without.

A recent nationwide series of 859 cases of myocardial infarction in pregnancy from the US[7] found a rate of 6.2 per 100,000 deliveries (95% confidence interval 3.0, 9.4). Although acute myocardial infarction is a rare event in women of reproductive age, this study found pregnancy to increase the risk three- to four-fold. The case fatality rate was 5.1%. The odds of acute myocardial infarction were 30-fold higher for women aged 40 years and older than for women less than 20 years of age. Other significant risk factors were pre-existing hypertension, thrombophilia, diabetes mellitus, smoking, blood transfusion and postpartum infection.

Quality of care

Care was considered sub-standard in seven of the sixteen *Indirect* maternal deaths from myocardial infarction and/or ischaemic heart disease. In some instances this involved doctors and midwives failing to recognise the classic symptoms of acute coronary syndrome/myocardial infarction, such as crushing chest pain radiating to the shoulder, or jaw, or a failure to identify obvious ischaemic changes on an ECG reading:

> *A socially disadvantaged women with type 2 diabetes and epilepsy, who had been advised to delay pregnancy until she had been formally counselled by her specialist consultants regarding her diabetes and epilepsy, became pregnant. She was admitted early in her third trimester with abdominal pain and vomiting and, although the pain was so severe to require morphine, no diagnosis was made. She may also have developed pre-eclampsia. When her condition deteriorated with further epigastric pain an ECG was finally performed but, although clearly abnormal showing an acute anterior myocardial infarction (MI), it was not reported as such. It is not clear who or how many people reviewed the ECG trace. She continued to be unwell and arrested four days later. Autopsy revealed an acute MI and a left anterior descending coronary artery that was occluded at its midpoint by atheroma and thrombus.*

The following vignette demonstrates another area of concern:

> *A parous woman who was a heavy smoker developed preterm pre-eclampsia. Labour was induced and she eventually required a caesarean section for fetal distress. She returned home three days later even though she remained hypertensive and felt unwell. She also complained of wind and nausea but none of her symptoms were investigated further. Eventually she was admitted with an acute antero-lateral myocardial infarction but the cardiologist advised against thrombolysis because of her recent operation. At cardiac catheterization, atheroma and thrombosis were identified in her left anterior descending coronary artery. She died shortly afterwards of a complication related to the coronary intervention.*

This mother should not have been discharged so shortly after delivery having had a history of pre-term pre-eclampsia, a caesarean section and on-going hypertension. Her symptoms should have been investigated further and the benefits of thrombolysis should have been balanced against the risks two weeks after surgery.

The RCOG study group on heart disease in pregnancy[2] concluded *"thrombolysis may cause bleeding from the placental site but should be given in women with life-threatening thromboembolic disease or acute coronary insufficiency"*.

Although there are few data relating to thrombolysis in acute coronary syndrome in pregnancy, a literature review[8] of 200 cases of thrombolysis for massive pulmonary embolism in pregnancy reported a maternal death rate of 1% and concluded that thrombolytic therapy is reasonably safe.

Outside pregnancy, primary angioplasty has been shown to be preferable to thrombolysis provided this is achievable within 90 minutes to 3 hours. In pregnancy urgent coronary angiography is even more important since not only does this allow differentiation between coronary artery dissection, thrombosis (relatively more common related to pregnancy) and atheroma, but also it allows for intervention with stenting to treat a dissection.

Box 9.1
Learning points: myocardial infarction

Ischaemic heart disease is now a common and increasing cause of death from myocardial infarction in pregnancy. This risk is higher in older women.

Current trends in lifestyle factors and increasing age at childbirth are likely to be contributing to an increase in incidence. All the women who died had identifiable risk factors including:

- Obesity

- Older age and higher parity

- Smoking

- Diabetes

- Pre existing hypertension, and

- Family history.

Myocardial infarction and acute coronary syndrome can present with atypical features in pregnancy such as abdominal or epigastric pain and vomiting.

There should be a low threshold for further investigation of ischaemic sounding chest pain especially in women with known risk factors.

There should also be a low threshold for emergency coronary intervention which will allow treatment of both acute atheromatous coronary occlusion with angioplasty +/- stenting and the less common coronary artery dissection with stenting.

Thrombolysis should not be withheld in the pregnant or puerperal woman.

Aortic dissection

Aortic dissection was, again, one of the leading causes of cardiac death. Nine women died from aortic dissection compared to seven in the last Report. A further woman, whose death is counted in Chapter 2, had an aortic dissection that contributed to her death from pulmonary embolism. Four of these deaths occurred late in pregnancy and five after delivery. Of the latter, three occurred within the first four days but the other two occurred a few weeks later. Three of the nine women were morbidly obese with a BMI over 35, and two were overweight. The dissection was type A (ascending aorta) in six cases, type B (descending aorta) in one case and type C (ascending and descending) in the two other cases. Of the nine cases, three women probably had Marfan syndrome although this was not realised.

Care was sub-standard in four of the nine cases. As highlighted in other Chapters in this Report there was, in some cases, an inappropriate emphasis on the diastolic blood pressure which led to a failure to treat systolic hypertension:

> *A pregnant woman with scoliosis was admitted with chest and epigastric pain radiating through to her back which did not settle with analgesia. A chest x-ray (CXR) showed an enlarged heart. She had systolic hypertension with a wide pulse pressure which was noted repeatedly during her subsequent antenatal checks. No action appears to have been taken until she presented in late pregnancy to a local hospital having been advised by a midwife to attend. A provisional diagnosis of pulmonary embolus was made and she was then transferred to another unit, unaccompanied*

by a doctor, with a systolic blood pressure of 170 mm/Hg and a heart rate over 130bpm. She arrested in the ambulance. At autopsy a Marfanoid appearance was noted with a high arched palate. There were two previous healed aortic dissections as well as the acute dissection leading to death.

Although the postmortem findings are very suggestive of Marfan syndrome this diagnosis should have been considered earlier in a tall woman with scoliosis. Her care was sub-standard because of the failure to make a diagnosis when she presented with severe chest and epigastric pain with a large heart on CXR, a failure to treat her systolic hypertension and also by transferring a tachycardiac, hypertensive woman to another unit without medical support. This would also have been inappropriate even if the diagnosis had been a pulmonary embolus. Worryingly, both her obstetrician and pathologist did not consider her death to be related to pregnancy despite the well known increased risk of aortic dissection in pregnant women. In another case:

A morbidly obese woman who died of aortic dissection was admitted in later pregnancy with severe chest, back and abdominal pain. She was referred to the surgeons but no diagnosis was made. Abdominal ultrasound was normal but no further imaging was undertaken despite her requiring repeated doses of intramuscular opiates. She was nursed in a low dependency area and suffered a cardiac arrest from which she could not be resuscitated. Her autopsy revealed aortic dissection with medial degeneration. She was very tall, over 180cm, so she may have had Marfan syndrome.

Box 9.2
Learning points: aortic dissection

Maternity professionals must remember that aortic dissection is a cause of chest or interscapular pain in pregnancy, particularly in the presence of systolic hypertension.

Women with Marfan syndrome are at high risk of aortic dissection, but previously apparently normal pregnant women may also suffer this complication, most commonly at or near term, or postnatally.

Marfan syndrome diagnosed at autopsy has implications for the family as it is possible to screen relatives for mutations in the fibrillin gene.

Women with severe chest pain requiring opiate analgesia must be investigated. Appropriate imaging includes a CT chest scan or MRI, or transoesophageal echocardiogram.

Other acquired cardiac disease

Cardiomyopathy

One woman died suddenly from cardiomyopathy due to new onset systemic lupus a few days after delivery. The diagnosis of fulminating dilated cardiomyopathy was made quickly but, despite appropriate management, she died within 24 hours of diagnosis.

There were twelve *Late* deaths from peripartum cardiomyopathy which occurred some weeks after delivery and four further *Late* deaths from arrythmogenic right ventricular cardiomyopathy and idiopathic dilated cardiomyopathy. There were also a further two where peripartum cardiomyopathy was a possible contributory factor. Although these twelve women are classified as having *Late* deaths, three presented antenatally, including one woman with previous unresolved cardiomyopathy, and six within six weeks of delivery. This highlights why this Enquiry believes it important to consider these *Late* cardiac deaths together with other *Indirect* cases. This is particularly so for peripartum cardiomyopathy which may present up to five to six months postpartum but is still directly related to the pregnancy. Similarly it may present antenatally or in the puerperium but death may occur many months later from the complications of heart failure. The assessors therefore recommend that the next revision of the International Code for the Definition of Diseases include all deaths from peripartum cardiomyopathy, at any point after childbirth, as *Direct* deaths.

The women who died

These deaths occurred predominately in parous women and eight were aged 35 or more. Most had other risk factors including previous peripartum cardiomyopathy, hypertension, pre-eclampsia, obesity and diabetes.

One woman who died from peripartum cardiomyopathy had no risk factors. Her care was judged as sub-standard because the diagnosis of heart failure was missed completely by several clinicians:

> A woman who spoke little English was admitted with breathlessness in later pregnancy. Despite clear documentation from the midwife on admission that she was "unable to lie down for abdominal palpation" both the obstetric and medical registrars, and a locum consultant obstetrician, missed the symptoms and signs of heart failure. Her "wheezing" was taken to be asthma, or possibly due to pulmonary embolism. She was left on the antenatal ward, tachypnoeic and tachycardic, and the severity of her illness was not appreciated. A combination of intravenous fluids and salbutamol nebulizers probably tipped her over into catastophic pulmonary oedema. Even when she arrested, frothing at the mouth, the working diagnosis was still pulmonary embolism. The diagnosis of peripartum cardiomyopathy was not made until she was on the Critical Care unit after having sustained a cardiac arrest and a perimortem caesarean section.

Whilst it is possible that her poor English contributed to the difficulty reaching a diagnosis and realising the severity of her illness, the failure to recognise heart failure represents gross sub-standard care. Another woman with no known risk factors also died:

> A multiparous women whose antenatal care had been uneventful complained to her midwife three days after delivery of leg oedema, chest and calf pain and breathlessness. She was tachycardiac and her midwife appropriately advised her to attend the Emergency Department (ED) from where she was discharged without a diagnosis. A few days later her General Practitioner (GP) prescribed diuretics but did not arrange any further investigations. She was admitted with severe heart failure some weeks later and found to have severe impairment of left ventricular function. She died some months later of a pulmonary embolus and worsening heart failure.

Here again the diagnosis of peripartum cardiomyopathy was not considered despite its presentation within the first few days after delivery. In a further case the diagnosis was also missed:

> A diabetic woman developed pulmonary oedema immediately after delivery, having been given two litres of fluid for an abruption. She was transferred to the ITU and then back to the postnatal ward. An echocardiogram showed global dysfunction but the diagnosis of peripartum cardiomyopathy was not made. She was discharged but readmitted a few weeks later with pulmonary oedema. She died of a pulmonary embolism, a well known complication of peripartum cardiomyopathy.

This women was given inadequate anticoagulation. No cardiologist seems to have been involved in her management and an ACE inhibitor was not prescribed.

Women in late pregnancy or within five months of delivery with symptoms of breathless, oedema or orthopnoea and the signs of tachypnoea and tachycardia may have peripartum cardiomyopathy and investigation with a chest x-ray and an echocardiogram are indicated.

The presence of a wheeze may not necessarily indicate asthma and may be a feature of heart failure.

Women with peripartum cardiomyopathy should be managed by cardiologists with expertise in this condition, and their care discussed, if appropriate, with the regional cardiac transplant centre.

Treatment with ACE inhibitors, beta blockers and full anticoagulation is appropriate for postpartum woman.

Myocardial fibrosis and myocarditis

Three women died from myocardial fibrosis, the same number as in the last Report. All died following sudden collapse and in all three the care was considered sub-standard. Two of these women had inadequate autopsies, which represents a degree of sub-standard care. One woman was inappropriately booked for midwifery led care despite a previous history of myopericarditis. Another woman who died of an unheralded cardiac arrest a few days after delivery, and who had been treated with a nasogastric tube for a postoperative ileus, had no monitoring of her urea and electrolytes and hypokalaemia could have been a contributory factor.

Two women died from myocarditis. One who became unwell in mid pregnancy received very good care. She had a timely and appropriate referral into hospital from her GP, but she died shortly after admission. An excellent autopsy made the diagnosis of widespread medium and small vessel vasculitis. Even if the diagnosis had been made before her death, and treatment with immunosuppression begun, this would have been very unlikely to have prevented death which occurred hours after admission.

Hypertensive heart disease

The following vignette describes the key learning points in relation to the planning and provision of care for women known to be at higher risk of medical complications, including hypertensive heart disease:

> A multiparous, obese woman was prescribed clomiphene for infertility. Her booking blood pressure was high and thereafter her hypertension was suboptimally controlled. She also developed gestational diabetes. Her general practitioner (GP) prescribed salbutamol for "wheezing" and she saw a cardiologist for breathlessness and dizziness. A suboptimal echocardiogram was reported as showing mitral regurgitation but no features of heart failure. Postnatally there was inadequate monitoring of her blood pressure and the midwives did not appreciate the significance of a "rattly" chest and chest pain. She died of hypertensive heart failure five days after delivery. Autopsy revealed a grossly enlarged heart with left and right ventricular hypertrophy, and evidence of longstanding back pressure on the lungs and congestive cardiac failure.

This case raises the issue of whether or not her GP or gynaecologist had checked her BP, or counselled her regarding the risks of obesity in pregnancy, prior to prescribing clomiphene. It is possible that her wheezing was due to heart failure and not asthma. Despite the diagnosis of "asthma", a betablocker was prescribed. Despite the presence of mitral regurgitation on her echocardiogram she did not receive cardiac antibiotic prophylaxis for delivery, and the possibility of left ventricular dilatation and poor function as an explanation for her symptoms and mitral regurgitation was not considered. Hypertensive heart disease is a long-standing condition and would not have appeared over days. There were warning signs antenatally and it is likely given the autopsy findings that the echocardiogram was abnormal. Perhaps the examination should have been repeated antenatally. Her postnatal care was also sub-standard.

Rheumatic heart disease

Until this triennium there had been no maternal deaths reported from rheumatic fever since the 1991-1993 Enquiry. However, in this Report, there were two maternal deaths from mitral stenosis; both in recently arrived immigrant women. This probably reflects an increase in the numbers of newly arrived immigrant mothers with a history of rheumatic heart disease. Since rheumatic heart disease has become so rare in the United Kingdom, and many maternity health professionals will not have seen a case, it is imperative that all pregnant women with rheumatic heart disease and/or mitral stenosis be referred to tertiary cardiac centres for advice regarding their management in pregnancy. The following vignette illustrates some of the many problems with the care of such women:

> *A previously well young immigrant woman, with little English, was booked for midwifery led care and only ever saw her midwife or her GP. She was admitted to an emergency department (ED) at the end of her second trimester with cough, breathlessness and chest pain. She was hypoxic and markedly tachycardic and, not unreasonably, the diagnosis was assumed to be a pulmonary embolus. Her chest was clear and no murmur was heard. The ED junior doctor discussed the case with the obstetric trainee, who did not review her personally but advised that heparin was safe in pregnancy, and with the medical trainee who advised against a chest x-ray (CXR). Her ECG showed P mitrale, suggesting an enlarged left atrium, but this was missed. She was given low molecular weight heparin (LMWH) but her condition deteriorated and she suffered a cardiac arrest from which she was resuscitated. She was then transferred to the Critical Care Unit. An echocardiogram was suggestive of only mild mitral stenosis but she had significant pulmonary hypertension (pulmonary artery pressure 55 + jvp mm/Hg) which should have raised concerns that the mitral stenosis was more severe, as was diagnosed at autopsy. She died the following day.*

Omitting to do a CXR was an error. This would have been an appropriate investigation even if pulmonary embolus was suspected. It may also have shown pulmonary oedema. A full physical examination by a doctor at her booking visit may also have revealed the murmur of mitral stenosis. Although the diagnosis was missed on her final admission, at this stage she was very tachycardic which would have made it harder to hear the soft diastolic murmur of mitral stenosis.

Box 9.4
Learning points: rheumatic mitral stenosis

Although extremely rare in the United Kingdom, rheumatic heart disease is still common in less developed countries, and mitral stenosis often complicates pregnancy. Newly arrived women from such parts of the world therefore require a full physical examination when they present for booking.

Although seemingly well in early pregnancy, women with mitral stenosis commonly decompensate at the end of the second trimester.

Symptoms of breathlessness, orthopnoea and the signs of tachypnoea and tachycardia, especially in an immigrant woman should raise the possibility of mitral stenosis and a CXR and an echocardiogram should be requested.

Pregnant women with mitral stenosis should be managed in tertiary centres with cardiological and obstetric services on a single site and by cardiologists and obstetricians with expertise in this condition.

Two women died from infectious endocarditis, both of which involved the mitral valve. One was in a mechanical valve replacement and the other in a woman who was known to be a substance abuser:

> *A young, excluded woman on a methadone maintenance programme booked early in her pregnancy but from then on was difficult to contact. She had a history of abscesses and deep vein thrombosis (DVT) related to injecting and although she was supposed to be on long term warfarin she had discontinued this. Late in her second trimester she felt generally unwell, which persisted for two weeks before her death. Several days prior to her death she was feeling hot and cold with abdominal pain and vomiting. In retrospect these were the symptoms of endocarditis/ bacteraemia. She had also stopped antibiotics prescribed by the GP.*

Her care cannot be classified as sub-standard even though it was only at autopsy that vegetations on the mitral valve and focal suppurative myocarditis were discovered. She also had infective thrombi in her kidneys and the organisms seen in other organs suggested an overwhelming bacteraemia. Although toxicology revealed therapeutic methadone, recent cocaine and very recent heroin, which also might have contributed to her death, she died of endocarditis and bacteraemia. Her attendance at the GP's surgery was a rare opportunity to treat her, but even if admission to hospital had been suggested she may well have declined. although theoretically intravenous antibiotics at this stage may have saved her. Her specialist midwives are to be congratulated for the efforts they made to contact her as the rare contacts she did have with them must have taken great persistence.

Sudden adult death syndrome (SADS)

SADS is defined as sudden death in an adult for which no cause can be found. Three mothers died of SADS during this triennium compared to two in the last Report. They all died before delivery, two in mid pregnancy and one at term. There were nine further *Late* deaths where no cause of death was found and these were therefore also classified as SADS. Of these twelve women, five were overweight or obese.

A French study[9] has demonstrated that circulating non-esterified fatty acid concentration is an independent risk factor for sudden death in middle-aged men. Hence, obesity may be relevant. A more recent study[10] has identified an inherited disease and likely cause of death in 17 of 43 families (40%) with one or more relatives aged 40 years or more with a history of sudden death. There is therefore a need to counsel family members of the possibility of a genetic component for this condition.

Acknowledgements

This Chapter has been seen and discussed with Dr Sara Thorne, Consultant Cardiologist, Birmingham.

References

1   Thorne SA, Nelson-Piercy C, MacGregor A. *Risks of Contraception & Pregnancy in Heart Disease.* Heart 2006; 92:1520-5.

2   Steer PJ, Gatzoulis MA, Baker P (eds). *Heart Disease and Pregnancy.* RCOG Press 2006.

3   Murphy JG, Gersh BJ, Mair DD, Fuster V, McGoon MD, Ilstrup DM, McGoon DC, Kirklin JW, Danielson GK. *Long-term outcome in patients undergoing surgical repair of tetralogy of Fallot.* New Engl J Med 1993; 329:593-9.

4   Khairy P, Ouyang DW, Fernandes S, Lee-Parritz A, Economy KE, Landzberg MJ. *Pregnancy outcomes in women with congenital heart disease.* Circulation 2006; 113: 517-524.

5   Knight M, Kurinczuk JJ, Spark P and Brocklehurst P. *United Kingdom Obstetric Surveillance System (UKOSS) Annual Report 2007.* National Perinatal Epidemiology Unit, Oxford.

6   Ladner HE, Danielsen B, Gilbert WM. *Acute myocardial infarction in pregnancy and the puerperium: a population-based study.* Obstet Gynecol. 2005; 105:480-4.

7   James AH, Jamison MG, Biswas MS, Brancazio LR, Swamy GK, Myers ER. *Acute myocardial infarction in pregnancy: a United States population-based study.* Circulation. 2006; 113; 1564-71.

8   Ahearn GS, Hadjiliadis D, Govert JA, Tapson VF. *Massive pulmonary embolism during pregnancy successfully treated with recombinant tissue plasminogen activator: a case report and review of treatment options.* Arch Intern Med. 2002; 162: 1221-7.

9   Jouven X, Charles M-A, Desnos M, Ducimetiere P. Circulating Jouven X, Charles M-A, Desnos M, Ducimetiere P. *Circulating nonesterified fatty acid level as a predictive risk factor for sudden death in the population.* Circulation 2001; 104:756.

10 Tan HL, Hofman N, van Langen IM, van der Wal AC, Wilde AA. *Sudden unexplained death: heritability and diagnostic yield of cardiological and genetic examination in surviving relatives.* Circulation 2005; 112:207-13.

Indirect deaths: Specific recommendations

Women, especially teenage girls, with pre-existing, serious, medical conditions should have pre-pregnancy counselling at every opportunity, even if they are not immediately seeking pregnancy. This is especially the case if they seek assisted reproduction.

As part of ongoing education, all medical and midwifery practitioners, particularly specialists in acute medical care, need some knowledge of the way in which common medical conditions interact with pregnancy.

The early detection of severe illness in mothers remains a challenge and the use of modified early warning scoring systems, adapted for obstetric patients, one of the top ten key recommendations of this Report, should help reduce the cases in which death has followed the late recognition of serious illness.

All women with serious medical conditions must be referred by their midwives or General Practitioners (GP) for specialist opinion as early in pregnancy as possible, even if this means breaking traditional rules about referral pathways and timing.

Effective pathways must be established so that physicians and obstetricians can communicate properly to treat pregnant women, both in acute illness and during regular antenatal care. The latter is best managed in a combined medical obstetric antenatal clinic.

Maternity trusts and other health care providers must ensure that pregnant women with neurological problems have early and ongoing access to combined neurology or medical/obstetric clinics to improve the care of pregnant women with neurological problems.

The consultant obstetrician on call should be told about all sick pregnant women in hospital whether they have a medical or an obstetric problem.

Maternity units should have on-site access to modern imaging facilities such as CT and MRI scans. There is no place for "isolated" consultant led maternity units.

Multiple attendances and/or readmission without diagnosis are danger signs of serious undiagnosed disease or a major health and social problem such as domestic abuse.

Epilepsy is dangerous because of the risk of sudden unexpected deaths in epilepsy (SUDEP). This risk may not be greater in pregnancy than in the non-pregnant state but for a variety of reasons, epilepsy may be more difficult to control in pregnancy thus increasing the risk of SUDEP. Mothers who stop anticonvulsant therapy in pregnancy must be made aware of the risk of SUDEP.

Introduction

Indirect maternal deaths are defined as those deaths which occur during pregnancy or up to, and including, 42 days after the end of the pregnancy and which result from previously existing disease, or conditions which develop during pregnancy which are aggravated by physiological effects of pregnancy. The introductory section of this Report describes the international definitions and classifications of maternal deaths in more detail.

Examples of *Indirect* deaths include those from epilepsy, diabetes, cerebral haemorrhage and HIV infection. Cardiac causes of death are also classified as *Indirect* but, such is their importance, they are discussed separately in Chapter 9 of this Report. The international definitions of maternal death exclude deaths from suicide due to perinatal mental illness and those from hormone dependent malignancies, both of which the UK assessors consider to be absolutely linked to the woman's pregnancy. These causes of death also have their own separate Chapters in this Report. The remaining deaths due to Indirect causes are counted and discussed in this Chapter and are classified as *Other Indirect*. However, in statistical terms, all these causes of *Indirect* deaths contribute to the overall UK *Indirect* mortality rate calculated for this Report.

Summary of key findings for 2003-05

Table 10.1 shows that in 2003-05, the deaths of 87 women who died from *Other Indirect* maternal causes were reported to this Enquiry, and Table 10.2 shows that their mortality rate was similar to that for 2000-02. In some cases very few details were available to the assessors. In addition, 35 other deaths have contributed to the learning points in this Chapter but are counted in the Chapters relating to their main cause of death. The deaths of a number of women who died much later after the end of their pregnancy, *Late* deaths, were also assessed as part of the learning points although they are not counted here nor do they contribute to the overall maternal mortality rate shown in Table 10.2. In future the majority of these *Late* deaths from causes unrelated to pregnancy, especially those which occur six months or more after delivery, will only be subject to minimal data collection.

Table 10.1
Causes of Other *Indirect* deaths; United Kingdom: 1997-2005.

Cause	1997-99	2000-02	2003-05
Diseases of the central nervous system	34	40	37
Subarachnoid haemorrhage	11	17	11
Intracerebral haemorrhage	5	3	11
Cerebral thrombosis	5	4	2
Epilepsy	9	13	11
Other	4	3	2
Infectious diseases	13	14	16
Human Immunodeficiency virus	1	4	5
Bacterial infection	8	6	5
Other	4	4	6
Diseases of the respiratory system	9	10	5
Asthma	5	5	4
Other	4	5	1
Endocrine, metabolic and immunity disorders	6	7	5
Diabetes mellitus	4	3	1
Other	2	4	4
Diseases of the gastrointestinal system	7	7	9
Intestinal obstruction	3	2	0
Pancreatitis	2	1	2
Other	2	4	7
Diseases of the blood	4	2	4
Diseases of the circulatory system	2	3	6
Diseases of the renal system	0	3	1
Cause unknown	0	4	4
Total	75	90	87

Table 10.2
Causes of **Other Indirect** deaths and rates per 100,000 maternities, United Kingdom 1997-2005.

	Number	Rate	95 per cent CI	
All *Other Indirect Deaths*				
1997-1999	75	3.53	*2.82*	*4.43*
2000-2002	90	4.51	*3.67*	*5.54*
2003-2005	87	4.12	*3.34*	*5.08*
Diseases of the central nervous system				
1997-1999	34	1.60	*1.15*	*2.24*
2000-2002	40	2.00	*1.47*	*2.73*
2003-2005	37	1.75	*1.27*	*2.41*
Infectious diseases				
1997-1999	13	0.61	*0.36*	*1.05*
2000-2002	14	0.70	*0.42*	*1.18*
2003-2005	16	0.76	*0.47*	*1.23*

The women who died

Given the disparate nature of the diseases to which the women whose deaths are counted in this Chapter succumbed, it is not possible to draw an overall picture of the type of woman likely to be at higher risk of an *Indirect* death. However, of these 87 women, five were aged less than 20, the youngest being 14, and five were over 40, the eldest being 43 years of age. Twelve were overweight with a body mass index (BMI) over 25. These included nine women who were obese with a BMI over 30 and five were morbidly obese with a BMI over 35.

Sub-standard care

Some of the most tragic cases in this Report are to be found in this Chapter, all involving extremely vulnerable women or young girls. And, as is the repeated pattern, the most vulnerable women who needed care the most received the least. Of the four women who died in later pregnancy or after delivery and who had no care at all, two were recently arrived non-English speaking illegal immigrants. One, a Bangladeshi girl of around 14 years of age, had been brought into the country as a new bride with forged papers and was only taken to the GP, at around six months of pregnancy, when her husband said she was "too ill to have sex". She died of tuberculosis a few days later. Another, trafficked, woman who had been lured to the UK under false pretences from an African country and kidnapped on arrival also spoke no English. She was thrown into the street in mid pregnancy when too ill to continue working as a prostitute. She was found by a passer-by and taken to the local hospital where she died of an HIV related illness a few days later. In another case an English woman concealed her pregnancy as her unborn child's father was a known sex offender and she did not want her baby taken into care. The final woman who died without having sought care had a history of non attendance in earlier pregnancies.

Of the seven women who were late in booking or who were poor attenders, several had chaotic lifestyles. Some were substance abusers with their other children in care. Two were subject to domestic abuse, one was needle phobic and the other was an HIV positive health care worker who did not want to reveal her status.

Fifty-eight of the eighty-seven women were White. Nine were Black African, four were Indian, four were Bangladeshi, three were Pakistani and three were of other Asian origin. The other six women came from a variety of other countries including Turkey, Afghanistan and Central Europe. Thirteen were recently arrived immigrants or asylum seekers and eleven spoke little or no English. Eleven other women were substance misusers and four were known to be subject to domestic abuse.

Overall, 30 of the *Indirect* deaths counted in this Chapter were associated with sub-standard care. Further details are given in the individual causes of death below.

Specific causes of *Indirect* deaths

Diseases of the central nervous system

Intracranial haemorrhage

Twenty-two women died from intracranial haemorrhage; eleven from subarachnoid haemorrhage and eleven from intracerebral haemorrhage, as Table 10.1 shows. Eight women bled antenatally, all in the second half of pregnancy. One subarachnoid haemorrhage occurred during labour and the other events occurred after delivery. The death in labour was due to a large middle cerebral artery aneurysm and presented as a seizure. This raises the possibility, discounted in the previous Report, that the stress of labour might provoke bleeding from pre-existing cerebral aneurysm.

Although subarachnoid haemorrhage may occur as a very sudden event, not necessarily associated with pregnancy, its management can be sub-optimal. Nine of the deaths from intracerebral bleeding were associated with sub-standard care as can be seen from the following example:

> *A multigravid woman was admitted near term with a very severe headache, nausea and photophobia. Both she and her midwife thought she was having a brain haemorrhage. Although her blood pressure was markedly elevated both at home and in hospital, there were no other features of pre-eclampsia. And, apart from testing her reflexes for imminent eclampsia, no neurological exam was recorded, neither was there any comment about neck stiffness. Her symptoms improved with analgesics. She delivered shortly after returned home. A few days later she collapsed and died from a ruptured basilar artery aneurysm. It is likely that the first episode of headache was caused by an initial small subarachnoid haemorrhage.*

This woman appears to have had very severe symptoms, which were unexplained. She should have had a full neurological examination and there should have been a request for either a neurological opinion or for neuro-imaging. This case is similar to those of another three women who were not offered imaging despite severe and incapacitating headaches.

Hypertension is a major risk factor for cerebral haemorrhage both in pregnancy and in the non-pregnant state. The cases of nine women who died from cerebral haemorrhage were associated with failure to control hypertension, a major cause of sub-standard care. For example:

> *A woman who had a cerebral haemorrhage due to an aneurysm in mid pregnancy had a coil inserted as a closed procedure to block the feeder vessels and to prevent further bleeding. Following an elective caesarean section, her blood pressure rose to 190 mm /Hg systolic but she was allowed home. Shortly after she was re-admitted with a further, fatal, intracerebral haemorrhage.*

This woman was at very high risk because of her previous subarachnoid haemorrhage and should not have been discharged with uncontrolled blood pressure. Poor control of blood pressure during and after pregnancy was also a factor in a number of other deaths in this Report, as noted especially in Chapter 3, Pre-eclampsia and eclampsia, as well as in the late death of a woman who died from stroke.

Five other deaths from cerebral haemorrhage are counted elsewhere. One, a rare but important death from chorioncarcinoma counted as a *Late Direct* death, is described in detail in Chapter 11 - Cancer and other tumours. Others are counted and discussed in the Chapters on haemorrhage, eclampsia and cancer. Cerebral haemorrhage was also the cause of death in a woman with thrombotic thrombocytopoenic purpura (TTP) and this case is described later in this Chapter.

Cerebral thromboembolism

Two women died from cerebral thromboembolism. One occurred in the puerperium in a woman who had had previous miscarriages and who at autopsy had a mural thrombosis in the her atrium as well as in the cerebral arteries. There was no evidence of endocarditis nor of any communication between the right and left circulations so she may have had antiphospholipid syndrome or a more generalised clotting tendency. The other death from cerebral thromboembolism occurred in a woman with ovarian hyperstimulation syndrome (OHSS):

> *A woman had repeated IVF cycles and had previous OHSS. In the last cycle many eggs were retrieved indicating further OHSS but, despite this, embryo transfer was carried out. She was later found unconscious and a scan showed a large cerebral infarct. Her gynaecologists were not involved immediately at the time of her admission and there was delay in recognising OHSS and in getting the brain scan. Earlier recognition of OHSS might have allowed effective treatment with fluids and thromboprophylaxis so care was judged to be sub-standard.*

Four women in this Report have died from different sequelae of OHSS but their deaths have been counted in the Chapters relating to the eventual case of death. These cases are also brought together in Chapter 1 to draw attention to this worrying rise.

Epilepsy

In this triennium 11 women died from epilepsy, a similar number to the 13 in 2000-02 triennium. Six deaths were classified as sudden unexpected deaths in epilepsy (SUDEP) along with a further two *Late* deaths. Deaths from SUDEP are usually not witnessed and may or may not occur during a seizure; the pathophysiology is not due to a complication of seizures such as aspiration. It is not clear whether pregnancy is an independent risk factor for SUDEP; it will, however, be an indirect risk factor since SUDEP is known to be more common in patients who do not take prescribed anticonvulsants and many women are reluctant to take anticonvulsants when pregnant or breast-feeding for fear of harming their babies. For example:

> *A woman died from SUDEP in mid-pregnancy. She had had epilepsy with tonic/clonic seizures for many years but had intolerable side effects from anticonvulsants which did not seem to affect seizure frequency. Because of this she had not taken any anticonvulsants for a year and was reluctant to try newer ones because she was concerned about teratogenicity. Although she attended the antenatal clinic at her GP's surgery very early in pregnancy she was not able to be fully "booked" until four weeks later because the midwives were too busy. Although she was referred to a neurologist she did not attend her appointment because she did not receive the appointment letter. As she was having regular fits she was referred again to the neurologist but, the repeat appointment was delayed by more than one month and she died before she could attend.*

Previous Reports have emphasised that women with epilepsy should have specialist care in pregnancy from a consultant obstetrician and a neurologist or specialist physician with interest in epilepsy and pregnancy. All members of the health care team both those directly concerned with pregnancy and specialists in other disciplines such as neurology, must ensure that women with life threatening conditions such as epilepsy are seen as early in pregnancy as possible.

Miscellaneous central nervous system disease

Two women died from acute hydrocephalus due to cysts in the midbrain. In one case:

> *A woman started to complain of new onset, persistent and severe headaches in mid pregnancy. No underlying obstetric cause was found and there was no record of a full neurological examination which should have included visualisation of her optic fundi. She had several admissions with headache, dizziness and visual disturbance but no abnormality was found and she was sent home. Eventually she developed unsteady gait and nystagmus, and rapidly deteriorated. She died after a CT scan at another hospital several miles away showed a cystic lesion in her midbrain.*

New onset headache is quite common in pregnancy and is usually benign. But this woman's headache seems to have been much more severe than most and should have been investigated further. As maternity services continue to reconfigure, consultant led maternity units should have on-site access to modern imaging facilities such as CT and MRI scans.

Infectious diseases

Bacterial infection

Five women died from bacterial meningitis. Two deaths were attributed to pneumoccocal meningitis, one to purulent meningitis where the organism was not found and two to tuberculous meningitis. Disseminated tuberculosis also caused one death and there was a further *Late* death reported that was attributed to tuberculous meningitis.

Tuberculous meningitis

Both the cases of tuberculous meningitis in pregnancy were diagnosed late, as often happens, and both occurred in women whose families were from the Asian sub-continent. In one case the diagnosis was delayed as the husband was acting as the interpreter, a recurrent feature of several deaths from a variety of causes in this and in previous Reports. There is still a great need for funding to be made available for suitably trained interpreters both in the community and in hospitals. The other case gave particular cause for concern:

> *A multigravid woman first complained of musculoskeletal pain in mid pregnancy for which her GP referred to her to an orthopaedic surgeon, who found nothing. She also attended the Emergency Department (ED) on a number of occasions. When she finally saw her obstetric consultant, by now also complaining of headache, she was referred for investigation to a tuberculosis clinic. Before she could be seen she was admitted via the ED to a medical ward with possible pulmonary tuberculosis. This admission, some weeks after her initial complaint of musculoskeletal pain, was precipitated by a few days history of fever and night sweats. Shortly after admission she became confused and a lumber puncture confirmed meningitis. She then went into labour, undetected, and had a live baby before the midwives were called. Subsequently she also had a postpartum*

haemorrhage. She continued to deteriorate and was looked by a number of different high dependency units before transfer to Critical Care for ventilation and died soon after. During her admission she was never cared for on any maternity unit.

As with another case of pneumoccocal meningitis this woman had numerous attendances before the diagnosis of tuberculosis meningitis was made. Multiple attendances without a diagnosis are a danger sign. If it was thought that this woman had tuberculosis in pregnancy she should have been admitted to hospital rather than sent to a tuberculosis clinic. Sub-standard care was also demonstrated by the lack of maternity staff input when she delivered and had a postpartum haemorrhage, and by the fragmented admission policy with her multiple sites of care. It was not clear who, if anyone, was responsible for her care.

Incidence of tuberculosis in pregnancy

As deaths from tuberculosis appear to be increasing a prospective national study of tuberculosis in pregnancy was undertaken by the United Kingdom Obstetric Surveillance System (UKOSS) from February 2005 to August 2006[1]. Over this period, there were 52 confirmed cases, representing an incidence rate of 4.6 per 100,000 maternities with a 95 % confidence interval from 3.4 to 8.0.

Pneumonia

Three women died from pneumonia, two from bacterial infection and one thought to be due to atypical organisms. There was also one *late* death from pneumonia. One of these women presented very late for antenatal care:

A young woman with needle phobia repeatedly failed to attend for care, despite reminders. Early in her third trimester she was admitted via the ED in labour and with fever, tachycardia and markedly reduced oxygen saturation. When transferred to the labour ward she was very unwell but initially refused intravenous access although intravenous antibiotics were started some hours later. She was delivered soon after and died of multi-organ failure a day or two later. It transpired that she had been ill for several days before her admission but had refused to come to hospital until she was in labour. Streptococcus pneumoniae was grown from her blood and sputum.

Fungal infection

In a very rare case, a woman died from septicaemia due to urinary tract infection and renal calculus, which caused a reactivation of a pre-existing peptic ulcer and subsequent blood vessel rupture further precipitated by fungal superinfection. A further death arising directly from fungal infection illustrates difficulties in obtaining specialised medical advice outside the remit of clinical obstetrics:

A multigravid asylum seeker had an uneventful pregnancy though she did attend the neurology clinic where "chronic daily headache" was diagnosed. Her young son always translated for her. She was admitted in late pregnancy with headache and objective evidence of weakness in the left arm and leg but discharged after a few days with no firm diagnosis being made. She was readmitted some days later with headache, pyrexia and photophobia, again seen by a medical registrar and quickly discharged. One week later she presented to the antenatal clinic unable to walk and was admitted to a neurology ward, a right-sided space occupying brain lesion having been found in a CT scan organised by the obstetricians via the ED. She was admitted via the ED because the neurology department could not or would not see her urgently even though she could not walk. She deteriorated rapidly and delivered by emergency caesarean section but a brain biopsy showed aspergillus and she died a few days later.

Aspergillosis usually occurs in immunocompromised patients. She was HIV negative but the CT of her chest showed mediastinal lymphadenopathy suggestive of lymphoma. In this case there were multiple communication problems not least because of her son acting as her interpreter. Her multiple admissions with headache and abnormal neurological signs should have provoked earlier imaging. Consultants did not adequately support the medical trainees working in the clinic and nor were the consultant obstetricians supported by their consultant colleagues in neurology. This case flags up yet again that multiple attendances without diagnosis are a danger sign, the issues around the provision of interpreting services and the need for combined neurology or medical / obstetric clinics which would improve the care of pregnant women with neurological problems.

There was one further death from overwhelming candida infection in a woman counted in the section on systemic lupus erythematosus.

Viral infection

Six women died from actual or presumed viral disease. Five were from HIV infection, in one of which earlier referral to a specialist HIV clinic would probably have improved the outcome. In at least one case a woman attended for care late in pregnancy for fear of stigmatisation. One case of presumed viral disease raises concerns about the quality of pathology that maternal deaths receive in that her autopsy was so inadequate a cause of death was hard to establish. As has been repeatedly stated in the Pathology Chapter (Chapter 15) of this, and previous Reports, the quality of maternal autopsies must be improved. They often do little more than exclude death from unnatural causes.

The death of another woman with HIV infection and tuberculosis who died of liver failure is discussed and counted in the section in this Chapter on gastrointestinal disease. There was at least one additional death from HIV where the notes have not been forthcoming and one *Late* death each from HIV and encephalomyelitis.

Diseases of the respiratory system

Asthma

There were four sudden and unpreventable maternal deaths from bronchial asthma. A further woman with asthma deteriorated throughout pregnancy and died of respiratory failure soon after a caesarean section. She has therefore been counted as an anaesthetic death and her case is discussed in Chapter 8.

Cystic fibrosis

There are always a few deaths for cystic fibrosis counted in these Reports as women with this condition have healthier lives, live longer and often wish to have children. In this triennium there was only one death from cystic fibrosis in a woman with severe disease who elected to continue with her pregnancy despite counselling about the very high risk of death in her case. She received excellent multidisciplinary care between the various specialist teams but eventually her respiratory infection flared and she started treatment with a home oxygenator. She died, despite excellent care, a few weeks after an early elective caesarean section. The outstanding care in her case shows how women with severe life threatening diseases but who elect for pregnancy can, and must, be supported in their choice.

Endocrine, metabolic and immunity disorders

The conditions in this diverse group are counted together for the sake of continuity with previous Reports and some are discussed more fully here.

Diabetes

Only one *Indirect* death was reported from diabetes in this triennium, and three additional *Late* deaths. One of the *Late* deaths occurred in a woman who developed diabetes in pregnancy which, in retrospect, was probably the first manifestation of type 1 diabetes. Unfortunately, she did not receive any medical follow up after delivery, insulin was stopped and she died of diabetic ketoacidosis.

Systemic lupus erythematosus (SLE) and antiphospholipid syndrome (APS)

There were four cases of lupus and/or antiphospholipid syndrome. In one of these cases, pulmonary hypertension was a contributing factor to the woman's death. In another:

> *A woman was diagnosed with APS following multiple pregnancy losses. She rapidly developed end stage renal failure but conceived while being dialysed. Pregnancy was not considered a cause for her amenhorrhoea until she had a routine pregnancy test taken for x-ray imaging but by then she was in mid pregnancy. She had good combined care but suffered an early placental abruption requiring an emergency caesarean section. She then developed coagulopathy, rapidly deteriorated and died from a haemopericardium.*

Pregnancies are still being missed in women on dialysis who have amenhorrhoea. In addition she should have had been offered pre-pregnancy counselling regarding the possible poor maternal and fetal outcome of pregnancy with women with APS, renal failure and on haemodialysis.

There were several other deaths in which SLE or APS played a part. One was a *Late* death from a stroke in a woman with APS and a poor obstetric history. Another woman, with severe SLE, died from cardiomyopathy and her death is counted in Chapter 9 - Cardiac disease. The death of a further woman with SLE is counted in Chapter 4 - Haemorrhage, because she died from postpartum haemorrhage due to placenta percreta which was almost certainly not connected with lupus. A woman with congenital adrenal hyperplasia who died from sepsis following prolonged rupture of membranes is counted in the Sepsis Chapter (Chapter 7). Her glucocorticoid treatment would have made her more susceptible to infection.

Gastrointestinal disease

Hyperemesis

There were three deaths in association with hyperemesis. One is counted in Chapter 2 - Thromboembolism, because she died from cerebral vein thrombosis; one is counted in Chapter 9 - Cardiac disease, because she died suddenly and unexpectedly though hypokalaemia from prolonged vomiting may have been a factor; the other is counted here:

> *A multigravid woman had hyperemesis again, having had it in each of her previous pregnancies. She was admitted to a gynaecology ward, given fluids and discharged some days later with instructions to attend her GP for follow up. A few weeks later she was found dead at home having suffered a massive haemorrhage from a tear in the oesophagus (Mallory Weiss syndrome).*

Mallory Weiss syndrome is a very rare complication of hyperemesis and it is even rarer for it to be fatal.

Liver disease

There were four maternal deaths from liver disease including one from liver rupture and three from liver failure. Liver rupture in pregnancy is usually a complication of severe pre-eclampsia, however one of these deaths was a complication of possible connective tissue disease thought to be Ehlers Danlos syndrome (EDS) type 4. Of the deaths in association with liver failure one was due to alcohol abuse and another due to chronic active hepatitis:

> *A woman had chronic active hepatitis which had caused acquired antithrombin deficiency, which in turn had increased her thromboembolic risk sufficient to have caused a previous pulmonary embolus. She also had oesophageal varices, ulcerative colitis, and had had several previous miscarriages. She sought IVF and became pregnant again which resulted in an unexpected vaginal breech delivery. She then required blood products for a postpartum bleed and soon became breathless. It was eventually thought she had pulmonary hypertension. She then deteriorated further, had a seizure and was considered to have had another pulmonary embolus for which she was given thrombolysis. This caused massive vaginal and generalised haemorrhage from which she died.*

Her autopsy confirmed pulmonary hypertension with characteristic changes in the heart and lung vasculature. There was no acute pulmonary embolus but it was thought that the pulmonary hypertension was consequent to her previous pulmonary thromboembolic disease. It is difficult to believe that this woman had adequate pre-pregnancy counselling before she had IVF. This case reinforces the recommendation that all women with serious medical problems must have adequate pre-pregnancy counselling even if they are not immediately seeking pregnancy and particularly before they have assisted reproduction.

The other case of pregnancy liver failure was in a woman with HIV infection being treated with anti-retroviral drugs who developed liver failure in the third trimester. This may have been due to acute fatty liver of pregnancy or to anti-retroviral drugs but since the latter seems more likely in her case it has been counted here. The case of a woman who died from fatty liver of pregnancy is counted in Chapter 3.

Pancreatitis

Two maternal deaths from pancreatitis are counted here. One occurred in very early pregnancy in association with alcoholism and, although the other woman who died may also have had an alcohol dependency problem she also had gall stones. There were also two *Late* deaths from pancreatitis, one of which is of concern because she was found dead a few hours after admission to a psychiatric unit. It appears that the staff there did not realise she was physically ill. This case is discussed in Chapter 11 - Psychiatric deaths.

Ruptured appendix and intestinal perforation

Two women died of the consequences of acute abdomen and/or surgical complications. In one case:

> *A young very obese primigravida attended with abdominal pain in mid pregnancy for which no reason could be found. She was readmitted with more pain and again no abnormality was found and she was discharged. It was only following a subsequent readmission, a few hours later still, that she was finally seen by a consultant. The consultant requested a surgical review and she had an urgent appendectomy. However her condition deteriorated and she died shortly afterwards of adult respiratory distress syndrome and sepsis.*

Here again is a lesson that is recurrent throughout this Chapter. Women who are readmitted very soon after discharge are a high-risk group and must be seen urgently by consultants. The diagnosis of appendicitis in pregnancy is notoriously difficult, particularly in obese women.

The woman who died from intestinal perforation was found at autopsy to have Ehlers Danlos Syndrome (EDS) type 4, the chief features of which are thin lax skin, joint hyper mobility, bleeding, blood vessel rupture particularly aortic dissection, intestinal rupture and preterm labour. This woman had been in hospital for several days with abdominal pain before she was found to have a perforated bowel, an incidental finding at caesarean section, when advanced faecal peritonitis was noted. She did not speak English well and this, and the unexplained abdominal pain, should have resulted in more aggressive investigation of her symptoms.

It is gratifying that no women died from Ogilvie's syndrome this triennium. These are *Direct* deaths from bowel perforation secondary to caesarean section. This compares with four *Direct* deaths and one *Late* death in the 2000-02 Report, which raised concern about postoperative care following caesarean section.

Diseases of the blood

Thrombotic thrombocytopenic purpura

Four women died from thrombotic thrombocytopoenic purpura (TTP) and one from erythrocytosis. TTP is disease that is rare in general but more common in pregnancy. It presents with thrombocytopoenia and neurological features. The blood film, which shows a microangiopathic haemolytic anaemia, is characteristic. Three of the women presented with fulminating disease:

> One woman developed neurological signs in mid-pregnancy and was referred to hospital where a routine blood film led to the diagnosis of TTP. She was quickly referred to a tertiary unit for plasmapheresis, the recommended treatment, but died within a few days from intracerebral haemorrhage. Another woman was admitted about a week after delivery with a 24-hour history of lethargy, jaundice and slurred speech. She was seen within one hour by consultants in anaesthesia and obstetrics and transferred straight to Critical Care. The diagnosis of TTP had also been made from the blood film but she died from circulatory failure due to cardiac necrosis (another feature of TTP) before plasmapheresis could be started. The third woman presented soon after delivery and was initially thought to have HELLP syndrome, which may have a similar blood film. However she did not have the other clinical features of HELLP syndrome and she also died before she could receive plasmapheresis.

The fourth woman collapsed at home while still pregnant. Her admission scan showed a cerebral infarct and her low platelet count and microhaemangipoathic haemolytic anaemia indicated TTP. She was transferred for plasmapheresis, and when her platelet count had risen somewhat she was delivered by caesarean section. However she bled heavily, required a hysterectomy and died.

Other haematological conditions

One woman with factor XI deficiency had exemplary care but died from a ruptured splenic artery aneurysm and is counted in the following section, Diseases of the circulatory system. A woman with haemoglobin SC died of amniotic fluid embolism and is counted in Chapter 5. One woman with sickle cell disease (Hb SS) who died suddenly at home also had epilepsy and her death has been counted with the other cases of SUDEP. Deaths from myeloid leukaemia or myeloma are discussed and counted in Chapter 13 - Cancer.

Diseases of the circulatory system

Four women died from a ruptured splenic artery aneurysm and one from a rupture of a pseudo aneurysm of the splenic artery. This latter case was complicated by autoimmune disease, secondary antiphospholipid syndrome and a previous bowel thrombosis. It was thought that the pseudo aneurysm related to a previous splenectomy. There were two deaths from rupture of the iliac artery, one counted here and the other counted in Chapter 5 - Amniotic fluid embolism, because it was thought that this was more likely to be the cause of her death. The tendency of blood vessels to rupture in pregnancy has been commented on in previous Reports and several of these cases gave cause for concern. For example:

> *A woman with an uncomplicated pregnancy required an instrumental delivery. Shortly afterwards she collapsed with pallor, hypotension and tachycardia. There was no revealed haemorrhage. Blood was taken for haemoglobin and cross matching. Over half an hour later the on-call anaesthetic team was called and fluids were started. The anaesthetic team performed a haemocue (near patient) estimation of haemoglobin, which was very low, and only then were the on call consultant obstetrician and anaesthetist called. An urgent laparotomy was performed with further hypotension at induction of anaesthesia. Massive intra-abdominal bleeding from the splenic angle was discovered and could not be controlled. Although the general surgeons were called to help, by the time they arrived she had died from haemorrhage from a splenic artery aneurysm.*

In addition one woman died from a pulmonary arterio-venous malformation:

> *A woman with no apparent past medical history was found dead in late pregnancy. At autopsy 2.5 litres of blood were found in her right pulmonary cavity. It had come from a pulmonary arterio-venous malformation arising because of plexigenic pulmonary arteriopathy. There was right ventricular hypertrophy but no other evidence of pulmonary hypertension.*

On reflection there were clues that she might have underlying disease. She had complained of breathlessness since mid-pregnancy but this was discounted as physiological. A relative had indicated she sometimes turned blue and this too was thought to be irrelevant. Her clinicians were falsely reassured by a haemoglobin level in excess of 13 G/litre when she first complained of breathlessness. This is relatively high for this stage of pregnancy and could have been related to chronic hypoxemia. Her GP incorrectly discounted a loud second heart sound as a feature of normal pregnancy. Breathlessness is difficult to evaluate in pregnancy and maybe a symptom of life threatening disease. Although it may be caused by pregnancy alone, this is a diagnosis by exclusion and any additional abnormality is an indication for further investigation.

The early detection of severe illness in pregnant mothers remains a challenge to all involved in their care. The relative rarity of such events combined with the normal changes in physiology associated with pregnancy and childbirth compounds the problem. Modified early warning scoring systems have been successfully introduced in other areas of clinical practice and systems appropriately modified for the obstetric patient have been described in Chapter 19 - Critical Care, These should be introduced for all acute obstetric admissions and should help to reduce the cases in which death has followed the late recognition of serious illness. This is one of the top ten key recommendations of this Report.

Other deaths

A number of women died from other conditions including one or two for whom the underlying cause could not be ascertained. These cases are traditionally counted here. One woman died from Moyamoya disease, a rare condition affecting cerebral blood vessels, and most frequently described in the Japanese. It tends to present in early childhood with symptoms of brain ischaemia or in later in adult life with cerebral haemorrhage. The appearance of cerebral blood vessels on MRI angiography is distinctive. Extracranial-intracranial bypass surgery is believed to improve the prognosis in those presenting with ischaemic symptoms but this is unproven. A Japanese review of up to 53 patients with Moyamoya disease in pregnancy concluded that pregnancy did not affect the outcome in those with previously known Moyamoya disease but not surprisingly those who presented in pregnancy with new onset disease, cerebral haemorrhage or ischaemia did badly, as was the case here.

Conclusions

Recurring themes in this Report which are also highlighted by the some of the cases in this Chapter are summarised in both the specific recommendations given at the start of this Chapter and in Box 10.1.

Box 10.1
Learning points: *Indirect* deaths

Epilepsy in pregnancy is dangerous because of the possibility of sudden unexpected deaths in epilepsy (SUDEP). Although the risk may not be greater in pregnancy than in the non-pregnant state, for a variety of reasons, epilepsy may be more difficult to control in pregnancy thus increasing the risk of SUDEP. If women stop anticonvulsant therapy in pregnancy they must be made aware of the risk of SUDEP.

Women who develop diabetes in pregnancy must have adequate assessment of their glycaemic status after delivery.

If a woman has new onset headache lasting for several hours and worse than she has ever had before she may have new intra-cerebral pathology. Brain imaging should therefore be considered.

Both systolic and diastolic high blood pressure should be controlled whether due to pre-eclampsia or to other reasons. A key recommendation of this Report is that systolic blood pressures of 160 mm/Hg or more require treatment.

References

1   Knight M, Kurinczuk JJ, Spark P and Brocklehurst P. *United Kingdom Obstetric Surveillance System (UKOSS) Annual Report 2007.* National Perinatal Epidemiology Unit: Oxford; 2007.

2   Komiyama M, Yasui T, Kitano S, Sakamoto H, Fujitani S & Matsuo S. *Moyamoya Disease and Pregnancy: Case Report and Review of Literature.* Neurosurgery 1998 43: 360-9.

11 Cancer and other tumours

Gwyneth Lewis, James Drife, Michael de Swiet

Introduction

It has been estimated that the incidence of cancer in pregnancy is 1 in 6,000 live births; half that for non-pregnant women of a similar age[1]. As the last Report demonstrated, pregnancy itself has a generally protective effect against medical conditions, thought to be due to the so called "healthy pregnant woman effect"[2]. Apart from this, there are several other possible reasons for the reduced overall incidence of malignancy. A woman with known cancer may avoid pregnancy, or a pregnant woman with occult cancer may have her diagnosis delayed because routine screening is not carried out, either because her symptoms are ascribed to her pregnancy or because investigation is less thorough.

For most malignancies pregnancy does not alter the incidence or prognosis compared with similar cancers diagnosed at the same stage in non-pregnant women. Pregnancy may, however, accelerate the growth of some cancers, particularly those which are hormone-dependent, for example cancers of the breast, cervix or reproductive tract, or those which occur in the blood, brain or skin. Choriocarcinoma, of which there were four reported cases this triennium, is the only malignancy known to be directly linked to pregnancy.

Although some 35 cases assessed in this Chapter are defined as *Indirect* or *Late Indirect*, because the course of the disease was modified or masked by the pregnancy, these would not be regarded as maternal deaths, or included in maternal death statistics, in other countries. As discussed in Chapter 1, the classification of maternal deaths in the UK, as determined by this Enquiry, is more inclusive than that used by countries who determine their maternal mortality ratios exclusively through the use of the International Disease Classification of Maternal Deaths (ICD 10). The inclusion of these extra cases in the overall maternal mortality figures helps to inflate the UK *Indirect* maternal death rate when compared to rates from other countries. An adjusted calculation for the UK rate, for comparative purposes, is given in Chapter 1.

Irrespective of the type of cancer, the stage when it was first identified or whether the woman died antenatally or postnatally, all deaths from malignancies are grouped together here because the lessons to be learned from their diagnosis and management are broadly similar. Evaluating these cases together strengthens the recommendations that can be drawn from them. This Chapter not only provides an overview of the remediable factors identified for some of the women who died but also serves to highlight other examples of outstanding care.

Summary of key findings for 2003-05

As shown in Table 11.1, the Enquiry assessors considered the deaths of 81 women who died of cancer during 2003-05, compared with 28 in 2000-02. This increase in the number of cases assessed is entirely due to a more intensive follow up and assessment of many more of the *Late Coincidental* deaths identified through the Office of National Statistics' (ONS) linkage system. The details of these are shown in Table 11.1. Thirteen of the 26 deaths from *Late Coincidental* tumours were reported through the ONS linkage system but were not assessed in detail.

Table 11.1
Numbers of deaths which were assessed by malignancy and type of maternal death; United Kingdom 2003-05.

Malignancy	Direct	Indirect	Coincidental	Late Direct	Late Indirect	Late Coincidental	Total
Choriocarcinoma	1	0	0	3	0	0	4
Breast	0	1	1*	0	7	0	9
Brain	0	2	2*	0	3	2	9
Blood	0	2	0	0	5	1	8
Melanoma	0	1	0	0	7	0	8
Ovary	0	0	0	0	2	0	2
Vulva or Uterus	0	0	0	0	3	0	3
Lung	0	2	2	0	0	7	11
GI Tract	0	1	6	0	0	6	13
Renal	0	0	0	0	0	3	3
Skeletal	0	0	1	0	0	2	3
Other	0	0	1	0	0	3	4
Unknown primary	0	0	3	0	0	2	5
Total	**1**	**9**	**16**	**3**	**27**	**26**	**82**

* Although these tumours may be aggravated by pregnancy, in these cases the assessors considered the deaths to be unrelated to pregnancy.

Overall the more intensive assessment of *Late Coincidental* cases carried out this triennium has shown that there are very few additional lessons to be drawn from most of these deaths, and such detailed assessments will not be routinely undertaken in future Reports.

In many cases, a high, sometimes outstanding level of care was given to the woman and her family once the diagnosis had been made. In a significant number of cases however, as has been discussed in many previous Reports, the opportunity to make the diagnosis earlier was missed despite overt symptomatology. Whilst this may not have affected the eventual outcome, earlier diagnosis would have enabled the woman to be made as comfortable as possible for the last months of her life as well as enabling earlier access to further medical care and the support services she and her family required.

The women who died

The ages of the women ranged between 17 and 46 years, with the median age being 31 years. About half who died were primiparous, but several were mothers with a significant number of children; a small number had more than ten previous live births.

Six women were immigrants or refugees/asylum seekers who had recently arrived in the UK. A further two appeared to have arrived late in their antenatal period seeking care for their pregnancy and/or their cancer. Six of these eight women spoke no English. One did not reveal her advanced breast cancer to her midwife at booking and had midwifery-led care until she revealed her history some months later, when terminally ill. The youngest of the refugees, a single, isolated teenager who had also recently arrived in the UK, was one of the four African women in this Report who was reported to be pregnant as the result of rape by soldiers in a war-torn country. It is likely that the stigma of rape delayed her seeking care until just before her delivery, but her case should have been picked up by those responsible for her welfare and she should have been referred to maternity services earlier.

Ten UK-born women were extremely poor attenders for care or delayed seeking their first antenatal appointment until they were several months pregnant. Two did not attend until shortly before delivery as they had deliberately tried to conceal frank malignancies:

> *Both of these women knew they were dying but did not, or could not, seek help. One died of fulminating squamous cell carcinoma of the vulva and the other of advanced cancer of the breast. Both cases were revealed only during birth. The women had highly complex social lives and multiple, but differing, features of vulnerability. Both had a history of concealed pregnancies with previous children in care. In one case the pregnancy was identified by a health visitor who made the referral to maternity services herself, and in the other the woman booked just prior to delivery. Both women had a fear of doctors and a history of refusing physical examinations. It is possible they concealed their obvious lesions because they thought they may have to have the pregnancy terminated. The care both received, once in the care of the maternity and oncology services, was exemplary.*

The woman who had concealed her cancer of the vulva, despite her fear and mistrust of the medical profession, consented to publication of her case so that others might learn from her misfortune. Cancer of the vulva is extremely rare, and a case such as this does not merit this Enquiry recommending a vaginal examination at booking for all pregnant women.

Of the other women who booked late, two were asylum seekers, two were substance abusers, two who died of lung cancer were smokers although they denied this at booking, and two were unaware they were pregnant.

Choriocarcinoma

Four women died of this rare, unpredictable and unpreventable cancer, which is the only *Direct* cause of maternal death from malignancy. Choriocarcinoma is a high-grade malignant tumour arising from fetal trophoblastic tissue. The disease tends to present suddenly a few weeks or months after a pregnancy which may have ended through miscarriage, unexplained intrauterine death, stillbirth or the safe delivery of a healthy infant.

Women who die of choriocarcinoma have no particular predisposing characteristics. In this triennium their ages ranged from the twenties to the late thirties and two were primiparous. One died within six weeks of delivery and the other three were *Late* deaths, the maximum period being four months after birth. Two of the pregnancies ended in intrauterine death and the other two in normal delivery. Only two of the four cases had the classic symptom of persistent vaginal bleeding after delivery and in one of these cases this led to very prompt diagnosis and referral, which nevertheless failed to prevent the fatal outcome. In another case there were unusual symptoms before delivery:

> *An obese woman with a past history of pulmonary embolism (PE) was admitted to hospital on several occasions with shortness of breath. A ventilation/perfusion (V/Q) scan ruled out PE and a diagnosis of pneumonia was made. She received thromboprophylaxis after delivery, yet she died*

suddenly a few weeks later and was found to have disseminated choriocarcinoma, with bleeding into a cerebral metastasis.

The assessment of chest symptoms in a woman with past history of thromboembolism who does not appear to have had a further PE is very difficult. VQ scans have a significant false negative rate and the pre-test clinical suspicion of PE for this woman should have been very high. An MRI or spiral CT scan might have shown chorioncarcinoma in her lung. In another case:

Following an intrauterine death at term, an externally normal infant was delivered. A detailed perinatal autopsy demonstrated a massive haemoperitoneum with a tumour on the liver which was shown to be choriocarcinoma. No primary site was identified in the placenta but eight weeks after delivery the mother was admitted to hospital with a brain haemorrhage. A brain biopsy demonstrated metastatic choriocarcinoma and, despite treatment, she died.

The results of the perinatal autopsy report were not sent to the family or any of her health professional carers. Indeed they were not known to them until the mother had been admitted with her fatal brain haemorrhage. Given that choriocarcinoma is curable if treated in time, this long delay represents substandard care. Sadly this may be a critical reflection on the paucity of paediatric pathologists that has now developed in the United Kingdom.

Quality of care

*"The midwifery commitment made me cry." ***

What has been most impressive since these Reports started to highlight the need for earlier detection, improved training and more coordinated multidisciplinary care for pregnant women with cancer and serious concurrent illnesses, is the level to which most of this care is now provided. In this triennium the assessors have seen yet more examples of outstanding multidisciplinary working or excellent personal care delivered by midwives or obstetricians in exceptional circumstances. Problems do remain, but many of the women who died, and their partners and families, were managed extremely sensitively once the diagnosis had been made:

A mother had a recurrence of a previous malignancy during pregnancy. The recurrence was quickly identified and she was managed jointly between her own named midwife, obstetrician and oncology team. Her midwife said "I took care to ensure that her visits were coordinated and if she had an appointment at the cancer day ward I attended there to perform the antenatal checks and to liaise with her oncologist and nurse. I undertook all of her routine maternity care, attended her delivery and visited her postnatally. I then maintained contact with her and her family until she died and attended her funeral together with her oncology nurse and obstetrician.

Remediable factors

Despite the high quality of care provided to these mothers in many cases, there were others which continued to demonstrate the repeated lessons from earlier Reports. For example, there were a worrying number of cases where pregnant women were not investigated for severe sustained pain, vomiting, shortness of breath, weight loss or other abnormal symptoms during pregnancy. Although earlier diagnosis would probably not have altered the course of the disease, appropriate pain relief and referral to the oncologists and support services could have been provided earlier.

*** A midwifery assessor's comment on one case.*

Severe abdominal and back pain, sciatica, urinary incontinence, haematuria, shortness of breath and significant weight loss continue to be under-investigated or attributed to other causes. Severe back pain, urinary incontinence and frank haematuria were put down to repeated urinary tract infections in some cases. A number of other women had pain and symptoms so severe that they repeatedly attended their GP or antenatal clinics or even the Emergency Department (ED). In some cases this necessitated one or more admissions for bed-rest and analgesia but no investigations were undertaken despite severe pain being recorded in the notes. Some women were not seen by a consultant obstetrician or physician, and others did not see a doctor at all:

> A woman who had had severe obstetric complications in a previous pregnancy booked for midwifery-led care. She developed back and shoulder pain, which was ascribed to anxiety even though it was so severe as to require weekly visits to the midwife, and her later breathlessness was ascribed to pre-existing asthma. She finally had a chest x-ray (CXR) after delivery, at which point her malignancy was finally diagnosed. As she was a known asthmatic and had had significant problems in an earlier pregnancy, midwifery-led care was, in any event, inappropriate.

> A woman who also had GP/midwifery-led care complained of increasing back pain which was ascribed to a urinary tract infection. The pain worsened but she was not referred to the hospital although it was suggested she could do so herself if she wanted. She was admitted to hospital later, through the ED, with increasing back pain requiring opiate analgesia, but this was ascribed to muscle spasm and she was discharged without being seen by a senior obstetrician. She was eventually readmitted in extremis having by this time lost a serious amount of weight. An immediate diagnosis of malignancy was made but she died shortly thereafter.

> A woman who spoke little English and booked late for care was admitted on numerous occasions for abdominal pain and vomiting. Little was undertaken in the way of investigations and she was eventually referred for a psychiatric opinion. She died of widespread carcinoma shortly after delivery.

In a few cases the diagnosis of malignancy of the reproductive tract was also delayed despite the rapid growth of what were assumed to be "fibroids" identified on the woman's booking scan. Malignancy must be ruled out if there is a rapid increase in the size of "fibroids" within a matter of a few weeks.

Pre-pregnancy counselling

A few women who had previous episodes of cancer sought pre-pregnancy counselling. One woman became pregnant despite being counselled of the immediate risks to her health as she believed that her radiotherapy would be an effective contraceptive.

Women planning pregnancies after a diagnosis of cancer, particularly of breast or cervix, should be counselled by an obstetrician with a special interest in oncology or an oncologist with specialist knowledge of obstetrics. Guidance from the Royal College of Obstetricians and Gynaecologists recommends that pregnancy should be deferred for at least two years after treatment for breast cancer as this timescale helps to differentiate those women with a better chance of long-term survival from those with more aggressive disease[3]. It further recommends that women with stage IV disease (with a five-year survival of less than 15%) should be advised not to have further pregnancies and women with stage III disease should consider deferring pregnancy for five years.

Cases where poor communications between professionals led to a delay in diagnosis and treatment

In several cases maternity staff were unaware that women were already being treated for cancer. In some cases the women assumed they knew but in others, the mother herself was the first to inform her midwife that she was being treated for cancer.

Box 11.1
Learning points: cancer

Although the practice of professional examination of the breasts as part of routine antenatal care has been discontinued, women should be encouraged to examine their own breasts regularly.

Pregnancy is not a contraindication for appropriate radiological investigations, especially for women with severe and unremitting pain or vomiting, including back, chest or epigastric pain, and particularly if the pain is so severe it requires management by major or epidural analgesia or prevents the woman from walking.

References

1   Drife, J O. The contribution of cancer to maternal mortality. In: O'Brien PMS, McLean AB (eds). "Hormones and cancer: proceedings of an RCOG study group". London: RCOG; 2000.

2   Ronsmans et al. Mortality in pregnant and non-pregnant women in England and Wales 1997-2002: are pregnant women healthier? in Lewis G (ed) Why Mothers Die 2000-02 . The Sixth Report of the Confidential Enquiries into Maternal Deaths in the United Kingdom. London: RCOG Press; 2004. 272-278.

3   Royal College of Obstetricians and Gynaecologists. Pregnancy and Breast Cancer. RCOG Guideline No.12: RCOG; 2004.

12 Deaths from psychiatric causes

Margaret Oates

Psychiatric deaths: Specific recommendations

New to this Enquiry 2003-05:

All professionals involved in caring for pregnant women who have been referred to child protection services should be alert to the fact that many of these women actively avoid maternity care despite being at high risk of medical or mental health problems. This risk is compounded by child protection case conferences and the removal of infants into care. Whilst the needs of the child must remain paramount, extra support and vigilance is needed for the mother and communication between all agencies involved in her care is essential. Further efforts are required to retain women who are substance misusers in treatment programmes after their child has been removed. Social workers should liaise with, and refer pregnant women in their care to, the local maternity services if necessary.

Extra vigilance and support is required for women who have requested a termination but, because of late gestation or other reasons, have to continue with an unwanted pregnancy. All women, but particularly the most vulnerable and excluded who have little money and a lack of transport, should have easy access to local facilities. Careful consideration should also be given to the method employed as medical terminations are particularly distressing for women who are home alone.

As in previous Reports:

All women should be routinely asked in early pregnancy about current and previous mental health problems including their use of prescribed and non-prescribed medicine and legal and illegal substances including tobacco and alcohol. Maternity staff should sensitively, but explicitly, enquire into the nature and severity of these problems. They should check with the woman's General Practitioner (GP) for further information.

During pregnancy, all women who are at identified risk of serious postnatal mental illness should be assessed by a psychiatric team. The woman should have a management plan which includes a system of close supervision following birth. Midwives should check on the continuing mental health of all their clients at least twice during pregnancy and following delivery.

Midwives should routinely inform the GP that their patient is pregnant and ask for any health or relevant social information. The responsibility of conveying previous psychiatric and medical history should not rest with the woman alone.

GPs should communicate not only with obstetricians, but also with midwives, details of their patient's previous psychiatric history including that of alcohol and drug misuse.

Psychiatric teams caring for women with serious mental illness, particularly bipolar disorder, should proactively discuss with all female patients of childbearing age the risks associated with childbirth and plans to manage this risk should they become pregnant.

Psychiatric teams should liaise with midwives and obstetricians about the management of pregnant women with mental health problems. Psychiatric teams should accept direct referrals from midwives.

The training programmes of midwives, general practitioners, obstetricians and psychiatrists should include perinatal psychiatric disorders.

Specialist perinatal psychiatric teams should be available to every maternity network or Trust to assist in the management of women who are at risk of becoming ill and to those who are suffering from serious postpartum disorders.

Psychiatric deaths: Specific recommendations continued

Women who require to be admitted to psychiatric hospital following delivery should be admitted to a specialist psychiatric mother & baby unit.

Substance abuse

Pregnant women with substance misuse problems should not be managed by GPs and midwives alone but by an integrated specialist service nested within the maternity services. This should comprise a specialist midwife and obstetrician, specialist drug treatment professionals who can manage both alcohol and drug problems, a social worker and other relevant agencies to ensure coordinated multidisciplinary and multi-agency care.

Close multidisciplinary and multi-agency care should be continued not only through pregnancy but also in to the postnatal period even if the infant is removed into the care of the local authority.

All drug and alcohol specialist services should enquire about domestic abuse at assessment and within ongoing treatment. Local protocols should be developed for effective collaboration between agencies and services.

All drug treatment agencies should record an agreed minimum consistent data set about the children of clients presenting to them and information should be shared between social services and health treatment agencies.

Introduction and background

This Chapter describes the key features of, and derives lessons from, those maternal deaths arising directly from a psychiatric condition, suicide or accidental overdose of drugs of abuse, as well as deaths from medical or other causes closely related to a psychiatric disorder. These latter deaths include those from the physical consequences of substance misuse and delays in diagnosis and treatment because of the presence of a psychiatric disorder, accidents and violence.

Perinatal psychiatric disorder

Psychiatric disorder during pregnancy and following delivery is common; both new episodes and recurrences of pre-existing conditions. Ten per cent of new mothers are likely to develop a depressive illness in the year following delivery[1], of whom between a third and a half will be suffering from a severe depressive illness[2]. At least two percent of new mothers will be referred to a psychiatric team during this time and four women per thousand will be admitted to a psychiatric hospital, of whom two per thousand will be suffering from a puerperal psychosis[3].

The majority of women who develop mental health problems during pregnancy or following delivery suffer from mild depressive illness, often with accompanying anxiety. Such conditions are equally prevalent in pregnancy and following delivery and probably no commoner than at other times[1]. In contrast, the risk of developing a serious mental illness (schizophrenia, bipolar disorder and severe depressive illness) is reduced during pregnancy. However, the risk of developing bipolar illness and severe depressive illness is markedly elevated following childbirth, particularly during the first three months[4].

The prevalence of all psychiatric disorders, including substance misuse, schizophrenia and obsessive compulsive disorder, is the same at conception as in the non-pregnant female population. Pregnancy is not protective against relapses of pre-existing serious mental illness, particularly if the woman has stopped her usual medication at the beginning of pregnancy.

Women who have had a previous episode of a serious mental illness, either following childbirth or at other times, are at an increased risk of developing a postpartum onset illness even if they have been well during pregnancy and for many years previously. This risk is estimated as at least one in two[5,6]. The last two Reports[7,8] found that over half of the women who died from suicide had a previous history of serious mental illness. It is also known that a family history of bipolar disorder increases the risk of a woman developing puerperal psychosis following childbirth[6].

Specialist perinatal psychiatric services

Serious psychiatric illnesses in the last few weeks of pregnancy and the first few weeks following childbirth have a number of distinctive clinical features including, importantly, the tendency of sudden onset and rapid deterioration. Half of all cases of puerperal psychoses will have presented by day seven postnatally, and 90% by three months postpartum[4], as highlighted in the last two Reports. This, together with other distinctive symptoms[9] and the special needs of women and their infants at this time, has led to national and international acceptance of the need for special services for perinatal psychiatric disorder[10,11]. This includes the recommendation that new mothers who require admission to a psychiatric unit following birth should be admitted together with their infant to a specialised mother and baby unit. The findings of the last two Enquiries underpin the importance of this strategy.

Maternal suicide

Until recently it had been thought that the maternal suicide rate was lower than would be expected[12], with pregnancy exerting a so-called "protective effect". However, the last two Enquiry Reports found that maternal suicide was more common than previously thought and was in fact the leading overall cause of maternal death. These Reports also called into question "the protective effect of maternity". However, suicide during pregnancy remains relatively uncommon and the majority of suicides occur following childbirth. Overall, the suicide rate following delivery is no different to that amongst women in the general population, but it may be that for a sub-group of women, those suffering from serious mental illness, the suicide rate is substantially elevated[13]. One of the reasons for the misunderstanding about maternal suicide is that suicide research over the last 40 years has consistently shown that rates based upon coroners' verdicts alone are under-estimates. For the last three triennia, the Office for National Statistics (ONS) has been able to link mothers' deaths up to one year after delivery with recorded births. This revealed that around half of all maternal suicides had not been reported directly to this Enquiry. Once this under-reporting was corrected, a more realistic estimate of maternal suicide was possible.

Summary of key findings for 2003-05

Suicide

The deaths of thirty-three women who, in the opinion of the assessors, committed suicide in the years 2003-05, were reported to the Enquiry. The circumstances surrounding two of these cases were suspicious of suicide but could not be proven. The ONS record linkage study, described in Chapter 1, only identified four more cases of suicide that appeared unknown to the Enquiry for this triennium. In total, therefore, it appears 37 women committed suicide whilst pregnant or during their first postnatal year in the UK for 2003-05. Twelve deaths from suicide occurred during pregnancy or shortly after delivery and these cases are counted as *Indirect* deaths in this Chapter. The other deaths, which occurred after the 42 day postpartum cut off point for maternal deaths, are counted in Chapter 14 as *Late* deaths. All but three of these later deaths were considered to be directly due to a postnatal mental illness and are counted as *Late Indirect*, the three others occurring in women with long standing mental health problems and were not considered related to pregnancy.

Substance abuse

An overdose of drugs of abuse was responsible for the deaths of twenty-two women, three of which occurring during pregnancy and three shortly after birth. These six cases are counted in this Chapter as *Indirect* maternal deaths as the circumstances surrounding the pregnancy and death meant the assessors could not rule out an intentional overdose. The others deaths were most probably accidental and occurred later after childbirth. These deaths are counted in Chapter 14, as *Late Coincidental* deaths.

Deaths from suicide and accidental drug overdose are considered to be psychiatric deaths and are described in this Chapter. However, they are counted either in this Chapter, or Chapter 14 depending on the timing of the mothers' death in relation to childbirth. The figures for this triennium are given in Table 12.1.

Table 12.1
Timing of reported maternal deaths due to or associated with psychiatric causes; United Kingdom: 2003-05.

Timing of death	Suicide	Substance misuse	Physical illness	Violence	All
In pregnancy or up to six months after delivery					
Before 28 weeks	5	2	5	2	**14**
28-33 weeks	0	0	1	0	**1**
34-41 weeks	3	1	1	0	**5**
Up to 42 days after delivery	4	3	11	2	**20**
All *Indirect*	**12**	**6**	**18**	**4**	**40**
Over six weeks after delivery					
7-12 weeks	2	1	4	0	**7**
13-18 weeks	4	2	2	0	**8**
19-24 weeks	1	3	1	3	**8**
Over 24 weeks	14	10	8	3	**35**
All *Late* deaths	**21**	**16**	**15**	**6**	**58**
All assessed	**33**	**22**	**33**	**10**	**98**
Not assessed	4	2	0	0	**6**
All	**37**	**24**	**33**	**10**	**104**

Violent deaths

Ten women died violently, including five murders, three falls, a suspicious road traffic accident and a house fire to which an underlying psychiatric condition contributed. These deaths are discussed here but counted in Chapter 14; Deaths unrelated to pregnancy.

Medical conditions aggravated by a psychiatric disorder

The deaths of 18 women who died from *Direct* or *Indirect* medical conditions that may have been influenced by the consequences of a psychiatric disorder are counted in the relevant Chapters of this Report, although the psychiatric lessons from these cases are discussed here. A further 15 women died later after childbirth from *Coincidental* causes which may have been affected by an existing psychiatric condition. In the main these deaths were associated with substance misuse.

As with the last Report in some cases physical symptoms were misattributed to psychiatric conditions. For example:

> A woman died from a subdural hematoma sustained having fallen down stairs. She had a new baby who had health problems. Her general practitioner (GP) was treating her for depression related to her concerns about her infant's progress and she was noted to be drinking to excess at the time. She fell down the stairs having consumed a large amount of alcohol, and was admitted to hospital with a subdural hematoma and evidence of a midline shift. Following her discharge from Critical Care her continuing agitation and behavioural disturbances were attributed to "postnatal depression" and she was referred for a psychiatric opinion. The psychiatrist noted fluctuating levels of confusion and neurological signs. She deteriorated rapidly and died 24 hours later.

In this case the misattribution of the mothers' confusional state to postnatal depression led to a delay in the appropriate treatment. This also highlights the importance of keeping women with an early onset postnatal depression with adverse circumstances under close review.

> A second case involved a woman who died in the early weeks following delivery from a pulmonary embolus and aortic dissection. She had been admitted in late pregnancy with severe upper back pain, thought at the time to be musculoskeletal in origin, overlaid with anxiety. Her pain continued following delivery and a few days later she was admitted with a history of breathlessness and chest pain and haemoptysis. She was agitated, frightened and thought she was dying. She was diagnosed with postnatal depression and referred to a psychiatrist. He found a frightened and physically ill woman who did not have a primary psychiatric disorder. The woman died shortly afterwards.

Timing of psychiatric deaths

The timing, in relation to pregnancy, of all deaths considered in this Chapter has been shown in Table 12.1.

The known epidemiology of perinatal psychiatric problems suggests that psychiatric disorder presenting in the last trimester of pregnancy is both unusual and predictive of problems following delivery. It is also known that the majority of women with serious mental illnesses will have presented by 12 weeks after childbirth. For this reason, together with the fact that deaths from psychiatric causes may occur some weeks or months after the onset of the condition, the deaths due to, or associated with, psychiatric causes were further analysed in six week periods relating to childbirth. As shown in Table 12.1, just under a half of all maternal suicides occurred during pregnancy or up to 12 weeks after delivery and a third of deaths due to substance abuse occurred in this period. Overall, the majority of deaths due to, or associated with, psychiatric conditions occurred after delivery.

Rates of maternal death

Table 12.2 compares the mortality rates for 2003-05 with those for 2000-02, the only previous triennium for which the methods and levels of ascertainment of psychiatric cases were similar. In the previous

Report, 26 deaths from suicide were reported to the Enquiry and assessed, and a further 32 suicides were identified by record linkage but were not included in the assessment process. This gave a total of 58 deaths from suicide counted in the last Report.

In this triennium 33 deaths from suicide were reported to the Enquiry and assessed. Only four additional cases were found by record linkage and were not assessed. This gives a total of 37 deaths from suicide this triennium. This decrease in the rate of deaths from suicide is just large enough to be unlikely to have occurred by chance. If this fall is sustained in the next Report the decrease may indicate that the recommendations made in the last two Reports about identifying women at potential risk in the antenatal period are having a beneficial effect. The increase of rates of death associated with substance misuse shown in Table 12.2 are not statistically significant and are compatible with random variation.

Table 12.2
Reported maternal deaths due to or associated with psychiatric causes; United Kingdom: 2000-02 and 2003-05.

Cause	Indirect up to 42 days post partum	Late 43 - 365 days post partum	Not assessed	All	Rate	95 per cent CI	
Suicide							
2000-02	10	16	2	58	2.9	2.3	3.8
2003-05	12	21	4	37	1.8	1.3	2.4
Change					-1.2	-2.1	-0.2
Substance misuse							
2000-02	6	5	0	11	0.6	0.3	1
2003-05	6	16	2	24	1.1	0.8	1.7
Change					0.6	0.0	1.2
Physical illness							
2000-02	15	1	2	18	0.9	0.6	1.4
2003-05	18	15	0	33	1.6	1.1	2.2
Change					0.7	0.0	1.4

Underlying psychiatric diagnosis

Overall, for 85 of the 98 women whose cases were assessed and who either died from a psychiatric cause i.e. suicide or substance abuse, or for whom a psychiatric disorder was a major factor, there was sufficient information to make a probable or definite psychiatric diagnosis. These are shown in Table 12.3. Two women had no psychiatric diagnosis. One was a woman who died from an overdose of recreational amphetamines but who had no other evidence of either psychiatric illness or substance misuse and the other died from a medical condition but whose physical symptoms were misattributed to a psychiatric disorder.

Table 12.3
Main psychiatric diagnosis by cause of death; United Kingdom: 2003-05.

Diagnosis	Cause of death				
	Suicide	Substance misuse	Physical illness	Violence	All
Psychosis	5	0	0	0	**5**
Severe depressive illness	7	0	2	0	**9**
Anxiety/depressive adjustment	3	0	2	1	**6**
Alcohol dependent	1	1	8	2	**12**
Drug dependent	5	20	15	5	**45**
Personality disorder	2	0	2	0	**4**
Learning disability	0	0	2	0	**2**
No psychiatric diagnosis	0	1	1	0	**2**
Unascertained	10	0	1	2	**13**
All	**33**	**22**	**33**	**10**	**98**

Suicide

Five women who were suffering from a psychotic illness committed suicide. One death occurred in late pregnancy and another shortly after delivery. Both of these women had a previous history of postpartum psychosis and bipolar illness. The three other women died later after childbirth, one of whom had a previous history of puerperal psychosis. There were no cases of psychosis in the other causes of psychiatric death.

Seven women who committed suicide were suffering from a severe depressive illness. One died in mid-pregnancy and the others later after childbirth. Four of these women had a previous history of severe depression. In addition, two women who died from medical conditions were suffering from a severe depressive illness: one died in early pregnancy from myocarditis and a second a few weeks after delivery from adult respiratory distress syndrome. In both cases it was felt that the women's mental health had delayed their access to medical care and that the antidepressants they were receiving had contributed to their condition.

Substance misuse

Substance misuse was either directly or indirectly associated with the deaths of 57 women. Twelve of these women were alcohol dependent and forty-five were illicit drug dependent. Most of the drug dependent women were using heroin, but a large number were also misusing amphetamines, cocaine, benzodiazepines and alcohol.

Six of the women who died from suicide were known substance misusers, five of whom used intravenous heroin. Four died by hanging and two died from an overdose of paracetamol, one in pregnancy and one later after delivery.

Twenty two substance misusing women died after a drug overdose, one of which was due to alcohol toxicity. Eight more women who were alcohol dependent and a further fifteen who were drug dependent died from medical causes directly or indirectly associated with their substance misuse. A further two alcohol dependent women died in house fires while intoxicated and five drug dependent women were either murdered or died in a road traffic accident as a consequence of their drug use.

Current psychiatric treatment

In the last two Reports the majority of women whose deaths were due to, or associated with, psychiatric causes were receiving some form of treatment for a psychiatric disorder during their maternity and over half of them were in contact with psychiatric services. Table 12.4 shows the highest level of psychiatric care provided for these women this triennium.

Table 12.4
Highest level of psychiatric care during index pregnancy: United Kingdom 2003-05.

| Level of care | Cause of death | | | | |
	Suicide	Substance misuse	Physical illness	Violence	All
Mother and baby unit	1	0	0	0	1
Inpatient general	1	0	2	0	3
Perinatal psychiatric team	1	0	0	0	1
General psychiatric team	4	1	5	0	10
Drug and alcohol team	0	8	9	2	19
GP only	14	7	4	3	28
None	8	5	9	4	26
Not known	4	1	4	1	10
All	**33**	**22**	**33**	**10**	**98**

As in the previous Report the majority, 62 (63%), of women who died were receiving some type of psychiatric treatment. However, the number admitted to a psychiatric inpatient unit has fallen. Only four women this triennium were receiving inpatient care compared to ten in preceding Report, and, as last time, only one woman was treated in a specialist mother and baby unit.

Twenty-eight women received no treatment for their psychiatric disorder and in ten cases no details were available. Less than half of the women who had substance misuse problems had been in contact with specialist drug or alcohol services during their pregnancy.

Risk identification and management

As shown in Table 12.5, 79 of the 98 women whose deaths are considered in this Chapter had a past psychiatric history and were at risk of a recurrence of their disorder, or a relapse of their condition, following childbirth. For 55 (70%) of these women this risk was identified in early pregnancy but less than half of these women had had a management plan developed and put in place. In only a few of these cases was the management plan either adequate or communicated between maternity and psychiatric services.

Table 12.5
Identification and management of past psychiatric history; United Kingdom: 2003-05.

	Cause of death				
	Suicide	Substance abuse	Physical illness	Violence	All
Past psychiatric history					
Number	21	21	30	7	79
Percentage of all deaths with a past history	*64*	*95*	*91*	*70*	*81*
Past history correctly identified during index pregnancy					
Number	10	18	20	7	55
Percentage of all deaths with past history	*48*	*86*	*67*	*100*	*70*
Past history managed during index pregnancy					
Number	2	8	12	2	24
Percentage of all deaths with past history correctly identified	*20*	*44*	*60*	*29*	*44*
All deaths	**33**	**22**	**33**	**10**	**98**

The following case highlights the findings and recommendations of the previous Enquiries:

> *A young woman living in stable circumstances killed herself in a violent manner several weeks after the birth of her baby. She had a previous history of bipolar illness with a number of inpatient admissions for mania. She had last been seen by psychiatric services shortly before the beginning of her pregnancy and appears to have stopped her mood stabiliser medication at this time. Although the General Practitioner (GP) mentioned her previous psychiatric history in his referral to the obstetrician, the midwife appears to have been unaware of this at booking. The woman remained well throughout the pregnancy but no steps were taken to monitor her mental health following delivery. Shortly after delivery she had non-specific mental health problems resulting in an assessment by a duty psychiatrist. No steps were taken to inform her GP, midwife or health visitor nor to refer her back to psychiatric care. A few weeks after delivery, she saw her GP for depression but he did not feel that she was mentally ill. The day before her death, relatives contacted the health visitor, but not the GP or psychiatric services, because of their concern about the woman.*

Because of her past history of bipolar disorder, this mother faced a risk of at least a 50% of a recurrence of her illness in the first three months after childbirth[7,8]. Her psychiatric team should have alerted her to the risk she would face if she had another baby and explained how it could be managed. She should have been asked at the booking clinic about her previous psychiatric history and her GP should have communicated this to the midwife. Further, she should have been seen by her psychiatric team during pregnancy and a management plan put into place should she relapse after delivery. She should have restarted her usual medication after delivery and been under close supervision during the postpartum period. Her illness was predictable and her death perhaps avoidable.

Specialist services

As shown in Table 12.4, one woman, who committed suicide whilst suffering from a puerperal psychosis, was cared for in a specialist mother and baby unit. Another woman who committed suicide was cared for by a specialist perinatal psychiatric team. The remainder of the 34 women treated by adult psychiatric services were under the care of general psychiatry or drug addiction teams.

There was no evidence in the ten deaths occurring in women with serious mental illness and cared for by general psychiatric services that advice or admission to a mother and baby unit had been sought from specialist perinatal psychiatric services. Sadly, this was evident even when such services were available locally:

> *A woman living in comfortable circumstances died from suicide a few weeks after the birth of her first baby. At booking she told the midwife that she had had counselling for some family problems previously but was currently well. This was not pursued further. It was not standard practice to enquire about a family history of psychiatric disorder. There was information in the GP records that this counselling had been about her father's suicide, related to bipolar disorder. The mother developed a depressive illness in the first few weeks following delivery which was initially treated by her GP. When she rapidly deteriorated and became psychotic, she was seen by a number of different psychiatric teams as her illness unfolded. She was taking antipsychotic medication and said to be improving immediately prior to her death.*

This death highlights a number of issues raised within this Report. There should be a greater awareness amongst both the public and health professionals of the risk associated with a family history of suicide and bipolar illness. Questions about family history of psychiatric disorder must be made routinely at antenatal clinic. If the midwife had checked with the GP it is possible that this family history might have been elicited during pregnancy. The significance of the early stage of her depressive illness could have been realised if information about her family history had been to hand. The elevated risk of suicide in women suffering from puerperal psychosis is well established, and is particularly true when there is a family history of suicide. Had this woman been admitted to a psychiatric mother and baby unit (there was none available in the region) then perhaps the outcome might have been different.

The children

The majority of mothers who died from suicide, as with other causes of psychiatric deaths, had existing children. In contrast to the last Report none of the women who killed themselves committed infanticide although the two who died in late pregnancy killed their babies.

Child protection

In all, 41 women died after a child protection case conference had been held. Thirty-four of these women were substance misusers.

In 23 cases the mother died shortly after her baby had been taken into care. Five of these women died from suicide, and 18 from substance misuse. Of the other 18 women, 15 died from medical conditions and three from other causes. More than half of these women were late bookers, or very poor attenders for care, as Table 1.26 in Chapter one has already shown. Their healthcare workers attributed this lack of engagement to fear of social services' involvement. In the majority of cases once the baby had been removed the level of support and care for the mother from both maternity and social services fell or ceased:

A young woman died from an overdose of opiates some months after delivery. She had a long history of heroin use and an older child was in the care of the local authority. Whilst she did not attend her hospital antenatal outpatient appointments, she did accept community midwifery care at home until a child protection case conference was held and a decision made to place the infant in care after birth. She then failed to keep any further maternity appointments until she gave birth at term. After delivery she received no support from addiction services or social services and her death took place shortly after she heard the decision to place her baby for adoption.

Termination of pregnancy

Three women killed themselves following a medical termination of pregnancy this triennium. Medical terminations may be very distressing, particularly for women on their own. There were no suicides associated with termination of pregnancy in the previous two Reports.

Sixteen other women whose deaths are discussed in this Report had requested, but not undergone a termination of pregnancy. Three of these women died of suicide, the rest from a variety of causes. Most of these cases involved a referral to a contracted non-NHS abortion service. Whilst in a minority of cases the woman changed her mind, the majority involved either too great a delay or a very late gestation on presentation:

An older woman died from an overdose of heroin in mid pregnancy. She had been an intravenous drug user for many years and had multiple long term physical sequelae. Her previous children had been taken into care. She presented to her GP requesting a termination of pregnancy at around six weeks gestation and an appointment was given for a month later, which she failed to attend. She received a second appointment when she was 20 weeks pregnant. She then attended, on the wrong day, explaining that she had been unable to afford the cost of travel to her previous appointment as the clinic was some distance away from her home. By the time she was finally seen she was 22 weeks pregnant and the clinic felt unable to proceed. She died a few weeks later.

Whilst there were other aspects of this woman's care which were sub-optimal, and her long term prognosis was poor, her termination could have occurred earlier had a local facility been available. It was unrealistic to expect someone so vulnerable, chaotic and socio-economically deprived to cope with the arrangements that were in place for that locality.

Communication

In half of the 98 deaths discussed here the assessors identified major deficiencies in communication between services and / or professionals. This was most notable between psychiatric services or drug treatment services and maternity services, and between child protection and mental health services. As in previous Reports, there were numerous examples of midwives not checking with GPs when a previous psychiatric history was elicited and GPs not informing midwives and obstetricians of a known psychiatric or substance misuse history.

Deaths from suicide

For many of the women who killed themselves later after birth there was no evidence that the death could have been predicted. It is probable that these suicides were triggered by social events out of the control of those caring for the woman. Nonetheless, there were many cases in which the seriousness of the mothers' condition appears not to have been appreciated and the timing and nature of the intervention was less than optimal.

Method

As first identified by this Enquiry, these women kill themselves by predominantly violent means as shown for this triennium in Table 12.6. Only nine women died from an overdose of a prescribed or over-the-counter medication, which is the usual method of suicide for non-pregnant women.

Table 12.6
Method of maternal suicide: United Kingdom; 1997-2005.

Method of suicide	1997-99	2000-02	2003-05	All
	n	n	n	n (%)
Hanging	10	8	14	32 (38)
Jumping from a height	5	4	4	13 (15)
Cut throat	4	1	0	5 (6)
Intentional road accident	1	2	0	3 (4)
Self-immolation	1	1	2	4 (5)
Drowning	1	1	2	4 (5)
Gunshot	1	0	0	1 (1)
Railway track	0	0	1	1 (1)
Overdose of prescribed drugs	3	9	9	21(25)
Total stated	**26**	**26**	**32**	**85 (100)**
Not stated	0	0	1	0

Age

The ages of the women who died from suicide ranged between 15 and 45 years of age, the mean and median age being 29 years. Although previous Reports have found that women who committed suicide tended to be older than those who die from physical causes of maternal death, this has not been shown for this Report.

Ethnicity

All but four women who killed themselves were White, the others being Indian, Black African or from Pakistan.

Social characteristics

Fourteen of the women were either single and unemployed or in relationships where both partners were unemployed. Several had professional occupations and two were health care workers. Ten mothers booked for maternity care after five months of gestation, or were irregular attenders for care. Twenty-two had had previous children. Fourteen were living with domestic abuse, eight were addicted to drugs and four were occasional drug users.

A summary profile of the women who died from suicide is shown in Table 12.7.

Table 12.7
Major social and clinical characteristics of the 33 mothers who died from suicide; United Kingdom: 2003-05.

Characteristics	Number	Percentage
Socio-demographic		
White ethnic group	29	88
Died following childbirth	27	82
Aged over 25	23	70
Had previous children	22	67
Unemployed and/ or had a partner unemployed	18	55
Living alone	12	36
Clinical		
Previous history of psychiatric disorder	21	64
Were seriously ill with a severe depressive illness or psychosis	14	42

Commentary on deaths related to drug and alcohol misuse

Judy Myles

Introduction

Fifty-seven women out of the 98 women whose deaths are discussed in this Chapter had problems with substance abuse. Forty five were misusing drugs and twelve were alcohol dependent. A further six cases of substance abuse were identified this triennium but have not been assessed in this Chapter. Although the majority of those who were drug dependent were using heroin, most were also using methadone, amphetamines, cocaine, benzodiazepines and some alcohol as well.

A small number died from suicide, the rest died from an "accidental" but lethal overdose of their drug of abuse, the physical consequences of their abuse or from related medical conditions. Some died from domestic abuse.

Many of these women were socially excluded and most were homeless or living in very poor circumstances. The majority were late bookers and poor attenders for antenatal care. Most had previous children in the care of the local authority and were subject to child protection conferences in their current pregnancy.

Substance misuse therefore makes a significant contribution to maternal mortality in general and to psychiatric causes of maternal death in particular. As shown in Chapter 1, 11% of all the women who died this triennium, of any cause, had problems with drugs or alcohol. Sixty per cent were registered drug addicts The care of these women during pregnancy and the postnatal period presents a challenge to maternity, drug treatment and social services.

Service delivery

Although pregnant women are fast tracked into treatment in the majority of drug and alcohol services in the UK, there is still a significant disparity in the numbers of women, in comparison to men, recruited into treatment services. The rate remains at a ratio of three males to one female, despite efforts to increase the number of women attending[14]. This is particularly of concern as the numbers of women misusing drugs and alcohol are rising. Women over the age of 16 have markedly increased their levels of harmful and hazardous alcohol consumption in comparison to men. Amongst women between the ages of 16 and 24, 24% have used an illicit drug in the previous year. Both drug and alcohol use in women of fertile age is becoming normative behaviour with a consequent increase in the numbers of exposed pregnancies and the reflected increase in maternal mortality either directly or indirectly associated with drug or alcohol misuse.

It is of utmost priority, therefore, that substance misuse services should provide environments that are acceptable to women of reproductive age, both for access and for retention in treatment. This is particularly an issue for women from ethnic minorities where drug or alcohol use is deemed unacceptable and consequently service access is particularly problematic:

> A mother of Asian origin died in early pregnancy from hepatic failure. She had been abusing alcohol for several years and had a long history of related gastrointestinal problems. She had not taken up the offer of help from her GP and the local alcohol services. Her GP did not convey this information to the maternity services and her family actively concealed her alcohol problem from those caring for her.

This case also illustrates the particular difficulties that women from an ethnic minority group may have in accessing substance misuse services and the importance of GPs informing maternity services about a previous psychiatric of substance misuse history.

Drug and alcohol abuse

The provision of drug and alcohol services varies across the country with some integrated services while in other areas there are separate drug services and alcohol teams. Given that poly-substance misuse i.e. alcohol and sedatives often in combination with opiates and alcohol has become the norm, it would be appropriate for this vulnerable group of women to have their drug and alcohol addiction treated in the same setting.

Need for integrated specialist care

Although there are examples of truly outstanding integrated care, in assessing these cases it is far more usual to find a lack of integration between community midwifery and specialist midwives and hospital-based obstetric care. Additionally, it is also evident that the continuing lack of integration between addiction services and maternity services also results in little or no information being passed between the two services. It is recommended that integration be achieved in each maternity service ideally by joint service provision between addiction services and maternity services for these vulnerable women but, where that is not possible, by joint discussion of care plans between services to improve the information held by each.

A number of women who died were managed by their GP and midwife without the involvement of drug treatment services and an obstetrician. The women's methadone was prescribed by their GP and often there was little awareness of the extent of their continuing use of street drugs. Women with substance misuse problems in pregnancy should not be managed by GPs and midwives alone. They should be fast-tracked to integrated care nested within maternity services, the so-called "one stop shop". This should comprise both specialist midwife and obstetrician, drug treatment professionals, social workers and other relevant professionals and resources so that multidisciplinary and multi-agency care can be provided on one site.

Identifying substance misuse

There remains an issue of under-identification of women with problematic substance abuse within maternity services. At the first visit maternity staff providing antenatal care for pregnant women should routinely ask for any history or present consumption of prescribed and non-prescribed, legal and illegal substances including tobacco and alcohol. Staff may require training in taking an addiction history as well as providing information on local specialist drug and alcohol services and ongoing support in managing this group of women.

All current guidelines recognise the need for an accurate assessment of drug and alcohol use, the need for associated social problems to be addressed and emphasise the importance of an integrated multi-agency approach. It is recommended that local protocols should be in place for effective collaboration between agencies and services, these should prescribe the arrangements for assessment and ongoing care with the ideal being that an integrated service should be available to these women.

Communication

In only a very few deaths does there appear to be any integration, communication or correspondence between addiction services and maternity services. Additionally, GPs are providing little or no information to obstetricians and midwives of a woman's past drug or alcohol history, with the history therefore not being revealed until late in the pregnancy. This further strengthens the recommendation made throughout this Report, that GPs actively inform obstetricians and midwives of any knowledge of a woman's past history of drug or alcohol misuse or addiction as early as possible in any pregnancy.

Co-existing mental health problems

It is known that women presenting with drug and/or alcohol misuse have a high incidence of mood disorders, estimated to be around 30%. On occasions the same woman may be receiving treatment from the addiction services, her GP and from generic mental health services and may be receiving anti-depressants whilst still using illicit substances that adversely affect her mood. Each such woman requires a lead agency to take responsibility for the overall management and co-ordination for further care as the combination of anti-depressants and stimulants in undesirable and treatment by several agencies may be confusing and lead to inappropriate prescribing of anti-depressants rather than treatment for stimulant misuse:

> *A young socially deprived woman, living in a hostel, died some weeks after delivery of her second child from an accidental overdose of heroin. She was being seen by the alcohol treatment service at the time and was awaiting inpatient detoxification. She died a number of days after her infant had been placed into care. The alcohol treatment services appear to have been unaware that she was also using heroin. In the past, she had been treated by alcohol services for her alcoholism, drug addiction services for her heroin addiction and adult psychiatric services as an inpatient and in the community. Her GP had been prescribing anti-depressants.*

This case also highlights the importance of communication between all those involved.

Care beyond pregnancy

Of all of the deaths due to, or associated with substance misuse, as reported earlier in this Chapter, it is noteworthy that the majority took place after 42 days after birth. It is a matter of concern that whilst drug and alcohol agencies actively recruit women into treatment whilst pregnant, the treatments are largely directed at stabilising the substance misuse during pregnancy. Post-delivery, particularly if the child is removed from the woman's care, many of these women then disengage themselves or are discharged from treatment. Therefore further efforts are required to retain substance misusing women in treatment programmes after pregnancy.

Occasional social misuse

Three women died by falling over when drunk, none of whom had evidence of an alcohol dependency. Two others died from amphetamine toxicity but there is no evidence that they had either previous contact with drug services or had any enduring drug problem. The third woman died from solvent inhalation. These deaths raise an issue as to how to better advise recreational substance users on the risks of social drug and alcohol use and whether services have a part to play in primary prevention of deaths from drug or alcohol misuse. For example:

A comfortably off employed older woman with other children died from acute amphetamine toxicity some weeks after the birth of her next child. She had no history of mental health problems and was well known to her health visitor and GP who did not suspect that she ever used illicit substances. Her mental health was said to be good during pregnancy and the postpartum period and she was seen by health professionals the day before she died and said to be very well. It appears that this woman was not a habitual drug user but merely an occasional recreational one.

Another older woman living in comfortable circumstances with older children, died from a head injury sustained after she had fallen downstairs when drunk. A few days earlier she had had a medical termination of pregnancy for a fetal abnormality. This woman had no history of previous mental health problems nor alcohol misuse. She had good compassionate care around the time of her termination but appears to have become distressed that evening and drunk to excess in order to get to sleep.

Domestic abuse

There is a clear association of domestic abuse with substance misuse, either as a reflection of lifestyle e.g. working in the sex industry, or as a consequence of living with a substance misusing partner. Again this strengthens the recommendation in this, and previous Reports, that all obstetric services and all drug and alcohol specialist services actively enquire about domestic abuse at assessment and within ongoing treatment. Attention to this is variable across addiction services in the UK:

A woman with longstanding heroin and alcohol misuse was murdered in late pregnancy by her drug misusing partner. She had been the victim of a number of serious assaults at the hands of her partner over the previous two years including one shortly before her death. She had presented to her GP late in pregnancy requesting a termination but her pregnancy was too advanced to proceed. She was seen only one occasion before her death by a drug liaison midwife but no mention was made by her GP or the woman herself of her domestic abuse.

Deaths from medical conditions

In addition to the deaths of substance misusers due to suicide or to accidental overdoses of illicit drugs, there were at least 23 further deaths in which substance misuse played a major role. Some of these deaths, particularly in those with alcohol dependency were directly caused by the psychiatric disorder, for example pancreatitis. Other deaths were due to the consequences of abuse, for example overwhelming infection or the failure of the woman and her carers to access timely medical help:

A woman died a few days following delivery from streptococcal septicaemia. She had a long history of intravenous heroin use and was in a poor physical state with multiple injection abscesses. After referral to social services in early pregnancy she failed to attend the majority of her antenatal visits and disengaged with the drug addiction services. A child protection case conference was held prior to delivery. She was admitted in labour at term, physically unwell but left hospital. The community midwife was unable to gain access to her home and presented just after birth in extremis some days later.

A young homeless woman died from bacterial endocarditis in late pregnancy. She had a long history of multiple drug abuse and had been using intravenous heroin for some years. She did not attend any maternity appointments after her midwife referred her to social services. A few weeks prior to her death, she saw a GP with fever and malaise and was prescribed antibiotics for a presumed diagnosis of a urinary tract infection. She did not complete the course of her antibiotics nor returned to her general practitioner. Her drug using boyfriend noticed that she was ill a few days before finding her dead in bed.

Both of these cases also highlight the additional risks that substance misusing women face when they avoid contact with health services following the involvement of child protection social services.

There were also a number of cases when the woman's heroin use led to the misattribution of physical symptoms or delay in the correct diagnosis. For example:

> *A young single woman with an older child in care died some months after delivery from cancer. She had a long history of heroin use and for some time had been living in very deprived circumstances and in a state of self-neglect. She did not reveal her heroin use until later in pregnancy following which she failed to attend for maternity appointments. She was admitted in late pregnancy with an antepartum haemorrhage and her premature baby suffered from a neonatal abstinence syndrome. Shortly after delivery she saw her GP, feeling unwell, and then continued to see him with complaints of weight loss and a chest infection. Her symptoms were attributed to her substance misuse and lifestyle. Her condition was not diagnosed until some weeks later when she presented as an emergency to hospital shortly before her death.*

Child protection

As is evident from the "Hidden Harm"[15] report, it is estimated there are between 250,000 and 350,000 children of problem drug users in the UK; this equates to one child for every problem drug user known to the services. This represents 2-3% of children under the age of 16 in England and Wales. This Report therefore recommends that all drug treatment agencies should record an agreed minimum consistent set of data about the children of clients presenting to them and further recommends that information be shared between the social services and health treatment agencies. This has undoubtedly already improved practice and has led to multi-agency planning meetings, being convened as early as possible in the pregnancy in an attempt to meet the multiple needs of the mother. However, paradoxically, the involvement of social services early in the pregnancy results in some of these women disengaging from treatment to avoid involvement from social services. It is therefore recommended that further work be done to improve attitudes towards pregnant women who misuse drugs or alcohol, to realistically address their multiple needs and to retain them in treatment.

Management guidelines

The care and management of pregnant women who are substance misusing, including alcohol, should be delivered according to best practice guidelines. National guidelines for Scotland were published in 2003[16], and suggested guidelines for England and Wales in 1997[17]. Guidelines for the management of the pregnant woman were included in "Drug Misuse and Dependence - Guidelines on Clinical Management", first published in 1997[18], which are currently being updated. Others can be found within the Evidence-based Guidelines for the Pharmacological Management of Substance Misuse, Recommendations from the British Association for Psychopharmacology[19]. This multiplicity of guidelines points to the need to synthesise these into one universal guideline, and this is a recommendation of this Report.

Discussion

Whilst the number of women who died from suicide in this triennium appears to be reduced compared to the last two Reports, it is evident that there are still problems with the identification of risk in early pregnancy and the appropriate management of that risk.

There has also been a reduction in the proportion of women who killed themselves with a previous history of psychosis, severe depressive illness and a previous history of serious postpartum illness. As serious postpartum illness is most likely to occur in the early weeks following childbirth it is not surprising that there has also been a reduction in the numbers of deaths from suicide taking place within three months of childbirth. It is hoped that these reductions reflect the recommendations of the two Reports concerning the identification and management of women with a past history of serious mental illness.

For many of the later suicides there was no evidence that the death could have been predicted and it is probable that the suicide was triggered by social events out of the control of those caring for the woman. Nonetheless, as in previous Reports, there were many cases in which the seriousness of the condition appears not to have been appreciated and the timing and nature of the intervention was less than optimal.

The majority of women who died from suicide, or whose deaths from other causes were associated with an underlying psychiatric condition and who were under the care of psychiatric services, were not receiving specialised care from perinatal mental health services or from substance misuse services integrated within maternity services. The evident lack of awareness of the special needs, distinctive clinical features and communication issues for women with perinatal psychiatric disorders leads to the conclusion that most of these women might have been better managed and perhaps some of the deaths avoided.

The majority of women who commit suicide continue to die violently. This finding was reported in the last two Enquiries and was thought to reflect the seriousness of the women's mental illnesses. In this Enquiry it is evident that violent death is also associated with less serious mental illnesses and persists throughout the postpartum year. This would suggest that severe but non-psychotic postnatal mental illnesses should also be taken seriously and that general practitioners and psychiatric teams should be alert to the possibility of sudden deteriorations and escalations in severity.

This Enquiry reveals that more women are dying from the direct or indirect consequences of substance misuse than from other psychiatric causes. Such deaths include accidental overdose as well as deaths due to overwhelming septicaemia and other physical causes related to substance abuse. For the majority of women their drug of abuse was heroin. With a few notable exceptions these women did not receive care from drug addiction services which were well integrated within maternity care. There was very poor communication between the two services and numerous examples of women with major addiction problems being managed by GPs and substance misuse midwives on their own. More of these women died from the physical consequences of their abuse than died from overdoses of their drugs or from suicide. This highlights the high risk nature of pregnancies in women who abuse substances particularly heroin and alcohol.

Whilst accepting that the needs of the child must always be paramount, the finding that so many deaths from psychiatric causes, took place shortly after a child protection case conference, or a child being removed into care, is striking. It is also striking that a third of the women who committed suicide and half of the women who were substance misusers appeared to be avoiding maternity care. This leads to the conclusion that additional support is needed for women in this situation. The removal of the child should not result in a removal of maternal care. There is a need for much closer working relationships and communication between drug treatment services and social services.

The commonest method of a first trimester termination of pregnancy is now a medical termination. The increase in the use of contracted abortion services involves organisation and a delay between referral and being seen, and, in many cases, a journey of some distance. For many vulnerable women, particularly substance misusers, this may be insuperably difficult and the termination does not take place. For others, particularly the young, the two stage process of a medical termination might be very traumatic and additional support is required.

It is still evident that there is a lack of distinction between mental health problems and mental illness, a lack of knowledge about the different types of mental illness and the distinction between mental illness and substance misuse and on occasion learning disability. This lack of differentiation led, on many occasions, to referrals to the wrong services and women not receiving appropriate care. Amongst those women who died from the physical consequences of psychiatric disorder it was evident that symptoms of physical illness were wrongly attributed to psychiatric disorder and states of distress or confusional states misidentified as functional psychiatric disorder. These findings would suggest that there is a need for basic psychiatric education to be included in the curricula for midwives, obstetricians and GPs and for psychiatric teams and drug addiction services to have a greater understanding of the physical problems that pregnant and recently delivered women may face.

As in the last Report all those involved in the care of pregnant and postpartum women should be reminded that physical illness can complicate or present as psychiatric disorder. Great care should be taken not to attribute physical symptoms to a psychiatric disorder without appropriate investigations.

References

1   O'Hara MW, Swain AM. *Rates and risk of postpartum depression - a meta-analysis.* Int Rev Psychiatry 1996; 8: 37-54

2   Cox J, Murray D, Chapman G. *A controlled study of the onset prevalence and duration of postnatal depression.* Br J Psychiatry 1993; 163: 27-41

3   Oates M. *Psychiatric Services for women following childbirth.* Int Rev Psychiatry 1996; 8: 87-98

4   Kendell RE, Chalmers KC, Platz C. *Epidemiology of puerperal psychoses.* Br J Psychiatry 1987; 150: 662-73

5   Wieck A, Kumar R, Hirst AD, Marks MN, Campbell IC, Checkley SA. *Increased sensitivity of dopamine receptors and recurrence of affective psychosis after childbirth,* Br J Psychiatry 1991; 303: 603-16

6   Robertson E, Jones I, Haque S, Holder R, Craddock N. *Risk of puerperal and non-puerperal (postpartum) psychosis.* Short Report Br J Psychiatry 2005; 186: 258-259

7   Lewis G, Drife J, editors. *Why Mothers Die 1997-199. The Fifth Report of the Confidential Enquiries into Maternal Deaths in the United Kingdom.* London: RCOG Press; 2001

8   *Why Mothers Die 2000-2002. The Confidential Enquiry into Maternal and Child Health.. Report on confidential enquiries into maternal deaths in the United Kingdom.* London RCOG Press 2004

9   Dean C, Kendell RE. *The symptomatology of puerperal illness.* Br J Psychiatry 1981; 139: 128-33

10 *National Service Framework for Children, Young People and Maternity Services.* Department of Health September 2004

11 NICE *Guidelines on Antenatal and Postnatal Mental Health National* DoH 2007

12 Appleby L. *Suicidal behaviour in childbearing women.* Int Rev Psychiatry 1996; 8: 107-15

13 Appleby L, Mortensen, PB, Faragher EB. *Suicide and other causes of mortality after postpartum psychiatric admission.* Br J Psychiatry 1998; 173(9); 209-211

14 *Living in Britain, General Household Survey No 31 (2002),* Office of National Statistics

15 *The Advisory Council on the Misuse of Drugs. Hidden Harm. Responding to the needs of children f problem drug users.* London, ACMD. 2003. www.drugs.gov.uk

16 Scottish Executive. *Getting Our Priorities Right: Policy and Practice Guidelines for Working with Children and Families Affected by Problem Drug Use.* Edinburgh: Scottish Executive 2003

17 Hogg C, Chadwick T and Dale-Pereira A (LGDF/SCODA). *Drug Using Parents: Policy Guidelines for Inter-Agency Working (England and Wales).* London: LGA Publications; 1997

18 *Drug Misuse and Dependence: Guidelines on Clinical Management of pregnant women* http://www.nta.nhs.uk/

19 British Association for Psychopharmacology (2004) *Evidence-based Guidelines for the Pharmacological Management of Substance Misuse, Addiction and Co-morbidity;* Recommendations from the British Association for Psychopharmacology.

13 Domestic abuse

Gwyneth Lewis

Domestic abuse: New and existing recommendations

Once multi-agency support services are in place this Enquiry continues to recommend that routine enquiries should be made about domestic abuse, either when taking a social history at booking, or at another opportune point during a woman's antenatal period.

Whenever possible, all women should be seen alone at least once during the antenatal period to enable disclosure more easily if they wish.

When routine questioning is introduced, this must be accompanied by the development of local strategies for referral to a local multidisciplinary support network to whom the woman can be referred if necessary.

Local trusts and community teams should develop guidelines for the identification of, and provision for further support for, these women, including developing multi-agency working to enable appropriate referrals or provision of information on sources of further help.

Information about local sources of help and emergency helplines such as those provided by Women's Aid should be displayed in suitable places in antenatal clinics, for example in the women's toilets or printed as a routine at the bottom of hand-held maternity notes or cooperation cards.

Clear, relevant and complete information must be passed from the GP to the antenatal care team, at booking, which accurately details any past current or past medical, psychiatric, social or family history.

It must be remembered that health professionals, too, are victims of abuse.

Women with known significant features of domestic abuse should not be regarded as "low risk" and should be offered multidisciplinary care in a supportive environment. If they choose midwifery led care the midwife should receive support and advice from an experienced superior.

All health professionals should make themselves aware of the importance of domestic abuse in their practice. They should adopt a non-judgemental and supportive response to women who have experienced physical, psychological or sexual abuse and must be able to give basic information to women about where to get help. They should also provide continuing support, whatever decision the woman makes concerning her future.

Background

Domestic abuse is defined by the Home Office as:

> *"Any incident of threatening behaviour, abuse or abuse (psychological, physical, sexual, financial or emotional) between adults who are or have been intimate partners or family members, regardless of gender or sexuality[1]".*

The term "domestic abuse" is now used in preference to "domestic violence", as the latter could be interpreted as relating to physical abuse alone. It also covers issues that mainly concern women from minority ethnic backgrounds, such as forced marriage, female genital mutilation/cutting (FGM/FGC) and so-called "honour crimes".

Honour crimes are defined by Human Rights Watch[2] as

> "Acts of abuse, usually murder, committed by male family members against female family members who are perceived to have brought dishonour upon the family. A woman can be targeted by her family for a variety of reasons including, refusing to enter into an arranged marriage, being the victim of a assault, seeking a divorce – even from an abusive husband – or committing adultery. The perception that a woman has acted in a manner to bring 'dishonour' to the family is sufficient to trigger an attack".

Domestic abuse occurs in all parts of society, and accounts for 25 per cent of violent crime in the UK. The estimated cost to the criminal justice system and the NHS, in 2004, was £3.1 billion[1]. However, its greatest cost is to the women and children who deal with its effects on their lives on a day-to-day basis, even long after the abuse has ceased. More key facts are summarised in Box 13.1.

Box 13.1.
Domestic abuse, key facts[1]

- In 2003/04 nearly all female homicide victims were killed by their current or ex-partner compared to 5% of male victims.

- 20% of women in England and Wales say they have been physically assaulted by partner at some point.

- More than 30% of cases first start during pregnancy.

- 40-60% of women experiencing domestic abuse are abused during pregnancy.

- More than 14% of maternal deaths occur in women who have told their health professional they are in an abusive relationship.

Where mothers are abused, children suffer too:

- In over 50% of known domestic abuse cases, children were also directly abused.

- About 750,000 children witness domestic abuse every year.

- Nearly three quarters of children on the `at risk' register live in households where domestic abuse occurs.

- Domestic abuse is a child protection issue. If a woman is being abused by a current or former partner and there are children in the home, they are likely to have experienced abuse by the same perpetrator.

Previous Reports have highlighted, as does this, the substantial number of pregnant or recently delivered women who died either as a result of murder or from medical or psychiatric causes but were known to be subject to domestic abuse. As a result, a number of local and national initiatives have been introduced. One, "Responding to Domestic Abuse, a Handbook for Health Professionals[1]" arose directly from the recommendations in the previous Report. This Department of Health for England handbook not only contains valuable information and advice but also includes a new national strategy for the identification and management of domestic abuse in pregnant women. A summary of the strategy is attached as an Annex to this Chapter and can be downloaded from www.dh.gov.uk/publications[1].

The mothers affected: 2003-05

During the three years 2003-05, 70 of the women who died from all causes had features of domestic abuse, including four women with genital mutilation/cutting (FGM/FGC). For the nineteen women who were murdered the abuse was fatal. The death of a woman who died of a placental abruption almost certainly caused by a blow to her stomach is counted in Chapter 4 – Haemorrhage, although she and her baby most likely died directly as a consequence of physical abuse.

Most of the other women, who died from a range of other causes, had proactively self-reported domestic abuse to a health care professional either before or during their pregnancy. None of these, or any of the other women whose deaths are considered in this Chapter, appeared to have been routinely asked about abuse, a previous recommendation in this Report. However, these deaths occurred prior to the introduction of routine enquiry during pregnancy.

Cases of murder are not routinely reported to this Enquiry although the association between pregnancy and increasing domestic abuse is well known. The cases described here should therefore be regarded as being representative of other cases of murder and domestic abuse that remain unknown to the Enquiry. However, from those that were reported, the warning signs were all too obvious in most cases. Several features of these reports illustrate the already described features of domestic abuse shown in Box 13.2.

Box 13.2
Indicators of domestic abuse, relevant to maternity care

- Late booking and/or poor or non attendance at antenatal clinics.
- Repeat attendance at antenatal clinics, the General Practitioners's (GP) surgery or Emergency Departments (ED) for minor injuries or trivial or non existent complaints.
- Unexplained admissions.
- Non compliance with treatment regimens/early self discharge from hospital.
- Repeat presentation with depression, anxiety, self-harm and psychosomatic symptoms.
- Injuries that are untended and of several different ages, especially to the neck, head, breasts, abdomen and genitals.
- Minimalisation of signs of abuse on the body.
- Sexually transmitted diseases and frequent vaginal or urinary tract infections and pelvic pain.
- Poor obstetric history:
    - Repeated miscarriage or terminations of pregnancy
    - stillbirth, or preterm labour
    - preterm birth, intrauterine growth retardation/ low birth weight
    - unwanted or unplanned pregnancy.
- The constant presence of the partner at examinations, who may be domineering, answer all the questions for her and be unwilling to leave the room.
- The woman appears evasive or reluctant to speak or disagree in front of her partner.

The mothers who were murdered

In this triennium the deaths of 19 pregnant or recently delivered women who were murdered were reported to this Enquiry. In the opinion of many assessors the death of another woman who died from obstetric haemorrhage was most likely directly related to the violence her partner had inflicted on her body. There are undoubtedly other deaths that have occurred and not been reported to this Enquiry so this is a minimum figure. Also because some of the cases in this Report are still *sub judice* it is not possible to obtain or give details of the exact circumstances, but the general lessons to be learnt from those cases that were available for assessment underline the need for vigilance, especially when there may be a high index of suspicion.

Fifteen of these women were already known to their local social services departments and nine had previous children in care. Three were sex workers and two others had recently been in prison. An extremely young pregnant schoolgirl, who was an occasional drug user and sex worker, was found raped and murdered in the local park whilst in the care of her local social services department. The care she had received from her teenage pregnancy midwife had been exemplary.

The ages of the women who died ranged from under 16 to their mid forties. Fourteen were White, four were Indian or Bangladeshi and the others were from a variety of other countries. Five could not speak English and in all cases the husbands acted as interpreters. In one other case however, the woman translated for her husband but still did not reveal her long standing history of abuse.

All of the women who were murdered also already had at least two of the identifiable risk factors of domestic abuse shown in Box 13.2, but none were referred for help or advice. Table 13.1 confirms previous findings that women who suffer from domestic abuse find it very hard to attend for regular and timely antenatal care. More than 80% of women who died from *Direct* or *Indirect* causes either booked after five months of pregnancy or received little or no antenatal care.

Table 13.1
Characteristics of the antenatal care received by women who were murdered or known to be suffering domestic abuse; United Kingdom 2003-05.

Type of death	Death in early pregnancy	Late or non attenders for antenatal care			Total number of deaths of women*
		Booked after 22 weeks or missed more than four visits	No ante-natal care	All	
	n	n	n	n (%)	n (%)
Direct	3	0	0	3 (75)	4 (100)
Indirect	1	6	3	10 (83)	12 (100)
All	**4**	**6**	**3**	**13 (81)**	**16 (100)**
Coincidental	2	4	3	9 (69)	13 (100)
Late deaths	0	15	2	17 (41)	41 (100)
Total	**6**	**25**	**8**	**39 (56)**	**70 (100)**

* Total number of deaths of women who were murdered or known to be suffering domestic abuse.

Of the women who were murdered:

- In all but two cases the perpetrator was a sexual partner or close family member.
- All but two of the women murdered by a partner or family member had a known history of domestic abuse.
- The majority of the women were murdered were either late bookers or poor attenders for care, as shown in Table 13.1.
- Many had "overbearing" partners or, as also seen in this Report, other family members who were present at all visits.
- More than half of the women were already known to social services and nine to the local child protection team; some had all their previous children in care.
- Three had family members or partners who were on the local sex offenders register.
- Some had histories of sexually transmitted diseases, multiple miscarriages or unexplained vaginal bleeding in pregnancy. The reasons for this were not followed up despite the known history of abuse.
- Some were regular attenders at the Emergency Department or antenatal clinics, complaining of non specific vague aches and pains.
- Four women had admissions with non specific abdominal pain, one women five times.
- In at least three cases there was family collusion and secret keeping.
- One woman seemed to have been forced to deliver at home.

In the majority of cases clear signs and symptoms of abuse were present but they were not followed up or acted upon:

> *In a widely reported case, and one of the most distressing reports ever to have been reviewed by this Enquiry, a young mother was effectively kept prisoner, starved and assaulted by her in-laws until she died of complications of her injuries some months after childbirth. Her autopsy report cited more than 60 recent assaults including sharp and blunt trauma, numerous broken bones and cigarette burns. She weighed just 45 kilos, having lost 22kg in weight since giving birth a few months earlier. Nine family members were convicted of her murder and/or perverting the course of justice.*

This young woman had married into a locally "notorious" family, well known to the local police and social services. Whilst she did manage to attend most of her antenatal visits she was always accompanied by a member of her husband's family. She was admitted several times for non-specific abdominal pains and also failed to gain any weight after 26 weeks' gestation. She had several episodes of vaginal discharge. She had an unplanned "born before arrival" delivery at home and was delivered by her mother-in law. Even though she required admission for a retained placenta, she discharged herself against medical advice and thereafter it became increasingly difficult for the community midwives or health visitors to maintain contact with her as the family became more and more obstructive.

Another woman who was obviously at very high risk also died:

> *This substance dependant older mother, with serious mental health problems and who had previously been stabbed by her abusive partner, sought a termination of pregnancy too late. She was then seen by a drug liaison midwife, who sent her for booking at a hospital clinic even though the woman had said she would refuse to attend a hospital but would accept care provided*

in the community. She was not offered an alternative and, predictably, did not attend. She was murdered by her known violent partner a few weeks later.

This woman was not only at high risk of abuse, she was also at risk of serious mental illness and suicide. She had made several previous suicide attempts and her sister had committed suicide whilst pregnant. She needed, but did not have, an individualised care plan. Not unsurprisingly she failed to attend her hospital appointment and was not given an alternative. To compound the risk, she was inappropriately booked to deliver in a local midwifery unit. Such an extremely high risk woman required intensive support and a clear management plan. Normal patterns and timescales for referral were bound to let her down. Perhaps more alarming still is that it appears that there was no serious investigation of her death despite major deficiencies in her care. It is therefore not clear what lessons, if any, have been learnt from her tragic and brutal death.

In other cases the comments of the health professionals concerned also demonstrated a complete failure to learn any lessons from these tragic events. As the regional assessor said of one case where the family of a woman with several broken bones and young children at home, were not referred to the child protection services despite the clear risk of the abuse being transferred to the children:

> *"The aspect of her care I really found most worrying was the lack of recognition of risk and a complete lack of reflection by the professionals involved".*

Discussion

Although the previous Report made firm recommendations concerning domestic abuse, repeated at the start of this Chapter, the timescale for their introduction and implementation means that they would have had little or no effect on the women who died during this triennium. It is hoped that the effects of the publication of *"Responding to Domestic Abuse, a Handbook for Health Professionals"*[1] and the recommendations of the National Domestic Abuse and Pregnancy Advisory Group for England, as summarised in the Annex to this Chapter may start to be seen in the findings of the next Report.

References

1   Department of Health. *Responding to domestic abuse. A handbook for health professionals.* London: Department of Health; 2006. www.dh.gov.uk/publications

2   www.hrw.org. (Last accessed 31/7/07)

Annex 13.1 The recommendations of the National Domestic Abuse and Pregnancy Advisory Group[1]

The Advisory Group's terms of reference were:

> "To advise Ministers on the practicalities of taking forward the commitment in the Children's, Young People's and Maternity NSF (National Service Framework) to provide a supportive and enabling environment within antenatal care for women to disclose domestic abuse."

An enabling environment is defined as:

> "An environment which ensures, at the very least, that all pregnant women know about the nature and frequency of domestic abuse, that those affected need not suffer in silence and will be listened to sympathetically, and all women are given information on how to access local and national sources of support and advice."

Recent NHS reforms were designed to meet the needs of patients more effectively. One outcome has been a shift of emphasis from Whitehall to the NHS frontline. It is the responsibility of local authorities, managers and professionals to set priorities in the light of their resources and the needs of their populations. The role of the Department of Health (DH) is to set out a clear national framework whilst providing resources, setting standards and looking at accountability.

Action points for local activity

1. Material concerning domestic abuse should be provided that meets the needs of the local population in a variety of easily accessible formats and media. Support should be available from the start in easy access formats for all, including in different languages and easy read format.

2. The numbers and website addresses of the national and local helplines should be automatically printed at the bottom of all NHS appointment cards and any other locally produced information.

3. The national and local helpline numbers should be printed on local hand held maternity and child health records as well as being made available in clinics by means of posters, videos etc.

4. New mothers to receive, as part of their baby record book, a laminated card with a complete list of useful national and local numbers of organisations that can help them and their babies, such as access to breast feeding advice, welfare foods etc but which will also include the domestic abuse numbers.

5. The national helpline numbers and website address should be printed on a standardised credit card sized leaflet freely available in clinics or elsewhere. These may be adapted for local use.

6. Regular surveys should be carried out to ascertain how many women recalled seeing the information, if they understood it and modifications made accordingly.

7. Policies should be audited locally as part of the monitoring process tracking implementation of the Maternity Standard of the Children's, Young People's and Maternity NSF.

8. NHS maternity services should move to include a routine question as part of the social history taken during pregnancy, but this should be introduced at a measured pace, and with appropriate training.

14 Deaths unrelated to pregnancy: *Coincidental* and *Late* deaths

Gwyneth Lewis

Introduction

This Chapter considers the lessons which can be drawn from the deaths of pregnant or recently delivered mothers which were not related to pregnancy. These are those women's deaths, apparently unconnected with pregnancy, which occur either in the antenatal period or up to one year after birth, miscarriage, ectopic pregnancy or a termination of pregnancy. Such deaths, which occur before or up to six weeks after delivery are internationally defined as fortuitous, although the authors of this Report prefer to use the term *Coincidental*. Deaths which occur after this period, but up to and including 365 days after delivery are classified as *Late*.

Although neither *Coincidental* or *Late* deaths, in international terms, are considered to be true maternal deaths and do not contribute to the calculations for any international maternal mortality rates or ratios, some contain important messages for the providers of maternity care. Clinically the lessons may include basic principles for the management of pregnant or recently delivered women with underlying medical or psychiatric conditions. From a public health perspective, the continuing assessment of such deaths re-enforces the need for information on the correct use of seat belts whilst pregnant, and, perhaps most importantly, the voluntary identification and management of pregnant women who suffer from domestic abuse. This is discussed in Chapter 13.

Summary of key findings for 2003-2005

Coincidental deaths

In this triennium, the deaths of 55 women who died of *Coincidental* causes either during their pregnancy or within 42 days of delivery were reported to this Enquiry compared to 39 for the previous triennium. This rise is due to better case ascertainment by the CEMACH regional managers and is not significant. As in the past, and as shown in Table 14.1, the largest overall category were deaths due to "unnatural" causes including murder and road traffic accidents. Deaths from cancer form the second largest overall category and the deaths of 16 women who died from cancers unaffected by their pregnancy are discussed in Chapter 11.

Table 14.1
Coincidental deaths occurring during or up to, and inclusive of, 42 days after, the end of pregnancy; United Kingdom: 2003-05.

Cause of death	Number
Unnatural deaths	
Road traffic accident	24
Murder	10
Overdose of street drugs	2
House fire	1
Cancer (see Chapter 13)	14
Medical condition	1
All *Coincidental* deaths	52

As with previous Reports, and other causes of death, many of the women whose deaths are counted in this Chapter were vulnerable and socially excluded. The general lessons to be drawn from this category of women have been discussed in Chapter 1. *Coincidental* deaths associated with domestic abuse and murder are considered in Chapter 13.

Road traffic accidents during and after pregnancy

Twenty-three women died from road traffic accidents, including pedestrian accidents, whilst pregnant or within six weeks of delivery. Another seven women are counted as *Late* deaths in that their accidents occurred two months or more after childbirth. Twelve women died undelivered and eight women died despite intense cardio-pulmonary resuscitation and perimortem caesarean section. None of the eight babies delivered in this way survived even though their gestational ages ranged between 24 and 38 weeks. One woman who died some weeks after childbirth may have intentionally killed herself in a road traffic accident, and her case is discussed in Chapter 11 - Psychiatric deaths.

Thirteen of the women who were drivers or passengers in moving vehicles were wearing seat belts, six were not and in two cases the evidence was not clear. The characteristics of the six women who did not wear seat belts are remarkably similar in that they were all vulnerable and had complex lives. Two of these six women, who died near term or shortly after delivery, had sought no care at all due to their chronic drug and/or alcohol misuse and domestic abuse, and another two women, with similar characteristics, had been seen only once or twice. Another woman, who had been repeatedly subject to domestic abuse, was killed by her drunken partner whilst in the front passenger seat of their car.

Eight of the women who died were pedestrians hit by oncoming vehicles. Of these, six also led socially complex lives and all but one were either regular or occasional drug users and most suffered domestic abuse. Several had high levels of street drugs at autopsy. One was an extremely young girl and another was a recent immigrant who spoke no English.

Twelve of the fourteen women who were either involved in pedestrian accidents whilst crossing a road, or who were not wearing seat belts whilst travelling in moving vehicles, had features suggestive of significant social exclusion. Seven of them were receiving support from social services and the four women who had not sought maternity care, or were very poor attenders, were also known to the Child Protection Services. Between these four women alone, 17 older children were already in care.

Box 14.1
Recommendations for the use of seat belts in pregnancy

"Above and below the bump, not over it"

Three point seat belts should be worn throughout pregnancy with the lap strap placed as low as possible beneath the "bump" lying across the thighs with the diagonal shoulder strap above the bump lying between the breasts. The seat belt should be adjusted to fit as snugly as comfortably possible, and if necessary the seat should be adjusted.

Late deaths

Late maternal deaths are defined as those deaths which occur in women more than 42 days, but less than one year after miscarriage, abortion or delivery. The International Classification of Maternal Deaths (ICD10) only classifies *Late* deaths due to *Direct* or *Indirect* maternal causes, whereas this report also includes *Late Coincidental* deaths from which educational, public health or other messages and recommendations may also be drawn. For this reason all *Late* deaths reported to the Enquiry are counted, and some are discussed in this Chapter, but none are included in the overall maternal mortality rate as defined in Chapter 1.

This triennium, the CEMACH regional managers have been proactively starting reviews on a large proportion, but not all, of the 273 *Late* deaths either notified to the Enquiry via the CEMACH regional managers or through the record linkage system derived by the Office for National Statistics (ONS). This system identifies all women who have died within a year of giving birth from whatever cause. Whilst this has meant an increase in the number of deaths assessed, it does not reflect an increase in actual numbers of maternal deaths and this has been discussed in detail in Chapter 1. The classification of these deaths is shown in Table 14.2. Apart from the *Late Direct* and some *Late Indirect* deaths related to pregnancy notably puerperal psychosis and cardiomyopathy, from which important lessons for maternity care can still be drawn, it is not the intention of the Enquiry to assess all *Late* cases in future.

When considering the findings of this Report it must be noted that the figures for the deaths counted in this Chapter, apart from the eleven directly associated with pregnancy in this triennium, cannot be compared to figures given in previous Reports due to an increase in extended case assessment.

Late Direct deaths

Some of the mothers who died 42 days or more after delivery actually died of maternal causes but, due to the limitations of the ICD 10 classification system for maternal deaths, cannot be counted as such in maternal mortality statistics. This is regrettable as they do contain important lessons for clinical care, especially in developed countries such as the UK, where these women often have prolonged support in a Critical Care unit before succumbing to their illness. There were 11 such *Late Direct* cases for this triennium, shown in Table 14.2 and discussed in depth in the relevant Chapters of this Report. Thus, for example, three *Late Direct* deaths from thromboembolism are discussed in Chapter 2, two from amniotic fluid embolism in Chapter 5, three from sepsis in Chapter 7 and three from choriocarcinoma in Chapter 11.

Late Indirect deaths

Similarly some 71 mothers who died later in their first postnatal year died from conditions that might have been aggravated by pregnancy. These are classified as *Late Indirect* deaths and the main causes in Table 14.2 are shown. The largest categories of *Late Indirect* deaths are those due to cancer, mental illness and cardiac disease. Lessons from deaths from cardiac disease or malignancies are discussed in Chapters 9 and 11 respectively. In this triennium 18 cases of suicide were reported and are discussed in full in the chapter on psychiatric causes. There appeared to be very few cases of substandard care in the other causes of Late Indirect deaths.

Late Coincidental deaths

The cause of deaths for the 125 women who died from *Late Coincidental* causes are also listed in Table 14.2. Where appropriate, the lessons for the Enquiry from these deaths are discussed in the relevant chapters of this Report. Three women who died from suicide were judged to have had a serious underlying, long-standing mental illness which was the precipitating cause, and these deaths were not associated with pregnancy or a puerperal mental illness.

Table 14.2
Late deaths known, or notified to, the Enquiry by the Office for National Statistics (ONS);
United Kingdom: 2003-05.

Underlying condition	Chapter	Cause of death	Assessed			Not assessed	Total
			Late Direct	*Late Indirect*	*Late Coincidental*		
Central nervous system	10	Cerebral haemorrhage	0	1	7	6	**14**
		Epilepsy	0	0	3	1	**4**
Cardiac	9		0	20	14	6	**40**
Respiratory	2, 10	Asthma	0	0	4	2	**6**
		Pulmonary embolism	3	0	1	2	**6**
Gastrointestinal	10	Pancreatitis	0	0	3	0	**3**
		Liver disease	0	0	3	1	**4**
		Peritonitis	0	0	0	2	**2**
Infectious	7, 10	Pneumonia	0	0	9	9	**18**
		Meningitis	0	0	4	2	**6**
		HIV	0	2	0	1	**3**
		Sepsis	3	0	0	0	**3**
		Other	0	1	0	1	**2**
Psychiatric	12	Suicide	0	18	3	4	**25**
		Substance Abuse/ Alcohol	0	0	21	2	**23**
Unnatural causes	13, 14	Accidents	0	0	6	0	**6**
		Murder	0	0	10	1	**11**
		Road traffic accidents	0	0	6	4	**10**
Endocrine/ Diabetes	10		0	2	1	0	**3**
Cancer	11		3	27	26	13	**69**
Autoimmune	10		0	0	0	2	**2**
Other	5, 10		2	0	4	7	**13**
Total			**11**	**71**	**125**	**66**	**273**

15 Pathology

Harry Millward Sadler

Pathology: Specific recommendations

Autopsies should be performed to the standards identified in the 2005 Royal College of Pathologists' Guidelines[1]: the fundamental principle of which states that *underlying everything is the need to satisfactorily answer the issues presented by a death.*

In all maternal deaths histology should be taken unless there are positive reasons against such an action.

Known reasons for failure to meet these standards should be stated in the clinicopathological summary.

Introduction

In this triennium, 2003-05, the pathology assessor reviewed 353 case report forms. Virtually all of the report forms for the *Direct* and *Indirect* deaths were assessed: 120 out of 132 and 161 out of 163 respectively. The remaining assessed deaths were from *Coincidental* or *Late* causes.

For 102 of the 353 deaths there was either no postmortem, or the postmortem report was not available or not released by the coroner. Some of these were documented biopsy-confirmed cases of progressive malignancy where an autopsy would not have added value, in others the reports could not be released as the deaths were *sub judice*. In a few cases the coroner refused to release the autopsy report. However, in at least 17 of the assessed cases there were clinical issues that should have been addressed by a properly conducted autopsy.

The quality of the autopsy reports

As in previous Reports, the quality of the autopsy reports fall into five categories: excellent, good, adequate, poor and appalling and these groups are used again here. It must be commented that although some reports are categorised as poor because they did not sufficiently address pertinent clinical issues or differential diagnoses, they were adequate for the purposes of a coronial autopsy as they identified the ultimate cause of death. The numbers of reports in each category are shown in Table 15.1.

Table 15.1
Quality of autopsy reports assessed; United Kingdom: 2003-05.

	Excellent	Good	Adequate	Poor	Appalling	Total
	n (%)	n(%)	n(%)	n(%)	n(%)	n(%)
Direct	28 (27)	27 (26)	25 (24)	19 (18)	3 (3)	**103 (100)**
Indirect	21 (18)	46 (40)	19 (17)	25 (22)	4 (3)	**115 (100)**
Coincidental	4 (12)	10 (30)	13 (39)	6 (18)	0 (0)	**33 (100)**
Total	53 (21)	83 (33)	57 (23)	50 (20)	7 (3)	**251 (100)**

Whilst it is gratifying that the proportion of "excellent" and "good" autopsy reports is increasing, it is still disappointing that there were seven appalling reports. Although the number was higher than in the previous triennium, because the overall numbers had risen, the proportion remained similar, as Table 15.2 shows.

Table 15.2
Quality of autopsy reports of *Direct* and *Indirect* deaths assessed; United Kingdom: 1997-2005.

	Excellent	Good	Adequate 2003-05	Poor	Appalling	Total
	n (%)	n(%)	n(%)	n(%)	n(%)	n(%)
1997-99	13 *(16)*	29 *(36)*	21 *(26)*	11 *(14)*	7 *(9)*	**81 *(100)***
2000-02	28 *(21)*	44 *(32)*	40 *(29)*	21 *(15)*	3 *(2)*	**136 *(100)***
2003-05	49 *(22)*	73 *(33)*	44 *(20)*	44 *(20)*	7 *(3)*	**218 *(100)***

The most consistent failings were a lack of correlation of the clinical history with the pathological findings, and to be satisfied with just establishing the immediate cause of death. Her Majesty's Coroners are empowered to establish how, where and when a death occurred. However, coronial practice seems to vary: most seem to accept that an understanding of the processes resulting in an untimely and unexpected death is necessary but other coroners will only accept investigations adequate to establish the immediate cause of death. In this review there have been several instances where the postmortem has given a final cause of death without determining the processes leading up to death. This is unsatisfactory not only for the purposes of critical clinical review of standards of care but also because the next of kin, not unnaturally, wish to know not only the cause of death but also to understand why it occurred. There are also instances cited in this Report where the available information suggests that the stated cause of death is wrong.

The fundamental point is that maternal deaths are often complicated and an accurate, detailed autopsy is required; a poor autopsy is at best unhelpful and at worst misleading. A poor autopsy satisfies no one despite fulfilling the technical legal requirements. As high quality autopsies can be conducted under the auspices of the coroner, it is difficult to know whether poor quality autopsies are created by the restrictions placed on the pathologist by individual coroners or whether the restrictions are a convenient smoke screen for poor performance. The assessors were also concerned about some cases where there was no autopsy at all:

> *A new mother who had had an uneventful pregnancy and birth telephoned a relative complaining of a very severe headache. She deteriorated rapidly and died before she arrived in hospital. A close family relative had had a subarachnoid haemorrhage in the past and because of this, and the clinical picture, the Procurator Fiscal allowed a certificate of death from subarachnoid haemorrhage to be issued without an autopsy.*

There were many other possible causes of her death, for example this could have been a direct death from cerebral vein thrombosis. It is not uncommon for deaths from cerebral haemorrhage diagnosed on imaging not to have an autopsy so unfortunately the underlying cause is not established. There are similar examples involving other disease categories in this triennium. Particular and detailed recommendations concerning specific types of maternal death have been made in previous triennial Reports[2] and publications[3]. Though still relevant they are not repeated here unless there is a particular need for emphasis from the current review.

Direct deaths

Deaths from pulmonary embolism were still the largest category of *Direct* deaths, but in this triennium there have been apparent increases in deaths from amniotic fluid embolism and from sepsis.

Pulmonary embolus

Death from pulmonary embolus was given as the cause in twenty-three autopsy reports, of which eight were excellent or good, nine were adequate but six were poor or appalling. Again there was a common failing not to search for evidence of previous episodes of pulmonary embolus:

> *A woman who had a termination of pregnancy presented to the Emergency Department (ED) with chest pain few weeks later. She had tachycardia and was apyrexial but, despite this, she was diagnosed as having pelvic inflammatory disease. She died one week later.*

Her autopsy report was less than one side of a sheet of A4. It identified impacted emboli in the pulmonary arteries of both lungs and stated there was no evidence of embolism (sic) in the pelvic veins. There was no histology or attempt, even macroscopically, to demonstrate previous pulmonary emboli. There was also no attempt to confirm or refute the clinical diagnosis of pelvic inflammatory disease. Pregnancy was not stated in the cause of death although in the opinion of the assessors it was a contributing factor of major significance.

This case contrasts dramatically with those who had excellent reports: in one, thrombi in the internal iliac vein and tributaries were histologically confirmed as recent in some veins and organising in others. Many small pulmonary vessels were undergoing extensive recanalisation but the major pulmonary emboli were confirmed as fresh thrombi with no organisation.

Box 15.1

Pathology learning points: pulmonary embolism

At autopsy:

Predisposing causes for thromboembolism should be identified.

The source of the emboli should be stated.

Evidence for episodes of thromboembolism preceding death should be sought.

Pre-eclampsia/ eclampsia

The case reports of 16 of the 18 women who died from pre-eclampsia or eclampsia were reviewed. Eleven were associated with cerebral haemorrhage or infarction, three with the HELLP syndrome and one was an anaesthetic death. The remaining woman had pre-eclampsia but her immediate cause of death was necrotising fasciitis involving the cervix and uterus. Three women who died from cerebral haemorrhage did not have an autopsy although they were referred to the coroner. Nine of the remaining 13 reports were good or excellent and there was only one poor autopsy:

> *A non-English-speaking woman was admitted for induction of labour. On admission her blood pressure was 136/83 mm/Hg and the diastolic remained at this level through most of her labour, which lasted around ten hours. Her raised blood pressure was not treated. During the second stage of labour she had a convulsion, at which point her blood pressure had risen and she had marked proteinuria. A CT scan revealed a cerebral haemorrhage and she died in intensive care. The postmortem report identified cerebral haemorrhage but there was no clinical resume, the macroscopic description of all organs was exceedingly brief and there was no attempt to perform any histology.*

In four other cases there was a very rapid rise in blood pressure during labour, leading directly to death. The rapid escalation and/or onset of fulminating hypertension in pre-eclampsia has been noted in previous Reports. No deaths from fulminating pre-eclampsia arising between antenatal reviews occurred in this triennium, but this is a possibility that may present as a sudden community death to be investigated by a pathologist. In such instances histology may be the only evidence for the sequence of events.

Haemorrhage

Thirteen of the seventeen maternal deaths from haemorrhage have been reviewed. Two were associated with placenta previa and two with abruption. The remaining nine cases were all postpartum haemorrhage. Of these, three women had refused blood products, one was associated with postoperative infection of the cervix and uterus, and one occurred several days postpartum.

No autopsy was performed in two cases although both were referred to the coroner. One of these cases was postpartum haemorrhage of unknown cause where amniotic fluid embolus could not be excluded from the differential diagnosis. The autopsy reports were good or excellent in seven, adequate in one and poor or appalling in three cases. This failure to address the clinical issues is apparent in all the poor reports and sometimes the quality of the autopsy report is such that the diagnosis still seems in doubt:

> A known drug user concealed her pregnancy until admitted in labour. Shortly after her delivery she left hospital. Lignocaine was then found missing from the ward trolley. Three days later she was found dead and the lignocaine was found beside her.

Her postmortem took place some days after death. The autopsy report contained no clinical history. In the report her liver was described as showing acute shock due to blood loss but the features were not identified. There was no description of blood loss on the external examination of the body and no source of bleeding was identified in the report. No histology reported. Toxicology was taken but lignocaine was not assayed. Nonetheless the cause of death was given as postpartum haemorrhage.

> A non-English-speaking woman had recurrent bleeding and was known to have a cervical fibroid. Heavy bleeding occurred in her second trimester and, although her husband said he would take her to hospital, he didn't. She collapsed at home the next day and required emergency admission. At this point she was unconscious, her wrists had been hurt and were bandaged, her haemoglobin was 7g and there was intrauterine death. At hysterotomy a partially organised retroplacental clot was found. She had severe disseminated intravascular coagulation (DIC) and a CT scan showed contusions associated with small undisplaced fractures of her temporal and frontal bones. She died despite neurosurgical intervention for subdural haematoma.

In the autopsy report there was no mention of her wrist injuries, no reference to the DIC or its possible causes, and no examination of her skull. The report then identified a swollen brain with no signs of raised intracranial pressure.

Amniotic fluid embolus

Seventeen *Direct* deaths plus two *Late Direct* deaths were attributed to amniotic fluid embolism this triennium, a considerable, though not statistically significant, increase. The possible reasons for this have already been discussed in Chapter 5 - Amniotic Fluid Embolus (AFE), and include variation by chance, increased case ascertainment, less stringent diagnostic criteria and increased use of prostins. Two of the deaths were *Late* deaths with mothers surviving in intensive care for prolonged periods after the precipitating event so that the diagnosis is of necessity based on the clinical features without pathological correlation. One other death was diagnosed clinically as AFE where autopsy was not performed. There were three other deaths in which the diagnosis was also made clinically but not confirmed at autopsy, for example:

> A woman was admitted in her third trimester because of hypertension and proteinuria; labour was induced. She had a rapid delivery but was transferred to theatre because it was thought she had delivered an incomplete placenta. At this stage her observations were stable but she suddenly collapsed with very low blood pressure. She was resuscitated but arrested again and died shortly afterwards.

At autopsy there were numerous petechial haemorrhages on serosal surfaces and pallor of the renal cortex. Extensive histology demonstrated the features of severe pre-eclampsia. There were no lacerations in her genital tract and no retained products were found, neither was any evidence of amniotic fluid embolism identified within the pulmonary vessels. Despite this, death was given as an anaphylactic reaction against amniotic fluid.

In 11 of the remaining deaths there was good clinicopathological correlation. In two there was an atypical clinical presentation and amniotic fluid embolus was not suspected clinically but was demonstrated at autopsy. For example:

> *A mother presented at term in spontaneous labour with fetal distress. Arrangements were being made for an emergency caesarean section when she became unrousable. She was resuscitated and at operation there was an excess of blood in her abdomen. An exploratory laparotomy revealed a two centimetre tear on the inferior aspect of the left lobe of the liver. Despite transfusion and blood products she continued to bleed from the site, though not elsewhere, and despite transfer to a liver unit, she died.*

A thorough and detailed autopsy confirmed the liver rupture with no underlying liver pathology on histology. Cytokeratin positive squames were found in her lung capillaries on immunochemistry. The cause of death was attributed to spontaneous rupture of the liver with the amniotic fluid emboli thought to be resuscitation 'artefact' but it is also conceivable that the vigorous resuscitation caused rupture of the liver in a patient with a bleeding diathesis from amniotic fluid embolus.

These cases illustrate our poor understanding of the underlying mechanisms surrounding AFE and the consequent difficulties for making an accurate diagnosis. There is evidence that foetal squames can be found in the maternal pulmonary circulation without initiating the clinical syndrome[4] suggesting that there is either an idiosyncratic response or a threshold effect. In the majority of cases the diagnosis will be obvious both clinically and pathologically and frequently foetal squames will be visible in the maternal pulmonary circulation on routine histological stains. There are obviously cases at both ends of the clinical and pathological spectrum when very careful clinicopathological correlation is a necessity. In these situations immunocytochemistry for foetal squames is mandatory and will usually resolve the dilemma. It is possible that foetal squames are a surrogate marker for other components of amniotic fluid that trigger an immunological reaction in a susceptible individual[5]. Consequently, in situations where the clinical and pathological findings lack concordance further investigations are indicated. An immunological reaction to the foetal sialyl Tn antigen has been found and the essence of this antigen can be demonstrated by immunocytochemistry[6, 7]. In the light of our current knowledge, this would be an appropriate further investigation for such diagnostic conundrums.

Box 15.2
Pathology learning points: AFE

The diagnosis of amniotic fluid embolism needs careful and critical pathological evaluation.

Difficult cases require detailed immunocytochemical studies for fetal squames and possibly for fetal mucins.

Sepsis

Puerperal sepsis is increasing in incidence. The Health Protection Agency's enhanced surveillance of all Group A streptococcal infections in 2003 identified a total of 2085 cases with an overall mortality of 27%. Three per cent of the total cases were women with puerperal sepsis[8]. In this Report the deaths of 19 deaths women have been directly attributed to sepsis. Overall the most common predisposing factor was an association with obesity as eight of the deaths were in women with a Body Mass Index (BMI) over 30. Review of the reports suggested that there was increased difficulty in diagnosing severe infections in such women.

The most common organisms were eight cases of streptococci and six cases of coliforms, often admixed with enterococci. There were also three exotic infections by citrobacter koseri and listeria monocytogenes as well as aeromonas subrea in an HIV positive patient. Two women had predisposing immunodeficiency states, one of whom was known to be HIV positive. The other had incontinentia pigmenti, a condition associated with the NEMO gene, abnormalities of which not only give rise to incontinentia pigmenti but can also be associated with immunodeficiency states[9].

Of the eight maternal deaths associated with streptococcal infection, one was due to ascending genital tract infection by strep pneumoniae but the other cases were all from Group A. Though not directly comparable with this review, the HPA's figure for streptococcal puerperal sepsis (3%) suggests that maternal death is a relatively rare complication of the infection. Coliform infections were usually associated with premature rupture of membranes or the insertion of cervical sutures.

The reports of 20 women who allegedly died from infection have been reviewed although not all of them are counted in Chapter 7 - Sepsis. In two cases no autopsy was conducted, one of whom died from necrotising fasciitis. Of the eighteen autopsy reports, nine were good or excellent and three adequate but six were poor or appalling.

All of the good or excellent reports had undertaken careful clinicopathological correlation and investigations relevant to the clinical circumstances. In most this involved appropriate microbiology and more specifically a search for the portal of entry. This search was inconclusive in several instances but in two cases there was clear histological evidence of inflammation centred on the genital tract and with a chorio-amniitis and funisitis in the placenta and cord. One other had not only demonstrated chorioamnitis due to enterococci and coliforms but had excluded streptococcal infection by polymerase chain reaction.

A frequent feature in the poor postmortem reports was inconsistency within the report itself. For instance, in one report the heart weighed 161 gm but was described as showing left ventricular hypertrophy. The most common deficiency however was a failure to address the clinical problems. In one death from streptococcal puerperal sepsis the woman had a preceding history of a sore throat and her lungs were described as consolidated but there was no histology taken to exclude either respiratory or genital tract infection. Furthermore, a laparotomy had revealed a dusky bowel and infarcted ovary but these features were not identified at the autopsy nor was there comment on the discrepancy. In another of the six poor postmortems there is serious doubt whether death was truly due to sepsis:

> A woman with congenital heart block had routine antenatal care by her midwife and General Practitioner (GP) until late in pregnancy when pernicious anaemia was diagnosed. Only then was she referred to a cardiologist. Labour was induced but a caesarean section was performed for fetal distress. She called her GP a day or so after discharge because of vomiting and was readmitted and received intravenous antibiotics. A few days after discharge, she suddenly collapsed with dyspnoea and quickly died.

At the autopsy, performed some days after her death, there was a duodenal ulcer and the incision into the uterus was gaping although the sutures were intact. There was no description of local inflammation or peritonitis. A suggestion of retained placental tissue within the uterus and of lung basal consolidation was not confirmed by histology and no definite focus of infection was identified either macroscopically or histologically. No microbiological samples were taken. Her heart was mildly enlarged but there was no detailed examination and there was no detailed histology. Although there was a history of puerperal sepsis this had clinically responded well to antibiotics and there was no evidence of continuing infection after her final discharge from hospital. There was no definite evidence of sepsis at the autopsy and the mode of death was much more indicative of a sudden cardiac arrhythmia rather than sepsis.

> **Box 15.3**
> **Pathology learning point:** sepsis
>
> Where possible the nature and portal of entry of the infection should be identified.

Other causes of Direct death

The cases reviewed in this category include nine deaths from ectopic pregnancy, two following miscarriage, two terminations of pregnancy, four anaesthetic deaths, three deaths from choriocarcinoma and a small number of individually rare causes. Autopsy confirmed the deaths from ectopic pregnancy and miscarriage, and one probable illegal abortion was identified. In this case a perforation was found in the lateral fornix in a woman who died of septicaemia from an unusual organism.

Autopsies for the anaesthetic deaths confirmed the absence of other causes of death and in one case demonstrated haemothorax from subclavian vein perforation during central venous line insertion. One death from choriocarcinoma deserves particular mention:

> *Following an intrauterine death at term, an externally normal infant was delivered. A detailed perinatal autopsy demonstrated a massive haemoperitoneum with a tumour on the liver which was shown to be choriocarcinoma. No primary site was identified in the placenta but eight weeks after delivery the mother was admitted to hospital with a brain haemorrhage. A brain biopsy demonstrated metastatic choriocarcinoma and, despite treatment, she died.*

The results of the perinatal autopsy report had not been sent to the family or any of her health professional carers. Indeed they were not known to them until the mother had been admitted with her fatal brain haemorrhage. Given that choriocarcinoma is curable if treated in time, this long delay represents substandard care. Sadly this may be a critical reflection on the paucity of paediatric pathologists that has now developed in the United Kingdom. Failure to demonstrate a primary site for choriocarcinoma is a rare, but well documented, event[10, 11].

Other miscellaneous *Direct* deaths include one death in a woman diagnosed as having fatty liver, but who probably had Ehlers-Danlos syndrome. There was no autopsy in another *Indirect* case of Ehlers-Danlos but the diagnosis was made on the bowel following resection for mesenteric vein thrombosis.[12]

Indirect deaths

The leading overall, and *Indirect* cause of maternal death, is cardiac disease. The second most common death from *Indirect* causes is suicide. This is a reversal from the last Report.

Cardiac disease

Obesity

Forty-eight women died from heart disease during pregnancy or within six weeks of delivery in this triennium and a further thirty four *Late* deaths occurring some months after childbirth were also considered by the Enquiry. Sixty-one of these deaths have been reviewed by the pathology assessor together with six cases of non-aortic dissections. Fifty four cases had available autopsy reports of which 29 were good or excellent, 11 adequate, 11 poor and three were appalling. As discussed later, they have been broadly subclassified into ischaemic heart disease and unascertained, arterial dissections, cardiomyopathies and miscellaneous.

Obesity was present in 55% of these cases and morbid obesity was present a quarter of women who died of ischaemic heart disease/myocardial infarction. A similar picture was seen for deaths from sudden adult death syndrome (SADS). Abdominal obesity is the form of obesity most strongly associated with the metabolic syndrome with its associated increased risk of cardiovascular disease. Clinically there is increased waist circumference with raised triglycerides, total cholesterol and low concentrations of high-density lipoprotein cholesterol in the peripheral blood. Non-esterified fatty acids are also frequently raised. Raised levels of non-esterified fatty acids have also been associated with sudden death from cardiovascular disease[13]. Measurement of non-esterified fatty acids at postmortem is unreliable but a good proxy is measurement of abdominal circumference particularly in ratio to the hip circumference[14]. For women an abdominal girth greater than 88 centimetres would be a criterion helping to define the metabolic syndrome[15].

Ischaemic and unascertained

Three of the 12 women who died from ischaemic heart disease and whose cases were assessed had no postmortem. Three autopsies were poor but the other six were good or better. All these women had clinical risk factors such as smoking, obesity or diabetes. The clinical history was often suggestive in the cases of women who died from sudden adult death syndrome (SADS). One woman, who had been investigated some years earlier for episodes of collapse that had been attributed to vasovagal faints, collapsed and died whilst talking to someone. Two other cases may have been due to SADS but cannot be adequately categorised; the coroner failed to release the autopsy report in one case whilst in the other the autopsy was so bad that an attributable cause may have been missed. Of the other cases of SADS where autopsy reports were available, one was adequate and another poor but the majority were very good and had clearly excluded other potential causes. For example:

> A young girl was found dead a few months after delivery and a thorough, detailed, autopsy failed to demonstrate a cause of death. Cardiomyopathy was suspected but excluded after referral to a cardiac pathologist and so a diagnosis of SADS was made. Subsequently cardiac tissue that had been submitted for genetic studies showed a mutation which was not in the European Society of Cardiology database.

The pathogenicity in this particular case is not known and can obviously only be determined when more cases are identified. This would require more detailed investigation of cardiomyopathies and SADS. It is, however, vital that there is further screening of the family members when a young woman under the age of 40 years has an unascertainable cause of death. In one study there were cardiac abnormalities in 40% of the families associated with such deaths. The causes included electrical conduction problems, cardiomyopathies of all types and hypercholesterolaemia[16].

Arterial dissections

There were 17 deaths from arterial dissection subject to pathological review. Of these eight were in the aorta, four in the splenic artery, three in the coronary arteries and one each in the external iliac and the basilar arteries.

All of the postmortems on the aortic dissections were performed to a high standard. Two women were morbidly obese, two had Marfanoid features, the father of another had died of aortic dissection and one had three separate aortic dissections with only the third rupturing. One further woman died of pulmonary embolus: the dissection had re-entered to create a double barreled aorta. In all but one case histology revealed features such as organisation of the blood within the aortic wall indicating that the dissection had started some days prior to final rupture though the duration of the clinical symptoms had rarely been greater than 48 hours. In one report on a woman with features of Marfan's, tissues were submitted for genetic analysis but no causative mutation was found in the Fibrillin-1 gene. However this does not exclude Marfan's as these mutations are only found in 77% of patients fulfilling the Gent diagnostic criteria[17].

There was no autopsy in three of the four cases of splenic artery rupture. All three had had surgery for haemoperitoneum but the histology reports on the resected spleens were only available in two. The site of rupture was not identified nor was the histology of the splenic artery described in one report. In the other the woman had some years previously had a splenectomy and rupture was attributed to a false aneurysm of the splenic artery. Myxoid degeneration of the media localised to the splenic artery was found in the one case referred for autopsy.

In two of the three cases of coronary artery dissection referred for autopsy the postmortem was poor with no attempt to perform histology or exclude systemic or inherited disease.

The case of the woman with a basilar artery rupture deserves mention if only because deaths from cerebral haemorrhage are now diagnosed on CT imaging and rarely come to autopsy even if the underlying cause is not known. The artery was described as abnormally tortuous close to its origin from the vertebral arteries and there was a 'tear' in the wall. There was no history of hypertension or pre-eclampsia (PET).

There are lessons from the case of a woman who died from a ruptured iliac artery associated with very friable tissues at surgery. The pathologist also commented on the difficulty with reconstruction as the sutures cut through the skin very easily. The histology of various organs was normal. Whilst Ehlers-Danlos Syndrome might have been the underlying cause, no tissue was submitted for genetic analysis and consent to retain the histology was refused. Consequently there is no possibility of any retrospective diagnosis should any other family members have problems in future.

Box 15.4
Pathology learning points: cardiac disease

Obesity should be identified and supportive evidence provided.

In unascertained and sudden unexpected cardiac deaths, the clinicopathological summary should strongly advise screening of close family members.

The possibility of inheritable causes of arterial dissection and rupture should be identified in the report and where appropriate investigated.

Cardiomyopathy

One of the anomalies of the international definition of maternal deaths is that it is restricted to death in pregnancy or within 42 days postpartum yet a peripartum cardiomyopathy, by definition, can arise within five months of delivery. Of the 17 deaths reported to this Enquiry, 16 were *Late* occurring more than 42 days postpartum. Four of these *Late* deaths were due to arrythmogenic right ventricular cardiomyopathy and the remainder were dilated/peripartum cardiomyopathy. There were no examples of hypertrophic cardiomyopathy. In all 13 of these have been reviewed for this Chapter but only nine had a postmortem. There was one poor and one appalling report and of the remainder two were adequate and five good or better. In one case citalopram probably contributed to death:

> *A woman collapsed and died a few months postpartum after multiple episodes of shortness of breath that had been attributed to her known agarophobia treated with citalopram and diazepam. At autopsy she had an enlarged dilated heart with numerous heart failure cells in the lungs. Toxicology showed non-lethal citalopram levels in the blood that can be associated with death when present with other pathology[18].*

Miscellaneous cardiac conditions

A total of 13 other deaths were reviewed, from nine different causes. There was no autopsy in two cases. In the others four were excellent, four adequate and three poor or worse. The most significant cases are the two deaths in Black or Minority Ethnic women from mitral stenosis due to rheumatic fever: a diagnosis that has not featured in previous triennial reports for some time.

Psychiatric causes of death

There were 98 assessed deaths caused, or contributed to, by a psychiatric disorder; 18 were due to suicide or substance abuse during pregnancy or in the first 42 days following delivery. A further 21 women died from suicide and 16 from an overdose of street drugs later in the first postnatal year. Ten other women died from violent causes and the rest from physical disease compounded by a psychiatric history.

The deaths of 29 women who committed suicide were considered by the pathology assessor. Only seven of these women died from an overdose of a prescribed or over-the-counter medication. As in previous Reports, the method of suicide was predominantly violent. Hanging and jumping from a height were the commonest methods of suicide, but there were also self-immolations, drownings and a death on the railway track.

These violent deaths usually occur in the community and the deceased will often no longer be in contact with the NHS maternity services. Consequently the pathologist may be the prime professional providing valuable information on the clinical circumstances surrounding the death relevant to the Enquiry. This of course has to be with consent of Her Majesty's Coroner which is usually, but not always given:

> *A prisoner had a miscarriage and, at her request, returned to prison a day later. The prison midwife was unable to see her straight away because of the prison rules and procedures relating to out of hours visits. She was found hanging in her cell some days later. The coroner refused access to the postmortem report apparently considering that the Confidential Enquiry was not an appropriately interested party.*

Box 15.5

Pathology learning points: psychiatric deaths

In any violent death in a woman of child-bearing age, details of any pregnancy within the preceding year should be sought and the information included in the report.

Other *Indirect* deaths

These cover a wide spectrum of diseases but the main conditions considered in this section are cerebral haemorrhage/infarction, epilepsy, infections and endocrine/immunity disorders. The exceptional esoteric case is also identified.

Cerebral haemorrhage

Of the 17 deaths from cerebral haemorrhage reviewed only six had a postmortem. The 'view and grant' Scottish example, in which alternative clinical diagnoses were not investigated, has already been identified but is not unique:

> *An obese multigravid woman with a long history of substance abuse including heroin, cocaine and amphetamines had pre-eclampsia controlled by labetalol. A few weeks after delivery her blood pressure was recorded as 130/90 mm/Hg but the following day she had a fit. Cerebral and*

subarachnoid haemorrhage was diagnosed on CT scan and she died shortly afterwards. Despite the known connection between cocaine and cerebral haemorrhage, no autopsy was authorised by the coroner.

All six autopsies were conducted to a very high standard. In half of the cases there were antecedent causes such as hypertension, primary erythrocytosis and haemorrhage into a vascular malformation. One death occurred some days after delivery in a woman with a two day history of worsening headaches. The pathologist carefully searched for and excluded features of pre-eclampsia and reviewed the literature around pregnancy-associated cerebral haemorrhage and stroke in the absence of pre-eclampsia[19, 20]. Another unique case had a family history of death from cerebral haemorrhage in pregnancy:

A first time mother booked saying that two close female family relatives had died from a brain haemorrhage in the latter half of their pregnancies. A thrombophilia screen of unknown detail had been negative. This history seems to have been ignored and she was not referred for assessment until she was admitted in the third trimester with vomiting, weakness and loss of balance. It was thought she had a neurological problem and she was transferred to a medical ward in another hospital where a CT scan showed brain swelling. She was then transferred to the local neurological centre where the cause of the swelling remained obscure even after a brain biopsy. A cerebral haemorrhage was thought to be the most likely diagnosis and despite intensive treatment she rapidly deteriorated and died.

At autopsy a cerebral vein thrombosis (CVT) deep in the thalamostriate vein was the cause of death. The superficial venous sinuses were patent confirming the imaging findings when she was alive. The pathologist was able to review material from one of the relatives' autopsy and concluded that a deep cerebral CVT, not cerebral haemorrhage was the cause of her death. It was not possible to examine material from the other relative though her death was confirmed as 'cerebral haemorrhage' in pregnancy.

Even if this family has an undetected inherited thrombophilia, the occurrence of a deep CVT arising in late in pregnancy in two, and probably three family members and without any other clinical manifestations of a thrombotic tendency is striking. It also demonstrates that the modern imaging techniques used to diagnose cerebral haemorrhage do not provide all the answers and a good autopsy can still add diagnostic value.

Epilepsy

Ten of the women who died from epilepsy in this triennium had a postmortem; only one was poor in its macroscopic description but this and two others lacked postmortem toxicology and therefore are considered deficient. Seven deaths were classified as due to sudden unexpected death in epilepsy (SUDEP). In this condition death is usually not witnessed and may or may not occur during a seizure but is not due to a complication of the seizure such as aspiration. It is not clear whether pregnancy is a direct risk factor for SUDEP. One reason for this is that there is only limited information on drug compliance during pregnancy. Clinically antiepileptic therapy was discontinued or only intermittently taken in at least two cases but only confirmed by postmortem toxicology in one of these.

In three cases there was no postmortem toxicology and the results were not detailed for a fourth. As both the SUDEP study and the College Guidelines[1] state, toxicology is indicated in these deaths. There was no underlying morphological abnormality in the brain in ten cases but detailed neuropathological examination was only performed in two.

Infection

Three deaths from tuberculosis, all in women from the Asian subcontinent, three other deaths from meningitis and four from pneumonia were reviewed for this Chapter. None of the women who died from tuberculosis had a postmortem. Two of the three deaths from meningitis were due to the pneumococcus and the organism was not ascertained in the third death. None had an autopsy.

Two of the deaths from pneumonia were due to the pneumococcus. One woman had positive blood cultures and classical lobar pneumonia after a two week history of a 'flu-like' illness. The other autopsy was poor in attributing the lobar pneumonia and her acute mitral and aortic endocarditis to meningitis. Histology was taken but no report was included and attempts by the regional assessor to obtain the histology report and slides failed. One death was due to a staphylococcal pneumonia complicated by invasive aspergillosis following an influenza B infection and the other an atypical pneumonia.

Endocrine and immunological causes

Apart from the diabetic women who died from ischaemic heart disease there were three other diabetic deaths. In one, a woman whose chaotic life style was associated with multiple episodes of ketoacidosis was found dead in bed a few days after discharge from hospital when her blood glucose had been 16mmol/L. Her baby had been stillborn. The poor autopsy excluded unnatural causes and the cause of death was given as unascertained but glucose and ketone sampling was not undertaken.

SLE/Antiphospholipid syndrome.

There were four deaths in this category. There was no autopsy for one and good autopsies addressed the clinical issues in two of the other deaths. The final case was a woman with a mid trimester stillbirth who was admitted with difficulty in breathing and chest pain. Clinical investigations suggested a diagnosis of SLE but the postmortem simply gave the cause of death as ARDS. As the local assessors comment: *'It is obvious that the question needing an answer is whether the death was directly due to systemic lupus......
the pathology report, albeit on a severely limited autopsy is substandard and does not give any evidence of attempting to elucidate the true nature of the underlying disease leading to death.'*

Miscellaneous Indirect deaths

Included in this category are deaths from a number of other causes as shown in Chapter 10, *Indirect* deaths. Of particular note were two deaths from liver rupture and bowel infarction related to Ehlers Danlos Syndrome (EDS). The chief features of EDS IV are thin lax skin, joint hypermobility, bleeding, blood vessel rupture particularly aortic dissection, intestinal rupture and preterm labour. If suspected then tissue from skin or aorta can be analysed for decreased type III collagen or skin for the mutation in the COL3A1 gene that is found in Ehlers Danlos type IV.

In another case a woman admitted acutely ill with epigastric pain and vomiting in mid pregnancy was initially diagnosed as having acalculous cholecystitis. It was later realised that she had serious alcohol dependency and she died soon after. Clinically this was the classic picture of acute alcoholic liver disease described over 40 years ago[21] but her inadequate autopsy gave the cause of death as acute liver failure secondary to disseminated intravascular coagulation and acalculous cholecystitis. No histopathology was performed and so the probable diagnosis of acute severe steatohepatitis was missed.

Coincidental deaths

The need to assess these deaths, which now mainly comprise those from malignancy and road traffic accidents, has been questioned. However suicides were previously in this category but because of their unusual characteristics in the first year postpartum, these are now considered to be *Indirect*. The possibility that other causes may be more closely related to pregnancy than is currently thought cannot be completely discounted and therefore they are kept under review. Although the postmortems have a variety of features and causes of death, the generic theme about the lack of correlation with the clinical circumstances remains pertinent. They also provide additional and valuable information on generic aspects of maternal health such as domestic violence, ethnic discrimination and language difficulties. These features are discussed in many of the Chapters in this Report.

Acknowledgements

Earlier drafts of this Chapter were seen and commented on by Dr Robert Nairn, Dr Laurence Brown, Dr Leslie Murray and Dr Grainne McCusker.

References

1   Royal College of Pathologists, 2005, *Guidelines on Autopsy Practice- best practice scenarios.* At http://www.rcpath.org/publications

2   Lewis G, Drife J (eds) *"Why Mothers Die 1997-9 " The Fifth Report of the United Kingdom Confidential Enquiry into Maternal Deaths.* London RCOG Press 2001.

3   Millward-Sadler GH, 2003, *Pathology of maternal deaths. In: Kirkham N, Shepherd N, editors. Progress in Pathology, Vol 6, 163-85.* London, Greenwich Medical Media Ltd.

4   Clark SL, Pavlova Z, Greenspoon J, et al. 1986, *Squamous cells in the maternal pulmonary circulation.* Am J Obstet Gynecol; 154, 104-6.

5   Benson MD, Kobayashi H, Silver RK, et al. 2001, *Immunologic studies in presumed amniotic fluid embolism.* Obstet Gynecol 97(4), 510-4.

6   Kobayashi H, Hidekazu O, Hayakawa H, et al. 1997, *Histological diagnosis of amniotic fluid embolus by monoclonal antibody TKH-2 that recognises NeuAc a 2-6GalNAc epitope.* Human Pathology, 28, 428-33.

7   Oi H. Kobayashi H., Hirashima Y., et al 1998, *Serological and immunohistochemical diagnosis of amniotic fluid embolism.* Semin Thromb Hemost., 24(5), 479-84.

8   Health Protection Agency. 2004, *First year of enhanced surveillance of Group A streptococcal infections. Commun. Dis. Rep. Wkly.* 14 (16)

9   Smahi A., Courtois G., Rabia SH., et al, 2002, *The NF-KappaB signalling pathway in human diseases: from incontinentia pigmenti to ectodermal dysplasias and immune-deficiency syndromes.* Hum Mol Genet 11, 2371-5.

10 Kishkurno S., Ishida A., Takahashi Y., et al, 1997 *A case of neonatal choriocarcinoma.* American J. of Perinatal 1997, 14, 79-82.

11 Tsukamoto N, Matsumura M, Matsukuma K, et al. 1986 *Choriocarcinoma in mother and fetus.* Gynaecological Oncology, 24, 113-9.

12 Jarmulowicz M, and Philips WG, 2001, *Vascular Ehlers-Danlos syndrome undiagnosed during life.* J. Royal Society of Medicine, 94, 28-30.

13 Jouven X, Charles M-A, Desnos M & Duciemetiere. 2001, *Circulating nonesterified fatty acid level as a predictive risk factor for sudden death in the population.* Circulation, 104, 756-61.

14 Ferns G. *Personal communication.*

15 Grundy SM, Brewer, HB Jr, Cleeman JI, et al., 2004, *Definition of Metabolic Syndrome: Report of the National Heart, Lung, and Blood Institute/American Heart Association Conference on Scientific Issues Related to Definition. Circulation; 109, 433-438.*

16 Tan HL, Hofman N, van Langen IM, et al. 2005, *Sudden unexplained death: heritability and diagnostic yield of cardiological and genetic examination in surviving relatives.* Circulation, 112, 207-13.

17 Halliday DJ, Hutchinson S, Lonie L, et al, 2002, *Twelve novel FBN1 mutations in Marfan syndrome and Marfan related phenotypes test the feasibility of FBN1 mutation testing in clinical practice.* Journal Medical Genetics, 39, 589-93.

18 Jonasson B & Saldeen T. 2002, *Citalopram in fatal poisoning cases.* Forensic Science International, 2002, 126, 1-6.

19 Geocadin RG, Razumovsky AY, Wityk RJ, et al. 2002, *Intracerebral haemorrhage and postpartum vasculopathy.* J. Neurol Sci. 205, 29-34.

20 Witlin AG, Mattar F, Sibai BM. 2000, *Postpartum stroke: a twenty year experience.* Am J Obst Gyn, 183, 83-88.

21 Edmondson H A, Peters R L, Reynolds T B, Kuzma O T, 1963, *Sclerosing hyaline necrosis of the liver. A recognizable clinical syndrome.* Annals of Internal Medicine, 59, 646-73 .

16 Issues for midwives

Grace Edwards[a]

[a] This Chapter was written in collaboration with Val Beale Local Supervising Authority Midwifery Officer NHS South West, Grace Edwards Consultant Midwife Liverpool Women's NHS Foundation Trust, Alison Miller, Programme Director and Midwifery Lead, CEMACH and Jane Rogers, Consultant Midwife, Southampton University Hospital Trust.

Midwifery practice: Specific recommendations

Professional competence and accountability

National

The Nursing and Midwifery Council (NMC) should audit the content of undergraduate and ongoing postgraduate midwifery programmes to ensure all staff have up-to-date knowledge and recognition of the warning signs of immediate collapse as well as the signs and symptoms of serious medical conditions and to know when to refer women for medical opinion.

Providers of post registration education and training must ensure that all midwives have up-to-date knowledge and are able to recognise the warning signs of immediate collapse. In addition, that all staff can recognise the signs and symptoms of medical conditions and are able to provide basic management and refer women appropriately for medical opinion.

Individual

All midwives should read, and adopt, the Action checklist for midwifery practice which can be found at the end of this Chapter. In particular:

- They must ensure they are competent to practice, identify, and address gaps in their knowledge base and skills, including recognising deviations from normal and act appropriately.

- Every midwife has a responsibility to ensure that s/he is familiar with all emergency procedures and attend regular updates appropriate to their needs and local recommendations.

- If a midwife is unhappy with a medical opinion s/he has a duty to take further action, seeking support from a Supervisor of Midwives or midwifery manager if necessary.

Raising standards through audit and review

Strategic

The Strategic Health Authority (SHA) or equivalent has a responsibility to share good practice. Since it also has a responsibility for the performance management of all trusts, it should evaluate every trust's response to the recommendations of the 'Why Mothers Die'/'Saving Mothers' Lives' Report. This could be linked to the response to serious untoward incidences (SUIs) and include the Local Supervising Authority Midwifery Officer and supervisor of midwives. This should include all Primary and Acute NHS Trusts or equivalents.

Local

It should be mandatory for all Trusts to disseminate and audit the uptake of recommendations arising from all external or internal reviews, or root cause analysis of a maternal death, SUIs or 'near misses', for educational purposes for all staff.

Midwifery practice: Specific recommendations continued

Supervisors of Midwives should contribute to every internal review and should share the key points through the Trust's Supervisors of Midwives forum.

Each Trust should have a clear, mandatory, induction process for all staff, including bank and agency staff. This should include clinical protocols, emergency procedures, how to summon medical aid, the location of resuscitation trolleys/equipment and the fire procedures. This should be subject to regular audit.

Communications

Strategic

Maternity services must be commissioned as part of a locally managed maternity network, which has clear pathways of care, and standardised protocols and guidelines, including rapid and effective communication between specialities, units and health professionals.

Local

Letters regarding a woman's care should be copied to all clinicians involved in the woman's care, including midwives.

Individual

Midwives should ensure that they have effective and clear communication routes with all other partners in a woman's care.

Midwives offering midwifery led care must include the woman's GP in all communications.

Introduction

The purpose of this Chapter is to inform all midwives of the key issues and implications for midwifery practice which have arisen from this Report and that need to be addressed. These findings and recommendations are based on the detailed assessment of all the relevant maternal deaths considered by the midwifery assessors for this Report. In many of the cases in this triennium midwifery care was exemplary and showed evidence of true partnership working. However, some of the cases mentioned in this Report highlight pregnancies where midwifery led care was inappropriate.

This Chapter cannot provide an exhaustive overview of all the key findings and recommendations contained within this Report. However, although many midwives will wish to read the Report in its entirety, all should read and act on the findings and recommendations contained in this Chapter, the key overall recommendations highlighted in Chapter 1 and also in Chapter 17 - Issues for General Practitioners, as they are remarkably similar.

The role of the midwife

In order to explore the issues surrounding midwifery practice it is useful to revisit the definition of a midwife and boundaries of practice. According to the International Confederation of Midwives[1], midwives are experts in normal childbirth, but also work in collaboration with other health professionals to ensure an effective service for women who may need to be referred for more specialist care. This emphasis on the midwife as an expert in normal birth is reiterated by the Royal College of Midwives, who state:

> "The role of the midwife is to ensure that women and their babies receive the care they need throughout pregnancy, childbirth and the postnatal period. Much of this care will be provided directly by the midwife, whose expertise lies in the care of normal pregnancy, birth and the postnatal period, and the diagnostic skills to identify deviations from the normal and refer appropriately[2]".

A midwife's skill and expertise lies not only in providing expert care for healthy women but also in identifying when a medical opinion is appropriate. Since the last Report[3] was published, in 2004, there have been many examples of midwives embracing its key recommendations by providing targeted and effective care for different groups of vulnerable women and their families. These include providing accessible, holistic, midwifery care for women through Children's Centres or other local facilities which currently provide services in the 30% most disadvantaged areas of the country. In addition, there has been an increase in the number of midwives providing specialist care for particularly vulnerable women e.g. teenage girls, women experiencing domestic abuse, those seeking asylum or who misuse substances and those who have suffered female genital mutilation/cutting (FGM/FGC). Examples of these responses can be found at the end of this Chapter.

Overarching themes for midwifery practice

Maternity Matters, the recent implementation plan for the National Service Framework[4] in England, describes two clear pathways of care that women may choose:

- midwifery care in the antenatal, birth and postnatal periods for healthy women with straightforward pregnancies, or

- maternity team care for women with more complex needs.

In both pathways the midwife will play a key role either leading care or working in partnership in maternity teams with obstetric and other colleagues. Similar initiatives exist in other countries of the UK. In Scotland the Scottish NHS Boards have embraced the principles outlined in 'A Framework for Maternity Services in Scotland' and 'Report of the Expert Group on Maternity Services' (2003)[5]. These reports endorse the promotion of pregnancy and childbirth as normal life events and advocate woman centred care, with service and care provider packages tailored to need. They recommend community focussed, midwife managed care for healthy women, with multidisciplinary maternity team care for complex cases. The All Wales Normal Birth Pathway[8] is mentioned later in this Chapter as evidence of good practice.

Several key issues discussed here and elsewhere in this Report have implications for midwifery practice in either pathway. These can be divided into two main overarching themes:

- Knowledge and skills

- Communication issues.

Knowledge and skills

Midwifery led care

During this triennium there were relatively few deaths of women who had midwife only or midwife/GP only antenatal care, and for many this care was entirely appropriate. However, in a few cases it was not.

Twelve women whose deaths were classified as being directly related to pregnancy had midwifery led care, of whom three were assessed to be substandard because of poor midwifery practice. A further five women whose deaths were classified as being directly related to pregnancy had care shared between the midwife and GP yet, although care was deemed to be sub-standard in three of these deaths, there was no evidence of poor midwifery care.

Fifteen women whose deaths were classified as *Indirect* had midwife only antenatal care, and although overall care was judged to be substandard care in three cases, in only one of these cases was there evidence of substandard midwifery care. In the other two cases the substandard care occured following appropriate midwifery referral to obstetric care. There was no evidence of sub optimal care in three other women who died from *indirect* causes and who had midwife/GP only care.

Of the eleven women who died later after pregnancy of direct causes, so called *Late Direct* deaths, one woman had midwife only care and two had had midwife/GP care. Although the latter two cases were considered to have suboptimal factors, these were not midwifery related. Of the deaths from *Coincidental* causes, eight women had midwife only care, one being associated with sub optimal midwifery care. There was no substandard care for the six women who died of *Coincidental* causes and who received joint midwife/GP care.

In summary, in only five of the 36 cases of women who had midwifery led antenatal care and who died of *Direct*, *Indirect*, *Coincidental* or *Late Direct* causes was midwifery care judged to be substandard. There appear to be no cases of poor midwifery care amongst the 16 women who died and who had received joint midwifery/GP led care.

However, these few case do highlight the problem of inappropriate midwifery led care being provided for known or potentially higher risk pregnant women. The last Report[3] highlighted the need for a national guideline to help identify those women for whom midwifery led care would be suitable. It is understood that, for England and Wales, the National Institute for Health and Clinical Excellence (NICE) are in the process of preparing this as part of their forthcoming update of the clinical guideline for the routine management of healthy pregnant women[6].

Another issue concerning midwifery care revolved around a failure to recognise deviations from normal, thus failing to refer the woman for medical opinion. In these cases a number of risk factors were identified which highlighted the need for joint medical and midwifery care and, although there were clear indications requiring referral to an obstetrician or other specialist, inappropriate midwifery led care continued. For example:

> *An underweight, young non English-speaking refugee who also had a low haemoglobin (Hb) was booked for midwifery led care. Her husband, who had very poor English himself, was used as her interpreter. She was admitted later in pregnancy with bleeding and abdominal pain. Constipation was diagnosed, despite abnormal liver function tests, and she was sent home under midwifery led care. She was readmitted some weeks later, late in pregnancy with abdominal pain and, despite a further abnormal blood assay, no senior medical opinion was sought and she was again discharged. Some days following this she was admitted, in extremis, in liver and multi-organ failure, her unborn baby having died in the meantime. Despite the severity of her condition, her care was still uncoordinated and, although she was visited by a critical care senior house officer (SHO) she remained on the delivery suite. The woman died two days later of disseminated intravascular coagulation related to fatty liver of pregnancy.*

Professional accountability and competence

In the majority of cases where the woman had a new or underlying medical or psychological problem, appropriate referrals for medical opinion were made. However, in many of these cases the midwives involved then appeared to consider that they had done enough and believed the woman was no longer their responsibility. On the other hand, some midwives were worried that their concerns were being ignored by medical staff. For example:

> *An older parous woman who was obese, smoked, had a long gap since her last pregnancy and a blood pressure (BP) of 150/89 mm/Hg was booked for midwifery led care. She presented with severe headaches and vomiting near term which required opiates for relief. On admission her midwife was unhappy with the junior doctor's lack of concern but "resigned herself to the fact that he knew best". A subarachnoid haemorrhage was eventually diagnosed but she deteriorated and died a few days later.*

This case illustrates an important point raised in many other cases as well. It is important that midwives should always seek a consultant opinion, and if necessary second consultant opinion, if they have continuing concerns about a woman in their care. If a midwife is still concerned following discussion with a medical consultant, support can be sought from a supervisor of midwives and the midwifery manager. Midwives have a duty of care for women, even when the pregnancy deviates from normal. This is reiterated by the Nursing and Midwifery Council, which states:

> *"You are personally accountable for your practice. This means that you are answerable for your actions and omissions, regardless of advice or directions from another professional[7]".*

Midwifery Learning Point

If a midwife remains worried following a medical opinion, s/he should have no qualms about contacting relevant senior medical personnel directly, such as the obstetric consultant on call. The Supervisor of Midwives is available for support and advice.

Midwives are also responsible for ensuring they are competent in their own practice and should highlight any perceived training needs during their supervisory reviews. This should be recorded for future reference. In some cases there were issues around midwives failing to recognise common, non-pregnancy related medical conditions, and/or failing to appreciate the severity of others. There were a worrying number of cases where, despite obvious symptoms, basic observations such as temperature, pulse and blood pressure were not taken, or ignored. In some cases, these simple measures would have alerted the midwife to more sinister pathology. For example:

> *A woman with a family history of hypertension had a BP of 140/90 mm/Hg at term. She had a straight-forward birth but complained of a severe headache a few days after birth. Despite the continuation and severity of the headache, the midwife did not check her BP or refer her for medical opinion. The woman collapsed and died of a subarachnoid haemorrhage a few days later.*

> *Another woman was transferred home a few hours after a straight-forward birth with a transient pyrexia, tachycardia and low BP which were recorded in the hospital notes but not recorded on the discharge summary. The first community midwifery visit was two days later when the midwife did not take the woman's temperature or record her pulse rate. The midwife also failed to realise the significance of a sore throat and red area on the woman's abdomen, despite the woman saying she felt "feverish". The midwife did not plan to visit for a further four days; the woman died from septic shock in the meantime.*

A young parous woman developed diabetes which warranted control by insulin. She was referred appropriately for joint medical and obstetric care. However, her blood sugars remained erratic and the baby was macrosomic at birth. After birth, without apparent discussion, her care was presumed to be midwifery led and no monitoring of her blood sugar or urine took place. There is no evidence of discussion or planning of her care with the diabetes team for postnatal care or preconception advice and no communication with the GP. She was discharged from midwifery care but died some weeks later from multi organ failure following diabetic complications.

However, it is important to reiterate that there were also examples of sensitive, holistic, care for women who were seriously or terminally ill, as evidenced below:

A young woman was diagnosed with a brain tumour in the second trimester following a short history of severe headaches. An inter-uterine death was diagnosed shortly after and the woman died a few weeks later. Her midwifery care was excellent and the midwife was with the woman when she died. The hospice staff commented about the excellent partnership working and communication from the midwifery team.

There were a number of cases where midwives showed a lack of experience and insight into the seriousness of the mother's condition. This lack of experience and knowledge was also evident in several cases of women with complex pregnancies. There were examples of lack of provision of adequate pain relief, lack of joined up care and a lack of engagement with other professionals e.g. oncologists, the palliative care team, surgeons and physicians. In some cases it seemed that both midwives and obstetricians had not ascertained the complete picture and so had not appreciated the severity of the woman's illness. For example:

A young healthy primigravida was admitted at term with reduced fetal movements. Hypertension was noted on admission but labour was not induced for some days. During this time severe anaemia was discovered and treated by transfusion but no senior medical advice was sought. During labour the woman became pyrexial and required a caesarean section for failure to progress. Following birth she was obviously ill but her care was given to an agency midwife. Despite involvement of the specialist registrars (SPRs) in obstetrics and anaesthesia there was no immediate action for her labile BP, tachycardia and rapidly falling Hb. It does not appear her temperature was recorded in the postnatal period despite being markedly febrile antenatally. The obstetric consultant was contacted, but did not attend until she suffered a cardiac arrest from which she could not be resuscitated. A hysterectomy was attempted but she died of heart failure following prolonged haemorrhage.

This case highlights factors seen in a number of other cases i.e. a lack of baseline observations, poor midwifery care, poor communications between professionals and a failure to appreciate the seriousness of the woman's condition.

Box 16.1
Key physical signs that may suggest serious illness, and that warrant immediate medical referral

The following signs should alert all health professionals including midwives, GPs, junior doctors and obstetric and other consultants that serious illness is a possibility:

- A heart rate over 100 beats per minute (bpm)

- A systolic blood pressure over 160 mm/Hg or under 90 mm/Hg and/or a diastolic blood pressure over 80 mm/Hg

- A temperature over 38 degrees Centigrade and/or

- A respiratory rate over 21 breaths per minute. The respiratory rate is often overlooked but rates over 30 per minute are indicative of a serious problem.

There have been questions raised as to whether contemporary midwifery education adequately prepares midwives for adverse pregnancy outcomes or serious unrelated problems in pregnancy. It is impossible to comment on this issue, but a recommendation will be made to the Nursing and Midwifery Council (NMC) that these questions may be investigated.

Adopting a care pathway approach

Care pathways, within a managed and functioning maternity and neonatal care network, are good examples of how care may be co-ordinated, woman centred and clinically driven. They may provide the best evidence based approach for the management of pregnant women, particularly those whose maternities are medically and/or socially complex. They are also useful for ensuring effective communication links across disciplines and may be used to underpin many key local and national agendas simultaneously. They are not rigid documents and clinicians are free to use their own professional judgement as appropriate.

A good example of a care pathway is the all Wales Normal Birth Pathway[8] which includes telephone advice, a patient information sheet, an active labour pathway and partograms. Initial findings have shown a marked increase in normal birth, with a corresponding reduction in caesarean section with no difference in mortality or morbidity[9].

A correct emergency response

The wrong emergency response was evident in several cases. In some cases the woman was taken by the paramedics to the nearest Emergency Department (ED) despite knowing she was pregnant. In other cases the midwife did not know the emergency telephone number to summon help or the paediatric emergency team were summoned to a maternal collapse, resulting in a crucial delay in resuscitation. In one case the cardiac arrest team was unable to get into the labour ward for a significant length of time because it did not know the security code for access. On several occasions the wrong emergency trolley, trolleys missing vital equipment or trolleys in the wrong place led to a delay in resuscitation. For example:

> *A morbidly obese woman with a BMI over 40 suffered from severe asthma. Her Hb fell to less than 7 d/l in pregnancy and although she was transfused, the cause for this was not investigated and it remained very low. She was delivered by elective caesarean section with no clear indication. After birth, despite severe breathlessness and evidence of oxygen desaturation, she was transferred from the theatre to the postnatal ward where she collapsed four hours later. There was a delay in resuscitation as the emergency trolley was not kept on the postnatal ward and time was lost in locating and fetching the relevant equipment. Resuscitation, once started, was unsuccessful.*

Several important issues arise from this case. There seemed to be no medical indication for the caesarean section; indeed, given her morbid obesity, a risk assessment should have been undertaken. Following the operation although it was evident that she had complex postnatal needs she was transferred from the recovery area too quickly. There was lack of an identified care plan and there appeared to be an inappropriate skill mix and lack of experience in caring for women with medical complications.

Some cases involved agency staff who seemed to be unaware of emergency drills. Midwives have a responsibility to ensure that they are familiar with emergency procedures, but it is acknowledged that this is often difficult to ensure.

Communication issues

Whilst most midwives are autonomous practitioners of normal birth, they do need to recognise professional boundaries and refer appropriately for advice to ensure true woman centred care. This was not always the case. In several of the cases reviewed there were communications issues across the primary/ acute care interface. In some instances this was because GPs failed to give midwives information about relevant medical or social histories, e.g. serious medical conditions or substance misuse. There were several comments from midwives who had gleaned most of their information from the women themselves. This often meant that the midwives were not completely aware of the prognosis, particularly for very rare conditions. For example:

> *A woman presented with a rare pre-existing blood disorder in early pregnancy. She was cared for by a consultant haematologist with substantial input from the community midwives. However, the midwives gained all their knowledge about this condition from the woman herself and she painted a positive picture of her prognosis. The midwives were shocked to learn from another source that the woman had died some weeks after birth and they had never been included in any of the communications concerning this woman's care.*

Although there were some very good examples of partnership agency working, particularly with substance abuse and teenage pregnancy teams, there were equally as many examples of poor communications between such agencies and midwives resulting in uncoordinated care for women. True woman centred care involves working collaboratively with other professionals and not working in isolation.

Maternity Matters[5] highlights the central role for midwives within maternity services with the statement "all women will need a midwife, but some need a doctor too". However, when midwives do refer for a medical opinion they are often not included in the subsequent discussion of care that takes place between the hospital staff and the GP. Midwives should be recognised as equal partners in care and should be included in all communications.

Although in many cases there were excellent examples of internal reviews following a maternal death, this was not always the case. It was also not always evident who was involved in such reviews. In some cases it was clear the review only involved those directly associated with the woman's care and lessons may not have been widely disseminated to others in the maternity service. If lessons are to be learnt it is important that all clinical staff are aware of the findings of such reviews, particularly those who may not readily access e.g. GPs and community midwives. The Supervisor of Midwives network is an opportunity to disseminate findings to midwives.

Midwives' responsibility for vulnerable or higher risk women

The number of deaths among women who are vulnerable and/or socially excluded remains unacceptably high. These include teenagers, women who are socially excluded, non English speaking women, refugees and women seeking asylum women with mental health problems and women who misuse drugs and/or alcohol. In addition there was evidence of uncoordinated care for women with complex pregnancies, women who are seriously ill or have a terminal illness and women who are obese.

As mentioned earlier, the use of any national guidelines or local protocols, and care pathways, will help focus care on the woman and her family, promote continuity of care and reduce fragmentation.

Chapter 13 discusses the issues raised by women who were subject to domestic abuse. Although often recorded in the notes there was little evidence to show that any support had been offered. Nineteen of these women were killed by their partners. Midwives should by now be routinely asking women about domestic violence during pregnancy, but should be appropriately trained to undertake this. As a result of the recommendations in the last Report[3], The Department of Health for England has produced an excellent handbook, 'Responding to domestic abuse: a handbook for health professionals'[10], which every midwife should familiarise herself with. A short summary of key recommendations for the identification and management of domestic abuse in pregnancy are given in the Annex to Chapter 13.

Obesity

There is growing evidence that obesity in pregnancy is associated with increased risk. In this Enquiry, for 2003-05, more than a half of all the women who died from *Direct* or *Indirect* causes, for whom information was available, were either overweight or obese. More than 15% of all women who died from *Direct* or *Indirect* causes were morbidly or super morbidly obese.

A BMI of below 18.5 is underweight, between 18.5 and 24.9 is an indication of healthy weight, 25 to 29.9 is overweight, a BMI of over 30 is referred to as obese, over 35 is known as morbid obesity, and over 40 indicates extreme obesity[11].

More than half of all the women who died from *Direct* or *Indirect* causes, for whom information was available, were either overweight or obese. More than 15% of all women who died from *Direct* or *Indirect* causes were morbidly or super morbidly obese.

Seventy three per cent of women who died from cardiac disease, seventy two per cent of those who died from sepsis and sixty five per cent who died from thromboembolism were overweight or obese. Conversely only 33% of women dying of ectopic pregnancies or other early pregnancy deaths, or from anaesthesia, and 38% who died from other *Indirect* causes were overweight or obese.

For many women with obesity or, particularly, morbid obesity there was no explicit care plan for birth, neither had a risk assessment been carried out. Such severe obesity not only compromises a woman's underlying general health but also causes logistical problems. Resuscitation was delayed in one case because the ambulance services were unable to remove the woman from her house and for other women a lack of suitably sized blood pressure cuffs led to delayed diagnosis of pre-eclampsia. In other cases the physical size of the mother masked clinical symptoms or caused problems with access at operation. And, as in previous Reports, there were several cases where caesarean sections had to be done on two beds pushed together as the weight of the woman exceeded the maximum safe weight for the operating table.

It is recommended that all obese women of child bearing age be counselled about this whenever possible, and offered advice and support to reduce their weight gain prior to pregnancy.

Smoking

The 2005 Infant Feeding Survey[12] found that 33 per cent of all women in the United Kingdom smoked at some time in the year before pregnancy or during pregnancy. These included 16 per cent who smoked before pregnancy but gave up, mainly on confirmation of pregnancy and 17 per cent who smoked throughout pregnancy. This was a slight decrease from 2000 when 35 per cent smoked at some time in the year before pregnancy and 20 per cent smoked during pregnancy.

The percentage who smoked at some time in the year before pregnancy ranged from 20 per cent of women in managerial and professional occupations to 48 per cent of those in routine and manual occupations and 35 per cent of those who had never worked. Linked to this was differences by age. The percentage of women smoking before or during pregnancy ranged from 68 per cent of women aged under 20 to 21 per cent of those aged 35 or over.

A smoking history was not documented for 67 percent of the women who died which makes further analysis of the increased contribution of smoking in pregnancy to maternal mortality impossible. It also highlights the need for better awareness amongst health professionals as well as better record keeping.

Accessing care

This Report demonstrates that late booking and poor or non attendance for antenatal care are absolute risk factors for maternal death. Table 16.1 shows some of the characteristics of the women who received less than optimal care this triennium.

The Recorded Delivery[13] Report reinforces these findings and indeed those of previous Reports where it was demonstrated that women from ethnic groups, a deprived background or who are single parents were more likely to recognise their pregnancy later, access care later and consequently book later for antenatal care.

There is a real need for midwives to identify the needs of these women and target and provide care appropriately. Sadly, and despite previous recommendations, only a handful of women in this Report, who were known to be at higher risk and who had defaulted from care were actively followed up.

Table 16.1
Poor or non attenders for maternity care by risk group. *Direct* and *Indirect* deaths whose pregnancy was equal to or exceeded 12 weeks' gestation: United Kingdom; 2003-05.

Characteristic	Women who were poor or non-attenders at antenatal care		Overall number of women	
	n	(%)	n	(%)
Domestic abuse	13	(81)	16	(100)
Known to child protection services or social services	26	(81)	32	(100)
Substance misuse	21	(78)	27	(100)
Black Caribbean	4	(57)	7	(100)
Single unemployed	19	(56)	34	(100)
Both partners unemployed	14	(47)	30	(100)
Black African	12	(40)	30	(100)
No English	9	(35)	26	(100)
White	31	(17)	183	(100)
At least one partner in employment	9	(5)	165	(100)

Conclusions

Although there are lessons to be learnt for midwifery practice, particularly around failure to recognise serious illness, a failure to act appropriately and lack of communication, there is also evidence of positive and innovative responses to the recommendations made in the last Report.

Some organisations have developed partnerships with local councils and children centres to develop targeted services aimed at support vulnerable families as shown in Box 16.2 and Box 16.3.

Box 16.2

Working in partnership

In Liverpool, close partnership working with statutory agencies has led to the development of locally based comprehensive services for women including:

- Four midwifery led centres in deprived parts of the city, offering holistic care including ultrasound scans, blood tests, parenting support and specialised midwifery support

- The National Society for the Prevention of Cruelty to Children (NSPCC) has financially supported the development of two midwifery posts to offer additional support for women who suffer from domestic abuse and women who misuse substances

- The local authority has supported the development of a specialist team of midwives to offer targeted support through local children's centres for vulnerable women and their families.

For further information contact Grace Edwards (Consultant Midwife)
Liverpool Women's NHS Foundation Trust
Telephone: 0151 708 9988
This response to the recommendations of the last triennium report is evident across the UK.

Box 16.3
Partnership working: Sure Start

The midwifery team in Southampton worked in conjunction with the Sure Start programme to enable women from vulnerable groups and their families to access Sure Start services with the aim of providing easier access to midwifery services in the community. The social model provided by midwives ensures that women have continuity of care throughout pregnancy, birth and afterwards for up to six weeks. One of the primary aims was to reduce the incidence of babies born with a low birth weight.

For women cared for by these teams there was a reduction in the incidence of babies with low birth weight from 12.6% in 2003 to 7.9% in 2006. Caesarean section rates decreased from 22% to 18% in the same period; smoking rates reduced from 34% to 29% and breastfeeding rates increased from 51% to 68%.

For further information contact Jane Rogers or Suzanne Cunningham (Consultant Midwives)
Southampton University Hospitals Trust
Telephone: (023) 8079 4209

Other examples of good practice may be found in 'Modernising Maternity Care - a commissioning Toolkit for England'[14] .

In Blackburn a dedicated caseloading team of midwives is successfully targeting vulnerable women as shown in Box 16.4.

Box 16.4
Caseload midwifery for vulnerable women

Blackburn Midwifery Group Practice are a team of caseload midwives who provide one to one care for the most vulnerable families in a deprived area of East Lancashire. The referral criteria include women who are abused or who have had severe perinatal mental health problems. The midwives aim to maximise health outcomes by providing intensive support to women in the antenatal and postnatal period.

The team promote normal, positive birth outcomes and frequently work with women who have had previous traumatic births. The statistics demonstrate higher than average normal birth rates and lower use of epidural and instrumental deliveries.

For further information contact Sheena Byrom (Consultant Midwife)
East Lancashire Hospitals NHS Trust
Telephone: 01254 263555

There has never been a more optimal time for midwives to re-establish the profession as the experts in normal birth. But it is essential that practice is evidenced based, woman centred and embedded in partnership with other health professionals. Practice parameters must be clear and communication pathways effective to ensure that care for each woman is appropriate, timely and effective.

Action checklist for midwifery practice

1. Every midwife should revisit and be familiar with, the Nursing and Midwifery Council (NMC) Code of Professional Conduct and the Midwives Rules and Standards.

2. There should be a comprehensive, accessible directory relevant to local needs and available in different mediums of the other key professional contacts for the care of vulnerable and high risk women.

3. All women should receive care that is embedded in the local maternity network, ensuring that they have an individualised care pathway throughout their pregnancy.

4. Mandatory and regular training should emphasise the importance of baseline observations and include the recognition of differential diagnoses in pregnancy and the appropriate action to be taken.

5. All clinicians have a responsibility to ensure they know how to contact appropriate help in an emergency and are competent to administer emergency treatment.

6. There should be explicit emergency systems in place which should include routine checking of emergency equipment, clear siting of equipment and knowledge of appropriate emergency responses.

7. The BMI should be recorded for all women and an explicit plan of care developed for women with severe obesity, i.e. a BMI of 35 or more. These women are unsuitable for midwifery only care.

8. Key personnel e.g. GPs, supervisors of midwives and other relevant agencies should be included on local review panels. Recommendations and lessons learnt from local reviews into maternal deaths and serious untoward incidents should be widely disseminated to all staff including community staff and GPs.

9. Letters and communications involving a woman's care should be copied to all clinicians, including midwives and GPs.

10. All trusts should ensure that the emergency telephone number 2222 is universally implemented.

11. The Strategic Health Authority (SHA) should develop a clear standardised process for sharing good practice and investigating serious untoward incidents.

References

1 International Confederation of Midwives (2005) *International Definition of a Midwife.*
   http://www.internationalmidwives.org/modules

2 Royal College of Midwives. Position Paper 26. *Refocusing the Role of the Midwife RCM.* London :
   RCM: .2006.

3 Lewis G (ed). *Why Mothers Die The Sixth Report of the Confidential Enquiries into Maternal Deaths in
   the United Kingdom 2000-02.* London: RCOG Press; 2004.

4 Department of Health. *Maternity Matters. Choice, access and continuity of care in a safe service.*
   London: Department of Health; 2007.

5 A Framework for Maternity Services in Scotland (2003): *Overview Report of the Expert Group on Acute
   Maternity Services,* Scottish Executive Board.

6 National Collaborating Centre for Women's and Children's Health (2003). *Antenatal care: Routine Care
   for the Healthy Pregnant Woman.*
   Available at www.nice.org.uk

7 Nursing and Midwifery Council .*The NMC code of professional conduct:, standards for conduct,
   performance and ethics.* London: NMC; 2004.

8 All Wales Normal Birth Pathway (2007).
   http://www.wales.nhs.uk

9 Langley C. *A pathway to normal labour.* RCM Midwives Journal, Volume 10, Number 2. London:Royal
   College of Midwives:2007 .

10 Department of Health. *Responding to Domestic Abuse: a Handbook for Health Professionals.* London:
   DoH;2006.

11 Department of Health. *Definitions of Overweight and Obesity.* London: DoH; 2007. www.doh.gov.uk

12 Bolling K, Grant C, Hamlyn B, Thornton A. *Infant Feeding Survey 2005.* Leeds: The Information Centre
   for Health and Social Care, 2007.

13 Redshaw M, Rowe R, Hockley C, Brocklehurst P. *Recorded delivery: a national survey of women's
   experience of maternity care.* Oxford: National Perinatal Epidemiology Unit; 2006.

14 The National Childbirth Trust, The Royal College of Midwives, The Royal College of Obstetricians And
   Gynaecologists. *Maternity Care Working Party : Modernising Maternity Care – A commissioning toolkit
   for England.* (2nd Edition). London: NCT; 2006.

Judy Shakespeare

General Practice: Specific recommendations

Communications

- GPs should ensure they undertake a careful risk assessment during telephone consultations with, or concerning, women who are or who may be pregnant. If they are in any doubt they should see the woman or arrange an appropriate referral for her.

- Whenever possible, the GP should give the woman's named midwife confidential access to her full written and electronic records.

- GPs should ensure that any significant letters are copied into the woman's hand-held maternity record.

- Midwives should ensure that all investigations that they initiate are copied to the GP.

Making urgent referrals

- There needs to be a routine system in every maternity service by which GPs, midwives and obstetricians can communicate rapidly with one another, and seek advice, if a woman's condition gives rise to concern. This might be phone, fax or email. For this purpose conventional referral letters are inadequate and take too long. Referral management systems must not impede access to urgent appointments.

- A GP should make "fast track" referrals directly to appropriate physicians if women have serious medical conditions such as congenital cardiac disease or epilepsy at the onset of pregnancy. They should not rely only on conventional referral pathways to an obstetrician or midwive as this introduces delays that may compromise the woman's health.

Migrant women and women who do not speak English

- A medical assessment of general health before or at booking of migrant women may prevent complications or even death in later pregnancy. This should include a cardiovascular examination, performed by an appropriately trained doctor, who could be their usual GP.

- Relatives should not act as interpreters. Funding must be made available for interpreters in the community, especially in emergency or acute situations.

Obesity

- GPs should record the Body Mass Index of pregnant women and those contemplating pregnancy, and should counsel obese women before and during pregnancy regarding weight loss or healthy eating.

- Women with obesity are not suitable for GPmidwifery-led care because their pregnancies are higher risk. These women should be referred for specialist care because of possible co-morbidity.

General Practice: Specific recommendations continued

Mental health and substance misuse

- GPs should take detailed histories from pregnant women about any previous psychiatric illness and its severity, enquire directly about substance misuse or addiction and check their previous records if there is any doubt.

- GPs should communicate details of their patient's previous psychiatric history, including that of alcohol and drug misuse, not only with obstetricians but also with midwives, preferably with the woman's consent.

- A GP should refer a pregnant woman with a significant mental health history to a psychiatric service, preferably a specialist perinatal service, during pregnancy, so a management plan can be developed.

- GPs should not work beyond their level of expertise in managing drug using women. They should refer or seek advice from specialists in drug misuse.

- Women who misuse drugs and alcohol should be managed by multidisciplinary teams involving GPs, specialists in substance misuse (who may be GPs), specialist obstetricians and midwives, health visitors and social workers. Each woman must have a lead professional, and agency, to take responsibility for the overall management and coordination of her care. This would not usually be the GP.

Social services and child protection

- Close multidisciplinary and multi-agency support must continue to be provided for women who have had their baby removed into care by social services.

Introduction

Although general practitioners (GPs) have been involved in the care of pregnant women for the fifty or more years of this Report, this is the first time it has been possible for a Chapter to be written by a GP for other GPs and staff working in family practice. Although this is rather late in comparison with most other specialties who care for pregnant women, this is to be welcomed because, despite the recent changes in maternity service provision, most mothers will still have contact with their GP at some point during and after their pregnancy. It is also the first time that it has proved possible for a practising GP to be assisted to find the time to review some of the maternal deaths considered in this Report in order to distil and promulgate those general lessons which are of particular relevance to primary care.

The aim of this new Chapter is to improve the care pregnant women or new mothers receive from primary care by drawing attention to the key messages contained within the overall Report that are of relevance to GPs and to highlight the key issues that affect all other staff working in community based family practice. It cannot provide an exhaustive overview of all the key findings and recommendations in the entire Report, but GPs should be aware of the major recommendations and act on the findings in this Chapter and the overarching risk factors, and key recommendations which are highlighted in Chapter 1.

In all, 66 report forms out of the 295 *Direct* and *Indirect* maternal deaths which occurred during this triennium were assessed by the GP assessor. These were cases selected as having particular relevance for general practice. As with all the other professional groups who care for pregnant women there were many examples of exemplary care and kindness provided by GPs for some very unfortunate women and their families. However, by the nature of things, the recommendations for improving practice contained here are developed largely from those cases when opportunities for excellent care were missed. Box 17.1 summaries the major issues that have emerged in relation to general practice for 2003-05.

> **Box 17.1**
> Summary of the key issues arising from maternal deaths in relation to general practice;
> United Kingdom: 2003-05.
>
> *Clinical issues*
>
> - Identifying seriously ill women
>
> - Recognising "red flag" signs and symptoms in women who need *emergency* referral
>   - Breathlessness may be due to pulmonary embolus
>   - Severe headaches may be suggestive of hypertension or subarachnoid haemorrhage
>   - Ectopic pregnancies continue to be missed, and can mimic gastroenteritis
>   - Puerperal fever is not a disease of the past
>   - Heartburn may be ischaemic heart disease
>
> - Recognising when women need "fast track" referral for urgent conditions
>
> - Mental health problems in pregnancy and after delivery
>
> - Substance misuse and its effect on pregnancy
>
> - The health of refugee and asylum seeking pregnant women
>
> - The risks of obesity in pregnancy
>
> *Communication issues*
>
> - Telephone consultations
>
> - Referral letters and providing complete information
>
> *Maternity Services reconfiguration*
>
> - The increasing emphasis on midwifery-led care
>
> - Changes in out of hours (OOH) primary care services

Clinical issues

Identifying seriously ill women

In many of the cases and conditions mentioned in this chapter there was a consistent issue with failure to recognise the signs and symptoms of seriously ill women. This does not just apply to GPs, but to all other medical, midwifery and nursing staff alike. As a result a key recommendation of this Report is the introduction and use of a modified early warning system for hospitalised women as described in Chapter 19, on Critical Care. This is not appropriate for primary care as women are not under constant observation. However, recognising sick pregnant or recently delivered women in the community is extremely important as the speed of referral and subsequent treatment can affect both their and their babies' lives.

In contrast to hospital doctors, family doctors often have the advantage of knowing the woman's normal health and appearance. However pallor, cold extremities or looking unwell alone may not alert the "sixth sense" that something is seriously wrong. All staff, including family doctors, need to rely on abnormal clinical findings and measurements: the more a measurement deviates from normality the more the doctor should worry and act on it. In these situations a GP should arrange for a woman's emergency admission to hospital, irrespective of the possible diagnosis. Some of the key physical signs and symptoms indicating a possible life threatening physical illness, which every health professional caring for pregnant women should be able to recite in their sleep, are given in Box 17.2.

| **Box 17.2** |
| Key signs and symptoms of possible serious illness in pregnant women or recently delivered mothers. |

The following signs should alert all health professionals including midwives, GPs, junior doctors and obstetric and other consultants that serious illness is a possibility:

- A heart rate greater than 100bpm,

- A systolic blood pressure of 160 mm/Hg or above or lower than 90 mm/Hg, and /or a diastolic blood pressure of 90 mm/Hg, or more.

- A temperature greater than 38 degrees Centigrade and/or

- A respiratory rate more than 21 breaths per minute. The respiratory rate is often overlooked but rates over 30 per minute are indicative of a serious problem.

Recognising "red flags" when pregnant women need emergency hospital admission

This section highlights the key clinical issues that have emerged in reviewing many of the maternal deaths discussed in this Report where there was scope for improvement in GP management, due to of a lack of either knowledge or skills. Further and fuller details are contained within the individual chapters relating specifically to each cause of death and these are can also be readily downloaded from www.cemach.org.uk.

Breathlessness may be due to pulmonary embolus (PE)

The number of women who died from thromboembolism, particularly in early pregnancy, has increased in this triennium despite the continuing decline in those following caesarean section which have continued to fall as thromboprophylaxis becomes routine. Most of the women who died of pulmonary embolus (PE) had the well-known risk factors for PE, especially obesity, and could have been identified as being at higher risk in pregnancy. The risk factors are given in Box 17.3.

Box 17.3
Risk factors for venous thromboembolism[a] in pregnancy and the puerperium[1]

Pre-existing	New onset or transient[b]
Previous VTE	Surgical procedure in pregnancy or puerperium
Thrombophilia	*eg. evacuation of retained products of conception, postpartum sterilisation*
Congenital	
Antithrombin deficiency	Hyperemesis
Protein C deficiency	Dehydration
Protein S deficiency	Ovarian hyperstimulation syndrome
Factor V Leiden	Severe infection e.g. pyelonephritis
Prothrombin gene variant	Immobility (>4 days' bed rest)
Acquired	Pre-eclampsia
(antiphospholipid syndrome)	Excessive blood loss
	Long-haul travel[c]
Lupus anticoagulant	Prolonged labour[c]
Anticardiolipin antibodies	Midcavity instrumental delivery[c]
Age over 35 years	Immobility after delivery[c]
Obesity	
(BMI >30kg/m2 either pre-pregnancy or in early pregnancy)	
Parity >4	
Gross varicose veins	
Paraplegia	
Sickle cell disease	
Inflammatory disorders	
e.g. inflammatory bowel disease	
Some medical disorders	
e.g. nephritic syndrome, certain cardiac diseases	
Myeloproliferative disorders	
eg. essential thrombocythaemia, polycythaemia vera.	

a   Although these are all accepted as thromboembolic risk factors, there are few data to support the degree of increased risk associated with many of them.

b   These risk factors are potentially reversible and may develop at later stages in gestation than the initial risk assessment or may resolve; an ongoing individual risk assessment is important.

c   Risk factors specific to postpartum VTE only.

The following vignette is typical of a death from PE considered in this Report:

> *An obese, parous woman had a home booking carried out by a midwife early in pregnancy. A few weeks later she telephoned her GP because of breathlessness and was told to contact the practice again if it got worse. The next day her husband telephoned the practice requesting a home visit as she had become worse and was told that the doctor would attend after morning surgery. The woman died a few minutes later.*

On reviewing this case it was clear that the woman's GP had failed to take an adequately detailed history of her symptoms; this is substandard care. The GP later commented that the woman's husband did not convey a sense of urgency, but all GPs should know that sudden and continuing breathlessness in an obese pregnant woman is a medical emergency. The risks of such telephone consultations are discussed later in this Chapter. This was not the only case where a GP's judgement was open to question:

> Another multiparous woman, of normal weight, had known thrombophilia. She was managed in a joint obstetric / haematology clinic throughout her pregnancy and received dalteparin prophylaxis both during pregnancy and for six weeks postnatally. A few weeks after she stopped dalteparin she presented with an extensive deep vein thrombosis (DVT) for which she was anticoagulated with warfarin. Some weeks later she saw her GP with a cough and shortness of breath: a chest infection was diagnosed and cough medicine prescribed. She had been poor in attending for her international normalised ratio (INR) tests and admitted to forgetting to take her warfarin. On the day before her death she attended the practice nurse for a blood test: her INR result was 1.3. The next day she collapsed and died of a massive pulmonary embolus.

This woman was known to be at high risk and was already on treatment for a DVT; her GP should have noticed that her compliance with blood tests and medication was poor. A diagnosis of a chest infection in this situation should only have been made once pulmonary embolism had been excluded by hospital investigations. This woman might have survived had she been referred promptly by her GP when she attended with a cough and shortness of breath.

Box 17.4
GP learning points: pulmonary embolism

A sudden onset of breathlessness in a pregnant or postpartum woman, in the absence of a clear cause, such as asthma, should raise the suspicion of pulmonary embolus, especially if the woman has risk factors.

Women with suspected pulmonary embolus should be referred as an emergency to hospital as the diagnosis of pulmonary embolus can only be made or excluded by secondary care investigations.

Severe headaches may be suggestive of pre-eclampsia or cerebral haemorrhage

Although, fortunately, in this triennium no women died from eclampsia because their GP had failed to identify headaches or hypertension indicative of pre-eclampsia or eclampsia, this has not always been the case. Severe headaches in pregnancy can also be indicative of intracerebral bleeding. During 2003-05, 21 pregnant or recently delivered women died from intracerebral haemorrhage, 12 of which were due to subarachnoid haemorrhage, a condition for which pregnancy, and hypertension in pregnancy, are risk factors. The following is a typical case:

> After a normal pregnancy and birth, a mother developed a severe headache with new onset hypertension early in her puerperium. Her headache was not relieved by analgesics and was described as very severe. The midwife reassured the mother but she still had a very painful headache two days later: no action was taken. Her midwife had planned to review her again four days later but, before that, she was admitted to the Emergency Department (ED) with a fatal subarachnoid haemorrhage.

Although she had not been seen by a GP, it is worth emphasising that a severe new onset headache, the worst a patient has ever described, must be taken seriously. This is especially the case for pregnant or recently delivered women. Patients with fatal subarachnoid haemorrhage often have preceding warning headaches. The indications for emergency referral of women with headaches given in the learning point box below are taken from the PRECOG guidelines[2] and are included as a brief reminder of good practice. The other recommendations are taken from the findings in the relevant Chapters, 3 and 10, of this Report.

Box 17.5
GP learning points: severe headaches in or after pregnancy/ pre-eclampsia and cerebral bleeds

Women with a headache severe enough to seek medical advice or with new epigastric pain should have their blood pressure taken and urine checked for protein as a minimum.

Women with severe incapacitating headaches described as the worst they have ever had should have an emergency neurological referral for brain imaging in the absence of other signs of pre-eclampsia.

The threshold for same day referral to an obstetrician is hypertension $\geq$ 160mmHg systolic and or $\geq$ 90 mm Hg diastolic or proteinuria $\geq$1+ on dipstick. The systolic BP is as significant as the diastolic.

Automated blood pressure machines can seriously underestimate blood pressure in pre-eclampsia. Blood pressure values should be compared with those obtained by auscultation (an anaeroid sphygmomanometer is acceptable).

Ectopic pregnancies continue to be missed, and can mimic gastroenteritis

Ten women died from ectopic pregnancy; care was sub standard for seven. The two previous Reports have highlighted the lesser-known presentations of ectopic pregnancy, especially with vomiting and diarrhoea in the absence of vaginal bleeding[3, 4]. It is important that GPs are aware of the possibility of ectopic pregnancy in all women of childbearing age. Avoidable deaths continue:

> *A young woman developed abdominal pains, diarrhoea and vomiting (D&V) with one episode of fainting and a history of amenorrhoea. She had telephone contact with an out of hours GP but was not visited. The next day she had a home visit as her D&V persisted but no action was taken and the possibility of an ectopic pregnancy was not considered. The following day a relative asked for another home visit as she had been "restless" overnight, although her diarrhoea had settled. She was found dead in bed by the GP when he visited later in the day. At postmortem she had a ruptured ectopic pregnancy.*

Gastroenteritis is common in the community, but clinicians should be aware that in women of child bearing age diarrhoea should raise suspicion of an ectopic pregnancy, especially if there has been abdominal pain, amenorrhoea or episodes of fainting. The absence of vaginal bleeding does not exclude an ectopic pregnancy. Once again, this case highlights the potential perils of telephone consultations.

Box 17.6
GP learning points: ectopic pregnancy

Clinicians in primary care need to be aware of atypical clinical presentations of ectopic pregnancy and especially of the way in which it may mimic gastrointestinal disease.

Fainting in early pregnancy may indicate an ectopic pregnancy.

Puerperal fever is not a disease of the past

For many years puerperal sepsis, "childbed fever", was a leading cause of maternal death and its signs and symptoms were widely known. The advent of antibiotics means that this illness has largely disappeared from the collective memory of health professionals and patients. However, women continue to die from puerperal sepsis in this, as in previous Reports. For example:

> *A woman had early discharge from hospital after normal delivery despite having pyrexia and tachycardia. Her community midwife visited daily for a few days but failed to recognise the signs and symptoms of developing sepsis. Despite the mother's continuing pyrexia, a tachycardia of 140 bpm, abdominal pain and diarrhoea, the midwife took no action and advised that she would phone the following day and visit again in a few days time. An emergency GP was called who advised analgesia and fluids. The woman was admitted to hospital a few hours later and died rapidly from septic shock.*

In this case both the midwife and GP provided substandard care. In the early stages of sepsis symptoms can be insidious in onset and non-specific. Fever and offensive lochia are not always present; diarrhoea is common. By the time sepsis is obvious clinically, infection is already well established and clinical deterioration into widespread septicaemia, metabolic acidosis, coagulopathy and multi-organ failure is very rapid and often irreversible. The best defence against this situation is awareness of the early signs of sepsis by routine basic clinical observations for several days after delivery; these should include pulse, temperature, BP, respiration, and lochia. The diagnosis of sepsis should always be considered in recently delivered women who feel non-specifically unwell. A white cell count, urine and vaginal cultures should be taken and the woman should be treated with antibiotics proactively while awaiting the results of investigations. There should be a low threshold for emergency admission for intravenous antibiotics if a woman fails to respond to treatment or has symptoms such as abdominal pain and fever or tachycardia. Good communication is essential between hospital and community carers.

Box 17.7
GP learning points: sepsis

Puerperal infection is not a disease of the past and health professionals are still failing to recognise its classic early symptoms and signs.

Puerperal sepsis should be considered in all recently delivered women who feel unwell and have pyrexia.

Women with sepsis can deteriorate rapidly, with the potentially lethal consequences of severe sepsis and septic shock. Abdominal pain, fever and tachycardia are indications for emergency admission for intravenous antibiotics.

Heartburn may be ischaemic heart disease

Sixteen women died from ischaemic heart disease, representing a continuing rise in the number of cases. This reflects both the trend towards older motherhood as well as public health risk factors such as smoking and the rising incidence of obesity. Therefore, although cardiac disease is rare in pregnant women, GPs need to consider the possibility in women with risk factors and typical symptoms. For example:

> *A parous woman who smoked and who had a family history of ischaemic heart disease presented late in the second trimester with a history of retrosternal pain radiating to the jaw. Her GP attributed the symptoms to heartburn. She collapsed and died the next day from a myocardial infarction.*

This woman's care was substandard: she had risk factors and classical angina pain. Her GP should have arranged for an emergency cardiological referral. Although heartburn is a common symptom of pregnancy it can mask serious pathology. Radiation of retrosternal pain to the jaw is rare in heartburn and should alert clinicians to the possibility of ischaemic pain.

Recognising urgent conditions when pregnant women need "fast track" referral to secondary care

Apart from the "red flag" conditions and signs and symptoms discussed above, there were other instances when women with serious medical conditions were not referred urgently by their GP and where such a referral may have changed the outcome.

Congenital cardiac disease

More women who have had surgery for significant congenital heart disease are reaching an age when they become pregnant. Fallot's tetralogy is the commonest form of cyanotic heart disease (1:3600) and surgically repaired tetralogy of Fallot is probably the commonest condition likely to be seen in general practice. A woman and her GP may not appreciate the cardiovascular risks of pregnancy:

> *A young woman had a repair for a congenital heart condition and was under paediatric cardiac follow up every few years. She was well and asymptomatic and due for transfer to adult congenital heart disease services. When she became pregnant she saw her GP early in pregnancy and was referred to the local specialist "teenage" midwifery service. She collapsed and died in the second trimester, probably from an arrhythmia.*

In this case the GP should have referred her urgently for a cardiological opinion at the start of pregnancy. And, although it would be helpful for her to have the specialist support that a teenage pregnancy service could provide, she clearly needed more specialist medical care. Paediatric cardiologists and GPs have a responsibility to counsel their teenage patients at any opportunity about the risks of pregnancy and to seek specialist care as early as possible should the patient wish to become pregnant. They should also be proactive in discussing the need for adequate contraception. A consensus view from the 51st RCOG Study Group on heart disease and pregnancy reads:

> *"A proactive approach to preconception counselling should be started in adolescence and this should include advice on safe and effective contraception. Proper advice should be given at the appropriate age and not delayed until transfer to the adult cardiological services[5]".*

Epilepsy

Eleven women died from epilepsy; six of the deaths were from sudden unexpected death in epilepsy (SUDEP). Previous Reports have emphasised that pregnant women with epilepsy should have prompt specialist care from a consultant obstetrician and a neurologist or specialist physician with an interest in epilepsy and pregnancy. Pregnant woman should also be seen as soon as possible after such a referral is made. In this triennium there were examples where urgent referrals were either not made by GPs or not responded to by neurologists:

> *A woman with a history of epilepsy since childhood had experienced intolerable side effects from anticonvulsants so stopped treatment. When she became pregnant she did not want to try newer drugs because she was concerned about teratogenicity. She saw her GP after she had a single fit, then again at the start of her second trimester, by which time she had had a few more fits. Her GP did not refer her back to her neurologist. She was referred urgently, by letter, by the obstetric registrar. He had found out about her fits because she reported them to the radiologist undertaking her routine fetal anomaly scan. The neurology appointment was given for a month later, by which time she had already died from SUDEP.*

Epilepsy is dangerous in pregnancy because it may be more difficult to control. This may be because therapeutic drug levels decline or because women may be reluctant to take their medication. Women who stop anticonvulsant therapy in pregnancy must be made aware of the risk of SUDEP. Here the GP missed the opportunity to refer her both at the start of pregnancy and urgently when her fits started. The obstetric registrar made an appropriate referral when he saw the woman, but a phone call would have been more effective than a letter. The neurologist did not recognise the urgency of the situation and responded too slowly.

Mental health problems during pregnancy and /or after delivery

Ninety-eight pregnant women or new mothers who died within a year of delivery, from whatever cause, were affected by or died as a result of a psychiatric disorder. These include deaths from suicide and drug overdose and violent deaths from murder, accidents etc. Although many of these deaths were not directly related to pregnancy these figures highlight the impact that ongoing mental health and substance abuse problems, particularly amongst the more vulnerable, have on maternal health. This Report has been recommending for the last few years that women are routinely asked in early pregnancy about significant severe past mental health problems, and, if necessary, referred to the local perinatal psychiatric services to develop pre-emptive care and management plans. These policies have been widely adopted and it is gratifying to see that the number of women who died from suicide from a perinatal mental illness is significantly reduced in this triennium.

It needs to be more widely known that women who have had a previous episode of a serious mental illness either following childbirth or at other times, are at an increased risk of developing a postpartum onset illness even if they have been well during pregnancy and for many years previously. This risk of recurrence is estimated at least one in two for women with previous puerperal psychosis, as discussed in detail in Chapter 12. It is also known that a family history of bipolar disorder increases the risk of a woman developing puerperal psychosis following childbirth. The last two Reports[3, 4] found that over half of those women who died from suicide had a previous history of serious mental illness. Even if this history is known it may be communicated poorly to other members of the team,

> *A young woman with existing children killed herself by violent means some weeks after the birth of her next child. She had a previous history of bipolar disorder with a number of hospital admissions for mania. She was last seen by psychiatric services shortly before the beginning of pregnancy and stopped her mood stabiliser medication at about this time. Her GP had mentioned her previous psychiatric history in his referral letter to the obstetrician, but the midwife was unaware of this history at the booking clinic. The woman was well during pregnancy, but no steps were taken to monitor her mental health following delivery.*

This woman faced a risk of recurrence of at least 50% in the first three months after delivery. Her psychiatric team should have made the woman, her family and her GP aware of this. When she became pregnant again her GP should have told her midwife and should have referred her back to the psychiatric team so that a management plan could have been put into place. She should have restarted her medication after delivery and been kept under close psychiatric supervision. If these interventions had been made, her death might have been avoided.

In other situations a pattern of escalating self harm may develop prior to suicide. Health professionals may be slow in offering interventions, they may not appear to take women's threats seriously or hospital based services may be inaccessible for a woman who is distressed:

> *A single mother with a number of children had a history of self harm and alcohol abuse. She had a miscarriage following which she repeatedly attended the Emergency Department (ED) with overdoses, alcohol intoxication and deliberate self harm. Her GP had received calls from her family expressing concern about her state. The severity of her self-harm escalated before her death, some months after her miscarriage. Shortly before she died her children were put on the child protection register after a case conference. Family members were so concerned about her that they rang the GP and he arranged for a psychiatric review the next day. She failed to attend and killed herself some days later. A subsequent psychiatric report said she found it difficult to engage with services, "maybe because of associated alcohol problems".*

Her care was substandard because the GP failed to recognise and act on her escalating self-harm despite concerns expressed by family and multiple attendances at hospital. This case is complicated by her dual diagnosis of psychiatric illness and alcohol misuse. The GP did not appear to involve other members of the team such as the health visitor. Whilst this may have made no difference to the outcome there was a sense from the case report that everyone thought she was a "hopeless" case in any event.

Another woman had poor care:

> *A vulnerable woman had a family history of suicide, was the victim of domestic abuse and found it hard to engage with services. Antenatally she only saw her midwife because she insisted on home visits. The community mental health team (CMHT) closed her case because she did not attend appointments. Her GP saw her once after delivery, made a diagnosis of postnatal depression and prescribed citalopram but did not arrange any follow up. The health visitor carried the burden of care, appeared to be working in isolation and was unsupported. The woman killed herself some weeks later.*

Here the CMHT did not recognise that the woman's failure to attend appointments might mean that she was so depressed that she was unable to leave the house. Failure to attend should be a "red flag" of severity requiring prompt outreach care rather than discharge. It is also possible that a specialist perinatal team may have managed this woman more actively. Her GP failed to recognise the severity of her depression when he saw her postnatally and failed to arrange follow up after starting antidepressants for her depression. Her health visitor was unsupported. Better team work may have built a support network around this woman and allowed her to access appropriate care that may have prevented her death.

Substance misuse and pregnancy

Around 11% of all the women whose deaths were assessed during this triennium, from any cause, had problems with substance misuse. They did not all die from the drug misuse itself, but also from associated physical problems and from accidents and murder. These women are vulnerable because they often have complex and chaotic social lives; they often suffer domestic abuse, are hard to engage in antenatal care and usually fail to develop trusting relationships with health professionals. There was also much evidence of good relationships and excellent care by GPs. However, there were also instances of GPs apparently working beyond their level of expertise which may have contributed to the outcome:

A young single parent with a history of polydrug misuse and psychiatric problems attended infrequently during her pregnancy but claimed to have stopped all her drugs by the third trimester. Although her baby was delivered prematurely and admitted to special care, the mother discharged herself immediately after the delivery. The GP then supervised her postnatal methadone prescribing, unsupported by a specialist in substance abuse. The administration of methadone was not supervised by the pharmacist. She died from a methadone overdose some weeks after delivery, shortly after a case conference at which the baby was placed on the "at risk" register.

This GP was working beyond his/her level of expertise and should have referred her to a specialist drug team. It may be that the woman refused such care, but their advice should have been sought at the very least. She may have left hospital immediately after delivery to re-establish her drug supply. Lack of supervised consumption postnatally may have contributed to an unreliable supply of opiates and diversion to the black market. In this case the involvement of social services may also have been a factor in her death and this risk factor for suicide is discussed in more detail in Chapter 12.

Box 17.9
GP Learning points: mental health and substance misuse

NICE have recently produced guidance on the management of antenatal and postnatal mental health and all GPs should be encouraged to read, and follow them[6].

It may be safer for women who misuse drugs to continue their maintenance treatment during and after pregnancy to prevent inadvertent overdose from street drugs.

Pregnant drug users may be difficult to engage in treatment. This may be because they do not recognise pregnancy, have chaotic lifestyles or have fears about the consequences of social services involvement.

Pregnancy in refugees and asylum seekers

Women who have recently arrived from countries around the world, particularly those from Africa and the Indian sub-continent, but increasingly from central Europe, tend to have poorer overall general health and are at risk from illnesses that have largely disappeared from the UK, such as TB and rheumatic heart disease. They are also more likely to be at risk of HIV infection. Some may also have suffered female genital mutilation/cutting (FGM/FGC). All of these conditions, alone or in combination, contributed to a number of the maternal deaths considered in this Report. If newly arrived women are unwell, GPs may need to consider unfamiliar possibilities in their differential diagnoses.

Rheumatic heart disease

No pregnant women have died from the consequences of rheumatic heart disease since the 1991-1993 Enquiry[7]. However, in this current triennium, two immigrant women died from mitral stenosis as a result of rheumatic heart disease. Rheumatic heart disease is likely to become even more common with increasing numbers of women who are asylum seekers or refugees, who may never have had a cardiac assessment[8].

A previously well young immigrant woman with poor English booked for midwifery-led antenatal care and was seen only by her midwife and GP. Her GP did not examine her heart. She was admitted to an ED at the end of her second trimester with cough, breathlessness and chest pain. Even though she was admitted, the diagnosis of mitral stenosis was not considered until she was moribund.

If she had been examined by her GP the murmur of mitral stenosis may have been picked up. It can be hard to hear the soft diastolic murmur of mitral stenosis if a woman is already sick and has a tachycardia.

Women with mitral stenosis may seem well in early pregnancy but they commonly decompensate at the end of the second trimester. Referring women with unexplained murmurs to a cardiologist early in pregnancy would enable earlier diagnosis of rheumatic heart disease and catastrophic deterioration may be prevented with proper assessment, monitoring and intervention.

Tuberculosis

Two cases of tuberculous meningitis in pregnancy were diagnosed late, as often happens, and both occurred in women whose families were from the Asian sub-continent. In one case the diagnosis was delayed as the husband was acting as the interpreter, a recurrent feature amongst other deaths in women who could not speak English. In one case her GP commented that this was a particular problem in his practice because there was no agreed source of funding for interpreters.

Box 17.10

GP learning points: refugees and asylum seekers

Newly arrived women, especially refugees and asylum seekers, are at higher risk of illnesses that are no longer familiar in the UK and this needs to be born in mind when caring for sick women from these communities.

A medical assessment of general health before booking of immigrant women may prevent death later in pregnancy. This should include a cardiovascular examination, performed by an appropriately trained doctor, who could be their usual GP.

The risks of obesity in pregnancy

Obesity represents one of the greatest and growing overall threats to the childbearing population of the UK. Fifteen percent of women who died from *Direct* or *Indirect* causes and who had a BMI recorded had BMIs of 35 or over, with half of these having BMIs exceeding 40. A further 12% of women had BMIs in the range 30-34 and and 24% had BMIs of 25-29. Obese women predominated among those who died from thromboembolism, sepsis and cardiac disease. There are many other aspects of the care of overweight women in pregnancy that cause concern beyond maternal risks, including the difficulties of prenatal diagnosis, the enhanced risk of gestational diabetes, the increased chance of caesarean section, and the challenges of analgesia and anaesthesia. The risks of obesity are discussed in more detail in Chapter 1.

Communications

Problems in communication are at the heart of many of the cases discussed in this Report and this Chapter has already raised issues about communication with patients, within the primary health care team and between GPs, midwives and specialists.

Telephone consultations

Telephone consultations are increasingly being used in medical contacts, including the triage of acute illnesses. They are acceptable to patients, and clinicians also value them but have anxieties about missing serious conditions[9]. There are cases described in this Report, and earlier in this Chapter, which underline this concern. The case of a woman who died from pulmonary embolus, described earlier, is an example where the quality of telephone assessment was poor and may have contributed to her death. There is evidence that telephone consultations are shorter than face-to-face consultations[10] but there is little evidence about the quality of care. Telephone consultations require an additional range of skills since the importance of verbal cues and focussed history-taking need to compensate for the inability to examine the patient. The BMA recommends that:

> "consulting over the telephone should normally be modified to allow the patient greater time to explain their problem. The doctor should also take a detailed history and seek the answers to all the relevant direct questions. There should be a summation and agreement with the caller/patient as to what exactly the problem is that the doctor is attempting to solve. The doctor should explain their assessment and detail the action s/he intends to take. If it is not possible to safely manage the patient over the telephone, the doctor should arrange a face to face consultation and make an appropriate referral[11]."

Doctors may need specific training in telephone consultations, an area that is currently neglected in the training and professional development of GPs[12].

Referral letters; providing complete information

General practitioners are the only professionals who have access to a woman's complete medical history and as such are the only health professionals able to provide a complete medical, psychiatric and social history. It is therefore crucial that all relevant information is included in referral letters to enable appropriate and planned care. These Reports have regularly highlighted examples of where inadequate information in referral letters led to adverse consequences for pregnant women and this triennium is no exception. A GP has a responsibility to ensure that any relevant history is conveyed in as much detail as possible to the midwife and/or obstetric team who will be caring for the woman during pregnancy.

Strategic changes in delivery of care

Increasing midwifery-led care

There have been several changes in service delivery over the period of the Enquiry which provide challenges in caring for pregnant women. The recent implementation strategy for the National Service Framework for Maternity Services[13], "Maternity Matters"[14] in England will result in all low risk women being offered a choice of midwifery-led care before, during and after childbirth. The lack of financial incentive for GP involvement in obstetric care under the 2004 GP contract has also led to many GPs becoming more distanced and less involved in maternity care. Maternity care has traditionally been a valued part of a GP's work, so they have often been unhappy about this change. For the period of this Enquiry only 3% of the women who died were reported to be receiving care "shared between midwife and GP" and this direction looks set to continue. This therefore raises some crucial issues for GPs and midwives in providing maternity care.

Booking low-risk women

One challenge is how a woman can be judged to be "low risk" at booking. Following a firm recommendation in the last Report about this, the National Institute for Clinical Excellence is preparing generic consensus guidance on this, which is due to be published in early 2008[15]. There may be medical, mental health or other problems that a woman may not appreciate, whose importance she does not understand, or that she fails to disclose. The GP is the only professional who has access to a woman's complete medical history. In addition a GP has particular skills in understanding and managing risk, handling uncertainty and recognising the early stages of disease. In order to undertake a proper risk assessment midwives need access to the electronic and paper GP record. If this is not possible GPs should be willing to give a copy of the medical summary to either the woman or the midwife and to discuss any issues that may be of significance in the pregnancy. It would be good practice for the GP and midwife to explain the reason for this in their discussions with the woman.

Woman-held records

Most maternity trusts enable women carry their own maternity records. It is important that all the correspondence relating to any woman's pregnancy should be available to every professional who is caring for her, particularly if the pregnancy is higher risk. It is now common practice for GPs to scan any correspondence into their records but they should ensure that any relevant scanned letters are also available in the hand-held record. Likewise, it would be good practice for specialists to send a copy of any letters to the woman and her midwife for inclusion in the patient-held record.

Communication of abnormal results

Midwifery-led care may mean that the results of investigations performed by midwives are not automatically reviewed by the GP:

> *A young refugee woman who had just arrived in the UK had a blood count that showed a pancytopenia which her GP thought was "cultural". She soon became pregnant, was booked and had bloods taken by the community midwife. The GP states that he never received copies of the antenatal results. At the end of her first trimester the woman developed an upper respiratory tract infection and was treated with amoxicillin. A few days later she was referred to the ED and admitted with a history of haemoptysis, fever and general aches and pains. She was found to have acute myeloid leukaemia and she died of overwhelming infection a few days later.*

If her GP had realised the significance of the initial abnormal result, or had received a copy of the antenatal results, he might have been able to refer this women earlier so that she did not develop a life threatening infection. With the shift to midwifery-led care it is important that the GP's name is automatically put on all bloods taken by the midwife.

Out of hours (OOH) care

There have been major changes in out of hours (OOH) care since the introduction of the new GP contract in 2004 when most registered GPs relinquished 24-hour responsibility for their patients. There are some indications that this could have consequences for the quality of maternity care. One problem may be communication with the woman's usual GP practice:

> *A woman in early pregnancy, with no past medical history, called an OOH doctor with a history of breathlessness, anorexia and vomiting. She also had a two-week history of pain in her left leg. She was reassured during the telephone consultation but collapsed and died of a pulmonary embolus a few days later. Her usual GP had received no record of this contact with the patient from the OOH service.*

The emergency GP should have considered the diagnosis of pulmonary embolus with the history obtained and the OOH organisation failed to pass information about the contact to her usual GP. This meant her usual GP had no opportunity to reconsider the diagnosis the next day.

Changes to OOH services also mean that patients may delay contacting a GP until they know their usual GP is available. This is a particular worry over weekends or Bank Holidays, when reassessment by the usual GP is impossible. The usual GP needs to ensure that s/he anticipates potential problems before long weekends:

A young pregnant woman who could not speak English was seen just before a Bank Holiday with bronchopneumonia and treated with antibiotics. Her GP thought he had "safety netted" by telling her husband to take her to the ED over the weekend if her condition worsened. The husband did not contact the OOH service and she was not seen again until four days later when she was seriously ill and admitted to hospital. She died shortly afterwards of fulminating pulmonary TB.

In this case the GP care was substandard; her usual GP, who saw her before a Bank Holiday failed to recognise how ill she was. He should have admitted her to hospital directly if early reassessment was impossible or communicated his worries about the patient directly to the OOH services. It is inappropriate to expect sick patients or their relatives to do this.

Box 17.11
GP learning points: out of hours (OOH) care

OOH services and usual GPs need to be able to communicate with each other rapidly and effectively, preferably electronically or by fax.

OOH services and usual GPs need to maintain records of all contacts with patients both within and between each service.

Conclusions

It is ironic that this Chapter, the first to be written specifically for GPs, comes at a time when GPs are no longer the main providers of antenatal care for women with low risk pregnancies. Nevertheless the contributions that they can make are still very significant: GPs are "experts" in managing uncertainty, the early presentation of illness and in managing and minimising risk. There is a risk that changes in midwifery care will lead to GPs becoming de-skilled, although they will still be the first to be involved if the family or midwife suspect something may be wrong. This role needs to be recognised and encouraged. They need to maintain their skills and professional development to be able to provide excellent care for all pregnant or recently delivered women, including those at higher risk or in emergency situations.

Even if they are no longer the lead carer, GPs still have a duty of care for pregnant women and should be interested in their health and well-being as they will be caring for these women, and their families, for many years to come. GPs should therefore not only make sure that the midwives or specialists caring for their pregnant women are as fully informed as possible of any past or current medical, psychological or social problems, but should also give them access to her complete case notes on request.

It is hoped that the learning points and recommendations in this Chapter will help to maintain and improve the care that GPs can provide.

References

1 RCOG. *Thromboprophylaxis during pregnancy, labour and after vaginal delivery.* Guideline No 37. London: RCOG; 2004. www.rcog.org.uk/resources/Public/pdf/Thromboprophylaxis_no037.pdf

2 APEC. *Pre-eclampsia community guideline (PRECOG guideline);* London: APEC; 2004. www.apec.org.uk/pdf/guidelinepublishedvers04.pdf

3 Lewis G (ed). *Why Mothers Die. The Sixth Report of the Confidential Enquiries into Maternal Deaths in the United Kingdom, 2000-02.* The Confidential Enquiries into Maternal and Child Health. London: RCOG press; 2004.

4 Lewis G (ed). *Why Mothers Die. The Fifth Report of the Confidential Enquiries into Maternal Deaths in the United Kingdom, 1997-99.* The National Institute of Clinical Excellence. London: RCOG Press; 2001.

5 Steer PJ, Gatzoulis MA, Baker P (eds). *Heart Disease and Pregnancy.* London: RCOG Press; 2006.

6 NICE. Antenatal and postnatal mental health. *Clinical management and service guidance. National Institute for Clinical Excellence. Clinical Guideline 45.* London: NICE; 2007. http://guidance.nice.org.uk/CG45/niceguidance/pdf/English

7 Department of Health, *Welsh Office, Scottish Home and Health Department, Department of Health and Social Services, Northern Ireland.* Report on the Confidential Enquiries into Maternal Deaths in the United Kingdom, 1991-93. London: HMSO; 1996.

8 Tan J, de Swiet M. *Prevalence of heart disease diagnosed de novo in pregnancy in a West London population.* Br J Obstet Gynaecol. 1998; 105: 1185-8.

9 Car J, and Sheikh A. *Information in practice: Telephone consultations.* BMJ, 2003, 326: 966-969.

10 McKinstry B and Sheihk A. *Unresolved questions in telephone consultations.* J R Soc Med 2006: 99; 2-3.

11 BMA. *Consulting in the modern world.* London: BMA; 2001. www.bma.org.uk

12 Car et al. *Improving quality and safety of telephone based delivery of care: teaching telephone consultation skills.* Qual Saf Health Care 2004; 13: 2-3.

13 Department of Health. Standard 11. *National Service Framework for Children, Young People and Maternity Services:* London: Department of Health; 2004.

14 Shribman S. *Making it better for mother and baby. The clinical case for change.* London: Department of Health; 2007.

15 National Institute for Clinical Excellence. *Antenatal care: Routine care for the healthy pregnant woman.* London: National Institute for Clinical Excellence; 2003. www.nice.org.uk

18 Emergency Medicine

Diana Hulbert

Specific recommendations for the management of pregnant women attending Emergency Departments (ED)

All ED clinicians must, at the start of their post and at regular intervals thereafter, have regular training in the identification and management of:

- The sick pregnant and postpartum woman

- Ectopic pregnancy, including the need to be aware of its atypical clinical presentations and especially the way in which it may mimic gastrointestinal disease.

Pregnant women with the following, otherwise unexplained, signs must be reviewed by an experienced doctor from the obstetric gynaecology team. If not available on site then arrangements should be made with the local maternity unit to discuss cases of:

- Abdominal pain

- Severe headache

- Hypertension

- Proteinuria

- Breathlessness

- Pyrexia

- Chest pain.

Pregnancy testing should be routine for all women of child-bearing age with a potentially pregnancy-related condition.

The woman's GP and midwife or obstetrician must be informed of the reasons for, and outcome of, every pregnant woman's visit to an ED.

The care of pregnant women with medical conditions requiring treatment, and particularly hospital admission, should be discussed and planned in conjunction with the local obstetric team.

Perimortem caesarean section should only be carried out when a maternal cardiac arrest has been witnessed within the previous five minutes; the outcomes of any other circumstances are universally poor. In addition the baby must be delivered within five minutes of the procedure being started to facilitate resuscitation.

Individual obstetric units should develop protocols for the management of pregnant women who are acutely ill / collapsed for non-obstetric reasons. This must involve liaison with emergency services and EDs regarding the most appropriate site (ED, local labour suite or another hospital) to ensure women receive speedy resuscitation.

Introduction

For the first time in the more than 50-year history of these Reports a summary chapter has been written specifically for Emergency Department (ED) practitioners. It is also the first time that a consultant in emergency medicine has reviewed the relevant maternal deaths to distil lessons and recommendations of particular relevance to staff working in emergency medicine services. Issues concerning the care provided for pregnant women in the ED have been highlighted in earlier Reports and this chapter endorses and strengthens these previous recommendations.

The aim of this new chapter is to draw attention to key messages in the Report of relevance to the emergency services and to highlight issues relating to pregnant or recently delivered women that particularly affect ED clinicians and other staff working in emergency medicine. It cannot provide an exhaustive overview of all the Report's findings but ED staff should be aware of the key recommendations and overarching risk factors highlighted in Chapter 1 as well as acting on the findings in this Chapter.

Emergency services

Emergency services in the UK are provided in the community by general practice and the ambulance services, in minor injuries units and in Emergency Departments (EDs). Minor injuries units are usually staffed by nurse practitioners working autonomously but some are also managed by local GPs or secondary care doctors. Some of these units are overseen by consultants in emergency medicine, but usually in a managerial rather than a clinical role. There are clear criteria and guidelines for the referral from minor injuries units to the local ED for any patient whose condition causes concern. Some have specific guidelines for pregnant women, but this is not universal.

In the ED various methods and levels of assessment are available for all patients depending on the severity of their presenting complaint. A patient can be seen entirely within the ED and discharged home, admitted to a short stay ward (also called a clinical decision unit or observation ward) for a period of observation and to await the outcome of specific tests or referred to an inpatient specialty team, usually for admission. In most EDs, pregnant women who need admission will be referred to a gynaecology ward up to a specified number of weeks of gestation and to the labour ward thereafter.

Occasionally a woman may be referred directly by her GP or midwife to an on-call team, usually the obstetric team but sometimes, as happened in one of the cases in this Report, to the on-call medical team. Most women who have been directly referred will not be seen in the ED but will be taken straight to the designated medical admissions centre to be seen by the on-call physicians. This centre may be called the Acute Medical Unit, the Emergency Medical Unit, the Acute Admissions Unit or the Medical Admissions Unit. For example:

> A new, older, mother was admitted to an acute admissions unit by her GP with breathlessness, pyrexia and hypotension two or three weeks after a normal delivery. A differential diagnosis of pneumonia or pulmonary embolism was made but a very few hours after admission she was transferred to a gynaecology ward where she later arrested and died. Autopsy showed a pulmonary embolism.

This mother was clearly very unwell and should have been managed in a high dependency area. It is possible that being pregnant or postpartum can cloud the issues for clinicians but it is important that a patient is treated in an environment appropriate to their medical status.

Pregnant women referred directly to the gynaecology or obstetrics team will generally be seen in a gynaecology admissions unit, an Early Pregnancy Unit, the triage area on the labour ward or on a general ward. This will depend on the round-the-clock availability of such facilities as well as the woman's gestation, presenting problem and apparent severity of the illness. Some women may be seen by the specialist teams within the confines of the ED but not by emergency medicine clinicians themselves. This was the case for a small number of the women whose cases were reviewed for this Report.

Summary of key findings for 2003-05

Of the women whose cases were assessed in relation to ED practice, the main diagnoses were:

- pulmonary embolism
- ectopic pregnancy
- intracerebral bleed
- sepsis
- road traffic accidents.

Fifty-two women who died from *Direct*, *Indirect* or *Coincidental* causes died in the ED. The majority of these women had either collapsed in the community and were already undergoing cardio-pulmonary resuscitation (CPR) on arrival or collapsed shortly afterwards.

Emergency care before arrival at the ED

The emergency services' response to a 999 call about a sick pregnant woman will usually consist of an ambulance staffed by a paramedic and an ambulance technician. Untrained personnel are not permitted to work in ambulances; the minimum training for an ambulance technician is equivalent to that of a nursing auxiliary. Additionally, in some areas, there may be a rapid response vehicle which allows early interventions to be carried out if this vehicle arrives first. These are staffed by paramedics usually in a car. In addition there are emergency care practitioners (usually with an ED nursing background) whose role is to manage the patient at home according to protocols. Regardless of type of vehicle, most paramedic crews act within very specific guidelines in terms of their resuscitation algorithms. Nevertheless, unanticipated problems can still occur:

> *A woman being transported to the hospital with severe abdominal pain was given nalbuphine en route for pain relief. This is an opioid which has become less commonly used with the advent of morphine into paramedic protocols. She had a profound anaphylactic reaction resulting in cardiorespiratory arrest and eventual death.*

In some areas a doctor will attend the patient in the community at the request of the paramedics. These doctors have undergone pre-hospital training (i.e. they are trained to manage sick patients outside a hospital environment) and most are GPs, ED doctors or anaesthetists. They provide a different set of skills for the patient out of hospital and a proportion of these patients are pregnant or peripartum women.

Women in extremis on admission

Fifty-two (18%) of women who died from *Direct* or *Indirect* maternal causes this triennium died in the ED, most of whom were brought in already undergoing cardio-pulmonary resuscitation (CPR). Several others were initially resuscitated and then moved to critical care. Overall, the level of care and the resuscitation measures were of a good or excellent standard with adherence to protocols. Even when the outcome is poor there can be a sense of satisfaction that these well researched guidelines are followed effectively.

Perimortem caesarean section

Thirteen of the women who died in the ED were delivered by perimortem caesarean section. A number of other women had a perimortem section in the ED but survived long enough to be transferred to Critical Care. Two of the women who had the operation performed in the ED, and who died there were only 20-22 weeks pregnant and only six women were more than 34 weeks of gestation. The median gestational age was 30 weeks. The only baby who survived was born to a mother at term who suffered a cardiac arrest after admission and for whom the operation could be performed within the recommended five minutes of collapse[1]. None of the babies of the women who were admitted already undergoing active CPR survived.

The total number of perimortem caesarean sections performed for all mothers this triennium, 52, has almost doubled since the last Report, where only 27 cases were assessed. In this Report twenty babies survived, including one set of twins, but their chances of survival were greatly improved with advanced gestational age. These findings indicate that with improved resuscitation techniques more babies are surviving perimortem caesarean sections particularly where the women collapsed in an already well-staffed and equipped delivery room or operating theatre. However they also highlight the very poor outcome for babies delivered in Emergency Departments, especially on women who arrive after having undergone CPR for a considerable length of time.

These findings underscore the guidelines from the Managing Obstetric Emergencies and Trauma course (MOET)[1] which make it clear that perimortem caesarean section should only be carried out when the mothers cardiac arrest has been witnessed within the previous five minutes. The outcome of any other circumstance is universally poor. In addition the baby must be delivered within five minutes to facilitate resuscitation.

The care the mothers received

A large number of women who died in 2003–2005 came into contact with emergency services including paramedics and on-call physicians in addition to those working in the ED. In the cases in which ED treatment has been implicated in the death, there are three clear themes for lessons to be learned:

- clinical practice
- education and training, and
- service provision.

Clinical practice

Recognition of the sick woman

One of the core skills of being a clinician is the recognition of a patient who is unwell. This is not the same as making a diagnosis. In fact the two skills are often independent of each other. Recognition of the seriously ill woman relies on taking a complete history (listening to the cues given by her or her relatives), measurement and understanding of vital signs such as heart rate, respiratory rate and pulse oximetry. It is not dependent on complex and time-consuming tests. Recognition of illness needs to be taught to clinicians of all grades on a regular basis. It is also important to make this teaching multi-disciplinary.

Scoring systems such as the modified early obstetric warning system (MEOWS) described in Chapter 19 - Critical care, and included as one of the overarching recommendations of this Report, can be used to elucidate the level of "unwellness". Essentially this adds together a score for heart rate, respiratory rate, blood pressure, GCS and temperature and gives an overall score. However early warning systems are only useful if they are regularly repeated and acted upon.

Shortness of breath and the diagnosis of pulmonary embolism

Pulmonary embolism (PE) continues to be a difficult diagnosis which is often made too late. Whilst some of the women who died from PE could not have been saved no matter when the diagnosis was made, a small number went unrecognised, mainly because PE was not considered early enough. The diagnosis of PE is already challenging in the non-pregnant patient but in pregnancy it becomes even more difficult. Of those women who died from a potentially salvageable PE many had felt breathless prior to admission. Traditional teaching allows clinicians to assume that isolated breathlessness is a normal feature of pregnancy and this can often reduce the awareness of its severity. It is unusual to be breathless at rest in pregnancy or in the postpartum period, especially in the presence of tachycardia:

> A woman presented to her GP with breathlessness, pyrexia and hypotension. She was referred to the medical registrar who saw her on the ambulatory medical unit (AMU) and made a diagnosis of pneumonia with a differential of PE. Intravenous antibiotics were commenced and a raft of tests done, all of which were abnormal. Although she was patently unwell she was transferred to a gynaecology ward where she suffered an arrest from which she could not be resuscitated. A postmortem diagnosis of PE was made.

The importance of tachycardia

Tachycardia is without doubt the most significant clinical feature of an unwell patient and is regularly ignored or misunderstood. Measurements of respiratory rate and heart rate are infinitely more important than measurements of blood pressure. A normotensive patient may all too often be unwell and compensating. A tachycardic patient is hypovolaemic until proved otherwise. A patient with tachypnoea has a cardiorespiratory cause until proved otherwise. Attributing tachycardia and tachypnoea to anxiety is naïve and dangerous. For example:

> A woman was seen three times in the ED with abdominal pain and diarrhoea. She was discharged on the first two occasions with a diagnosis of gastroenteritis, even though she had a history of collapse and measured heart rates of 130 and 144 beats per minute. She arrested and died on her third presentation. At postmortem she was found to have had an ectopic pregnancy.

Ectopic pregnancy

Mismanaging ectopic pregnancies has always been easier than making the correct diagnosis, partly because cases present infrequently (1 in 100 pregnancies) but mainly because their presentation may not be classical. The triad of symptoms described in textbooks of emergency medicine is bleeding, abdominal pain and amenorrhoea, but many of the women who died, as well as some who survive, have a variety of non-specific symptoms including diarrhoea, vomiting and collapse. Many of the women who come into the ED with symptoms from ectopic pregnancy do not know or volunteer that they are pregnant. It is disappointing that occasionally these women do not have a pregnancy test done as a routine. Without a pregnancy test it is hard to include ectopic pregnancy in the differential diagnosis. It is crucial that the risk factors for ectopic pregnancy are taught and recognised. The following case is an example of the consequences of misdiagnosis:

A woman collapsed at home following an episode of diarrhoea. On admission to the ED she was tachycardic, hypotensive and IV access was difficult. No pregnancy test was carried out. She arrested and was resuscitated after a very prolonged period of CPR. On the return of spontaneous circulation she was noted to have a haemoglobin of 8 dl. An ultrasound scan was carried out, which led to further delays, and free fluid was noted . At her eventual laparotomy a ruptured ectopic pregnancy was revealed but she suffered a further, fatal, cardiac arrest.

Box 18.1
ED learning points: ectopic pregnancy

ED clinicians need to be aware of atypical clinical presentations of ectopic pregnancy and especially of the way in which it is often associated with diarrhoea and vomiting and may mimic gastrointestinal disease. Fainting in early pregnancy may also indicate an ectopic pregnancy.

There must be a low threshold for ßhCG testing in women of reproductive age attending the ED with abdominal symptoms.

Pregnant women with abdominal pain should be reviewed by staff from the Obstetrics & Gynaecology department.

Education and training

Teaching of ED staff

All departments have formal teaching for medical and nursing staff in addition to the shop floor teaching to which EDs particularly lend themselves. EDs see a huge range of patients including children, surgical emergencies, patients with mental health needs, medical emergencies and major and minor trauma. Thus pregnancy-related complications form a small but important component of the daily workload. The ability to organise a teaching programme which encompasses all eventualities is crucial. In addition the teaching has to be delivered early in the clinician's post, repeated to those who are unavailable, and competency tested. This challenge is made more complex by the changing nature of job applicant experience and length of post in the ED.

"Red flag" teaching is usually carried out early on in the post or on induction days. This highlights conditions not to be missed, their recognition and management. The red flag signs and symptoms are those which call out for early attention due to their importance and reflection of life-threatening illness. Early teaching about the pregnant woman must include recognition of the sick mother, PE and ectopic pregnancy.

Locums/Agency staff

There is little point in having perfect systems in place if they fall apart when locum or agency staff are working. Many Trusts have a policy whereby locums cannot get paid until they go through an e-learning exercise which should contain important departmental protocols. At the very least new clinicians should be closely monitored.

Service provision

Availability of senior help

In most EDs the majority of medical staff are in the SHO-equivalent grade (F2) and therefore most patients are seen in the first instance by a relatively inexperienced clinician. If the patient is collapsed, however, or otherwise unwell the middle grade doctor or consultant should be involved from the outset, as will senior nurses. Thus, in addition to teaching trainees how to pick up subtle clinical signs there must be a clear chain of command which is easy to access and is understood. The importance of being able to access senior help cannot be over-emphasised.

Usually if the diagnosis is clear the specialist team is sought; and if the diagnosis is unclear a more senior ED opinion is requested. All EDs have a 24/7 senior on-call rota; many (especially the larger departments) have 24/7 resident middle grade cover and a few have consultant availability on site. Most labour wards have a consultant obstetrician present during the day as well as one being on call during the night. Often, however, the labour ward is in another hospital and this can cause logistical challenges. From an ED perspective it is most efficient if all services are on one site.

Protocols for referral to specialist teams

In some centres specific groups of patients are not seen by ED clinicians unless they require resuscitation. Instead they are seen directly by specialist in-patient teams. Such groups include children under one, who are seen by paediatricians, and pregnant women, who are seen by the obstetric team. Clearly there are some groups, for example those in active labour, those with second or third-trimester bleeding, those who are unwell who should always be see by an in-patient team.

Transfer of women

In general the safest place for someone who needs resuscitation is the resuscitation room of an ED, whether or not they are pregnant. The best place to give birth, however, when there are obstetric complications, is in a delivery suite with trained clinicians on hand. Cardiac arrest in pregnancy generally does not have a good outcome for mother or baby and optimal management is needed to avoid it.

Thus there should be clear and agreed pathways of care for where collapsed mothers go. First, a pre-emptive call should be made from the pre-hospital team to alert the hospital team of her imminent arrival. Senior staff should be on hand to meet the collapsed woman. Taking an unwell woman straight to a busy ward is rarely helpful, and it is usually a mistake to transfer a sick mother to another hospital which is smaller and less well staffed just "because it is the maternity hospital". If necessary the team can come to the patient. Local knowledge is essential in knowing where to take the patient to access the best care.

Conclusions

A wide variety of underlying factors may have contributed to the deaths reviewed in this Chapter. Nevertheless when misdiagnosis occurred there was often a failure to understand the altered physiology of pregnancy and a failure to ask for senior and/or specialised help.

Emergency Departments are getting busier all the time and the expectations of the general public are quite rightly getting higher. More interventions are being carried out in the ED by more senior staff but this must never preclude requesting opinion from obstetric colleagues. It is important that Emergency Departments know whom to call in an obstetric emergency and how to call them.

Not all the deaths reviewed for this chapter could have been avoided, even with better training, but there were a significant few which resulted from a poor understanding of basic clinical signs. There is a great need to ensure that teaching, training and retraining in the recognition of the sick pregnant woman should be mandatory in all medical and nursing training programmes, at induction and throughout their careers. This applies to junior and senior doctors and nurses working in the ED as it does to other clinical staff and to locum staff.

Excellent training is available in many centres, and in others the introduction and routine use of an obstetric early warning score card, a key recommendation of this Report, will be of great benefit. There should be watertight procedures in place for ensuring all staff are aware of the importance of basic clinical signs and symptoms.

References

1   The Advanced Life Support Group. The Managing Obstetric Emergencies and Trauma course. www.alsg.org

19 Critical Care

Tom Clutton-Brock

Critical Care: Specific recommendations

The early detection of severe illness in mothers remains a challenge to all involved in their care. The relative rarity of such events combined with the normal changes in physiology associated with pregnancy and childbirth compounds the problem. There is a need to introduce education, training and other processes which will improve detection rates.

Modified early warning scoring systems have been successfully introduced in other areas of clinical practice and systems appropriately modified for the obstetric patient have been described. These should be introduced for all acute obstetric admissions including early pregnancy.

Changes in medical training and work patterns have reduced the exposure of junior medical staff to life threatening illness. This should be addressed by the introduction of simulation training, preferably as part of a nationally accredited scheme.

The management of obstetric emergencies such as massive haemorrhage is necessarily team based. Maternity teams should be expected to demonstrate their competency in scenario based training and protocols for the management of obstetric emergencies should be subjected to regular review.

In the future, all staff, including temporary staff, involved in the care of seriously sick women should have undertaken appropriate competency-based training and have a record of success.

Introduction

A chapter on Intensive Care is now a well established feature of this Report and for this triennium the name has been changed to Critical Care in order to bring it into line with internationally accepted definitions. A common criticism levelled at this type of publication is that similar messages are repeated from one report to another and Critical Care will be no exception. The very fact that similar conclusions appear is in itself a salutary message; we are of course dealing with rare events and will never achieve a rate of zero. Every death remains a tragedy and any lessons that can be learnt deserve repetition and reinforcement.

A further criticism is that denominator data are missing for many of the causes of death investigated. Until recently the largest Critical Care obstetric dataset from the UK was that reported by Hazelgrove et al[1], who collected data on admissions to 14 general Critical Care Units in the South West Thames region. They identified 1.8% of all admissions (210 out of 11,385 cases) to be related to pregnancy. More recently, in 2005, the Intensive Care National Audit and Research Centre (ICNARC) published a study looking at the case mix, outcome and activity for obstetric admissions to adult, general Critical Care Units[2].

Of 219,468 admissions in the ICNARC Case Mix Programme Database (CMPD), 1452 (0.7%) were identified as *Direct* obstetric admissions. A further 278 admissions were identified as *Indirect* or *Coincidental* obstetric admissions by the presence of an obstetric code in the 'Other conditions relevant to the admission' or a partially completed obstetric code in any field. Additionally, 175 admissions matched one or more of the terms used in the text field search. Of these, 164 clearly met the condition of 'being pregnant or having recently been pregnant' and the remaining 11 were excluded. This left a total of 450 *Indirect* or *Coincidental* obstetric admissions (0.2% of all CMPD admissions). The comparison group of all non-obstetric female admissions aged 16–50 years consisted of 22,938 admissions (10.5% of all CMPD admissions). In total, the 1902 obstetric admissions represented 0.9% of all CMPD admissions and 7.7% of all female admissions aged 16–50 years. After adjusting for the changing units participating in the CMP, there was no significant trend over time. On average only 7 per 1000 intensive care admissions will be obstetric patients and even a large unit will only see five to six women each year. It is hardly surprising then that very few intensivists will have had much exposure to the critically ill obstetric patient.

Similarly only a very small proportion of obstetric patients will end up in an Intensive Care Unit (ICU). A study of 435 obstetric patients admitted to ICUs in France[3] estimated that the frequency was 36 per 100,000 live births. The mortality was lower with scheduled cases. In a Canadian study in 1999[4] over 14 years, between 1980 and 1993, 0.7 per thousand women required transfer for critical care. The main reasons for transfer were hypertensive disease (25%), haemorrhage (22%) and sepsis (15%). Wheatley et al.[5] reviewed the predictability of admissions to their ICU; they found that 67% of women had no previous medical or obstetric history. As in other series, the major reasons for admission were hypertensive disorders of pregnancy (66%) and haemorrhage (19%); 79% followed caesarean section and 40% required ventilatory support. Using these figures as an estimate a busy obstetric unit with say 6,500 deliveries per year will on average only send five women to intensive care each year. This number will include both survivors and non-survivors.

Another important finding from the ICNARC review of obstetric patients on intensive care was the low mortality observed in obstetric patients. The South West Thames study had reported a mortality of 3.3%. The ICNARC study found only 2.2% of patients with *Direct* obstetric admissions dying before ultimate discharge from hospital, versus 6.0% among *Indirect* or *Coincidental* obstetric admissions and 19.6% among female non-obstetric admissions aged 16–50 years ($\chi 2$ test, $P < 0.001$). In summary then 96% of obstetric admissions to intensive care survive. Combining this with the figures above we can roughly estimate that a busy obstetric unit will have a death in a Critical Care Unit approximately once in every five years.

Obstetric patients may well be a fitter and younger group than the aged matched control group. The ICNARC study showed that the widely used Acute Physiology and Chronic Health Evaluation (APACHE) II severity scoring and mortality prediction model was poorly calibrated for the obstetric patients and significantly overestimated their risk of death. This would support the view that this group of patients do better than predicted by any existing model.

These data also support the view that, overall, the care of the critically ill obstetric patient both before and during their stay in Critical Care must be of a high standard and that reports dealing only with mothers who have died must be set in this context.

Summary of key findings for 2003-2005

One hundred and ten reports of mothers who were admitted to Critical Care and who died were reviewed in detail. Of these, 63 deaths were attributed to *Direct* causes and 47 to *Indirect* causes. As in previous Reports the types of presentation were very varied. Some mothers suffered a sudden intra-cerebral event without warning and were admitted to a Critical Care Unit for a short period of ventilation prior to brain stem death tests. Almost without exception this process was well documented and in many cases appropriate organ donation was discussed. Other mothers suffered out-of-hospital cardiac arrests and despite extensive resuscitation attempts did not survive. For example:

> *A previously healthy woman in mid pregnancy developed severe one-sided back pain at home and collapsed. She arrived at the emergency department (ED) in cardiac arrest. The ED had been pre-warned by the paramedic crew and the critical care specialist registrar had already asked the consultant on call for critical care to attend. Shortly after admission an emergency*

caesarean section was performed by the emergency medicine consultant. Massive transfusion, tracheal intubation, external cardiac massage and defibrillation restored her cardiac output and she was transferred to the operating theatre by a consultant anaesthetist for a laparotomy by a consultant obstetrician to investigate continued bleeding. At operation she was found to have an aneurysm of the splenic artery which had ruptured. She received large amounts of blood including O negative, fresh frozen plasma (FFP) and aprotinin in an attempt to control the bleeding. Postoperatively she was transferred to the Critical Care Unit where a femoral arterial and a pulmonary artery catheter were inserted and she was started on continuous veno-venous haemofiltration. Despite the use of inotropic, ventilatory and renal support she developed multiple organ system failure and following a further bleed she died less than two days after admission.

It is difficult to fault any aspect of her management from the time of her collapse to her death. While no less of a tragedy to all involved, these cases probably represent a group of mothers in whom a significant reduction in mortality remains a difficult challenge. In contrast were a number of cases where, as in previous Reports, both the recognition and the subsequent management of a variety of life-threatening illnesses were considered to be sub-optimal.

Recognition of life-threatening illness

Delays in the recognition of life-threatening illness as a contribution to avoidable mortality are certainly not confined to maternal deaths. Controlled trials will always be difficult, if not impossible in this area, yet it seems intuitive that, in some cases at least, the earlier detection of severe pathology must lead to a better chance of survival. It is a common activity for critical care consultants to review a patient's observation charts and criticise the delay in recognising that something serious was developing. This must however be interpreted with care, the benefits of hindsight are easy to overlook:

A woman with a past medical history of mild asthma presented to her local gynaecology unit early in her second trimester with a history of increasing shortness of breath. She was pyrexial on admission at 38 oC and with a C-reactive protein (CRP) level of 300 mg/l (normal < 10 mg/l), a provisional diagnosis of influenza was made and she was admitted for observation. Twenty-four hours later she was seen by a junior medical trainee who recorded that she had a silent chest, a markedly reduced peak expiratory flow rate and was coughing up green sputum. The medical team were not prepared to take over her care because she was pregnant. She was started on intravenous steroids, antibiotics and inhaled bronchodilators. Several discussions between junior medical staff and a consultant physician ensued and she was eventually seen by a medical specialist registrar and admitted to the Critical Care Unit. Shortly after admission she began to miscarry and rapidly developed septic shock and multiple organ failure leading to death a few days later. Sputum samples subsequently grew streptococcus pneumoniae.

Despite clear evidence of a severe systemic infection, none of the medical staff initially involved in this woman's care appreciated just how sick she really was; antibiotics were started late and senior staff were either not involved in her care at an early enough stage or also failed to appreciate the severity of her illness.

Box 19.1
Critical care learning points: identifying very sick women

The recognition of life threatening illness is challenging.

Physiological reserves increase in pregnancy and may further conceal the development of serious pathology.

Modified early warning scoring systems

The well recognised problems of recognising life threatening illness has led to the introduction of a number of early warning scoring systems (EWS), also known as patient at risk scores (PARS) or modified early warning scores (MEWS)[6]. An EWS is calculated for a patient using five simple physiological variables: Mental response, pulse rate, systolic blood pressure, respiratory rate and temperature. For patients who are postoperative or unwell enough to be catheterised a sixth variable, urine output can also be added. The principle is that small changes in these five variables combined will be seen earlier using EWS than waiting for obvious changes in individual variables such as a marked drop in systolic blood pressure which is often a pre-terminal event. Of all the variables, respiratory rate is the most important for assessing the clinical state of a patient but is the one that is least recorded. Respiratory rate is thought to be the most sensitive indicatory of a patient's physiological well-being. The changes in physiology seen in normal pregnancy mean that any scoring system may need to be modified for this group of patients as pregnancy progresses. The poor calibration of scoring systems for obstetric admissions supports this theory[2] but does mean that the error will be on the safe side, i.e. mothers will be referred earlier than may be necessary.

Modified early obstetric warning scoring system (MEOWS)

Some units have produced their own scoring systems modified for obstetric patients and the one reproduced in the Annex to this Chapter has been developed by Aberdeen Maternity Hospital and is reproduced with their kind consent.

Box 19.2
Critical Care learning points: early warning scores

Modified early warning scoring systems improve the detection of life threatening illness.

Some modification of the physiological limits set may be required later in pregnancy.

However, the detection of life threatening illness alone is of little value. It is the subsequent management that will alter the outcome.

On their own, though, MEOWS can only be part of the solution, as it is the response to the abnormal score that will determine any real change in outcome:

> A woman was admitted with a diagnosis of ovarian hyper-stimulation syndrome (OHHS), and was pyrexial and tachycardic on admission. A couple of days later she was short of breath at rest with pulse oximeter saturations of 89%, a blood pressure recorded as 146/34 mm/Hg and a reduced urine output. She was found to have bilateral effusions and ascites. The nursing staff placed her under increased observations and used a MEWS chart. Critical care referral and blood gas analysis were suggested to the junior medical staff who decided to do neither. Shortly afterwards, with her decline carefully charted but no action taken, she had a pulse rate of 176 bpm and an un-recordable blood pressure. She died of her pneumonia on the Critical Care Unit.

Management of life-threatening illness

Haemorrhage

Examples of the poor management of haemorrhage in obstetric patients have been raised in this, and previous Reports. Obstetric haemorrhage continues as one of the major reasons for admission to Critical Care and so overall its management must be good if the low mortality amongst obstetric admissions is to be easily explained:

> *A woman suffered a postpartum haemorrhage after a normal vaginal delivery and, following an examination under anaesthesia, went on to have a hysterectomy during which her estimated blood loss was 3,000 mls. She received 1,000 mls of Hartmann's solution, 1,000 mls of normal saline, 1,000 mls of a gelatine based plasma expander, six units of re-suspended red cells and 2 units of FFP. There was no Critical Care bed immediately available so anaesthesia was reversed and she was admitted to the high dependency unit (HDU). She remained tachycardic for the next four hours but maintained her blood pressure at 110/60 mm/Hg. Over the next few hours she became increasingly tachycardic up to 160bpm and hypotensive down to 90/28 mm/Hg. During this period she received a further seven units of re-suspended red cells, 1,000 mls of Normal Saline, two units of FFP, one pack of platelets and five units of cryoprecipitate. She was eventually admitted to Critical Care some hours after the end of her surgery where she was intubated and ventilated because of poor blood gases and appeared to develop a disseminated intravascular coagulopathy (DIC). She had a cardiac arrest some hours later and subsequently died.*

There are lessons to be learnt from several aspects of this case. 3,000 mls is a major loss of blood during a hysterectomy and the junior staff involved should have asked for senior help earlier. Although her circulating volume was reasonably well replaced during surgery this was almost entirely with a mixture of red cells and saline with little or no appreciation that this would inevitable lead to a serious dilutional coagulopathy.

Recently the whole question of transfusion regimens for significant bleeding has been questioned. The American military have moved to using a ratio of one FFP to every unit of packed red cells and have apparently demonstrated an improvement in battlefield mortality. Using a pharmacokinetic model of clotting factor levels Ho et al[7] concluded that in major haemorrhage the equivalent of whole-blood transfusion is required to prevent the development of a coagulopathy and whole blood transfusion remains a widely used practice in combat situations. The exact requirement for FFP replacement will never be known but the availability of increasingly reliable point-of-care testing devices for haemoglobin estimation and clotting tests will help in the management of bleeding patients.

Many units have massive transfusion protocols and these should be regularly reviewed as new evidence becomes available. Effective management requires experience, the ability to predict likely requirements, good communication with, and cooperation from, haematology and blood bank services and appropriate fluid delivery and warming equipment.

The management of massive obstetric haemorrhage is included in commercially available advanced life support courses[8] although at present these are primarily directed at medical staff only. There is perhaps a need to develop a nationally approved, scenario based team training in the management of major obstetric haemorrhage that is available and affordable to all members of theatre, recovery and high dependency unit teams.

The delay in obtaining a critical care bed has been discussed before and overall the provision of critical care beds has improved since the last Report. Despite this, delays will on occasion be inevitable but are no excuse for poor quality care.

> **Box 19.3**
> **Critical care learning points:** haemorrhage

Massive haemorrhage protocols should be used early and adhered to.

The development of a dilutional coagulopathy should be avoided if at all possible by the early use of FFP and other blood products as required.

Teams should practice the management of massive haemorrhage on a regular basis.

Sepsis

Severe systemic sepsis especially when accompanied by septic shock remains a challenge to all those involved in the care of critically ill patients. The onset of severe sepsis can be alarmingly rapid and once established difficult to treat as demonstrated by the woman with streptococcal pneumonia discussed above. There were other cases reported where there were reasonably clear signs of severe sepsis which were initially ignored:

> *A woman presented at early in her third trimenster with a low grade pyrexia and contractions and was treated with ritodrine, steroids and augmentin. Her CRP level rose from 16 to 152 mg/l during the first day of her admission. She underwent a caesarean section under general anaesthesia. Her arterial saturations by pulse oximetry were 66% at the start of the procedure rising with an increase in inspired oxygen. Despite this she was extubated at the end of the procedure with saturations of 75-88% on eight litres per minute of oxygen by facemask. A blood gas taken at that time showed a base excess of -11.9 mmol/l. She was referred to the critical care team because of increasing shortness of breath before she was commenced on continuous positive airway pressure (CPAP). Due to a lack of beds she was transferred to the theatre recovery suite and was managed on CPAP with direct arterial pressure monitoring. She was eventually transferred to the Critical Care Unit a few hours post operatively where she steadily deteriorated and died some days later from severe acute respiratory distress syndrome (ARDS). Her blood cultures grew listeria.*

While it is impossible to say whether earlier, more aggressive, intervention might have saved her, the development of such a severe metabolic acidosis early on in her treatment was indicative of septic shock.

Although our understanding of the complex processes underlying severe sepsis increases year on year, the search for "silver bullets" remains largely unproductive. Recently a different approach has been proposed with the introduction of the Surviving Sepsis Campaign[9]. This is an initiative of the European Society of Intensive Care Medicine, the International Sepsis Forum, and the Society of Critical Care Medicine, which has been developed to improve the management, diagnosis, and treatment of sepsis. The approach has been to develop evidence based guidelines, delivered as bundles of care, the first two bundles cover resuscitation and management of severe sepsis and are delivered as a continuum. The inclusion of a considerable quantity of locally dictated protocols supports the view that there remains uncertainty in some areas of care. The bundles of care proposed are reproduced in Box 19.4.

Box 19.4 Surviving sepsis campaign

Sepsis resuscitation bundle

- Serum lactate measured.

- Blood cultures obtained prior to antibiotic administration.

- From the time of presentation, broad-spectrum antibiotics administered within three hours for emergency department (ED) admissions and one hour for non-ED ICU admissions.

- In the event of hypotension and/or lactate >4 mmol/L (36 mg/dl):

  – Deliver an initial minimum of 20 ml/kg of crystalloid (or colloid equivalent)

  – Apply vasopressors for hypotension not responding to initial fluid resuscitation to maintain mean arterial pressure (MAP) ^{3}65 mm Hg

Sepsis management bundle

- Low-dose steroids administered for septic shock in accordance with a standardised ICU policy

- Drotrecogin alfa (activated protein C) administered in accordance with a standardised ICU policy (See note below)

Although at first sight these seem complex, and indeed the management bundle is applied differently from one unit to another, the resuscitation bundle is applicable to both ward and HDU based patients as well. The failure to respond to fluid resuscitation should trigger an urgent critical care referral.

The use of activated protein C is associated with an increase in bleeding in some groups of patients and trials in children have been halted. The balance of risks and benefits at present remains unclear.

Box 19.5 **Critical care learning points:** severe sepsis
Severe sepsis can develop quickly and when accompanied by septic shock kills previously fit women.
Serum lactate, blood gases and blood cultures should be measured early in suspected cases of systemic sepsis.
Fluid resuscitation should be prompt and the effect noted without delay.
Failure to respond to 20mls/kg of intravenous fluids should trigger an urgent critical care referral.

Resuscitation

In the majority of cases reviewed where cardiopulmonary resuscitation took place this was delivered to a very high standard and current advanced life support (ALS) guidelines were followed, although there were exceptions:

A woman had labour induced for post dates. This was accompanied by a marked rise in blood pressure, a sudden reduction in her conscious level and twitching of her limbs. Her observations were recorded as blood pressure 200/106 mm/Hg, pulse 20 bpm and saturations of 64% on 4 lpm of oxygen. An in-and-out urethral catheter was inserted following which her saturations fell and the on call anaesthetist was fast bleeped. An assisted delivery failed. Shortly afterwards her observations became unrecordable and an arrest call was put out. She was transferred to HDU with a blood pressure of 71/58 mm/Hg and saturations of 58%. Approximately an hour after her initial collapse she was transferred to the operating theatre for intubation and section, and subsequent transfer to a nearby Critical Care Unit. She died some days later and her autopsy showed a recent subarachnoid and mid brain haemorrhage.

Her intracerebral bleeds and subsequent death may have been unavoidable but the management of her airway, breathing and circulation was below an acceptable standard. A new ALS algorithm has recently been introduced and should be adopted in all clinical areas.

With the inevitable pressures to contain the costs of healthcare and the changes in working patterns amongst both junior and senior staff the attainment and renewal of appropriate resuscitation competencies is becoming a major challenge. A recent announcement[10] by the Resuscitation Council (UK) states "We are investing considerable resources in the development of e-learning materials to enable resuscitation training to be delivered more efficiently and cost-effectively. This will reduce the time that NHS staff need to be away from their workplace. Training will remain standardised and the quality preserved." This blended learning approach in which e-learning is combined with practical demonstrations and assessment should make the completion of nationally recognised ALS courses a more efficient process.

Box 19.6
Critical care learning points: staff training

All staff involved in the care of acute obstetric admissions should have current ALS or ILS certification.

The introduction of blending learning for ALS will improve its uptake.

Conclusions

Reviewing case after case of often previously fit young women who, despite critical care, have gone on to die is a sad and depressing process. It is all too easy with the knowledge of hindsight to criticise the care they received. Some would have died however excellent their care, some would not. The excellent survival rates for obstetric patients admitted to Critical Care Units supports the view that the vast majority of these sick women receive care of the highest quality. There are nevertheless important lessons to be learnt from those who did not survive. Many of these lessons and messages have been discussed before but there is clearly still room for improvement and complacency should be avoided.

References

1 Hazelgrove JF, Price C, Pappachan VJ, et al.: *Multicenter study of obstetric admissions to 14 intensive care units in southern England.* Crit Care Med 2001:29;770-775.

2 Harrison DA, Penny JA , Yentis SM , et al. *Case mix, outcome and activity for obstetric admissions to adult, general Critical Care units: a secondary analysis of the ICNARC Case Mix Programme Database.* Critical Care 2005, 9(Suppl 3):S25-S37.

3 Bouvier-Colle, M.H., Salanave, B., et al. *Obstetric patients treated in intensive care units and mortality.* Eur J of Obstet, Gynecol and Reproductive Biol 1996; 65: 121-5.

4 Baskett TF, Sternadel J. *Maternal intensive care and near-miss mortality in obstetrics.* Br J Obstet Gynaecol. 1998, 105(9):981-4.

5 Wheatley, E., Farkas, A. & Watson, D. *Obstetric admissions to an intensive therapy unit.* Int J of Obstet Anaes. 1995; 5:221-4.

6 http://www.nda.ox.ac.uk/wfsa/html/u17/u1710_01.htm

7 Ho AM, Dion PW, Cheng CA, Karmakar MK, Cheng G, Peng Z, Ng YW. *A mathematical model for fresh frozen plasma transfusion strategies during major trauma resuscitation with ongoing haemorrhage.* Can J Surg. 2005 Dec;48(6):470-8.

8 www.alsg.org

9 www.survivingsepsis.org

10 www.resus.org.uk/pages/ALSequiv.htm

Chapter 19 Annex A

CHAPTER 19 ANNEX A : AN EXAMPLE OF AN OBSTETRIC EARLY WARNING CHART. REPRODUCED WITH THE KIND PERMISSION OF ABERDEEN MATERNITY HOSPITAL

OBSTETRIC EARLY WARNING CHART   (FOR MATERNITY USE ONLY)

Name: _____   DOB: _____

_____   Ward: _____

NHS
Grampian

CONTACT DOCTOR FOR EARLY INTERVENTION IF PATIENT TRIGGERS ONE RED OR TWO YELLOW SCORES AT ANY ONE TIME

Date :				>30
Time :				21-30
RESP (write rate in corresp. box)	>30			21-30
	21-30			11-20
	11-20			0-10
	0-10			
Saturations	95-100%			11-20
	<95%			95-100%
Administered O₂ (L/min.)				%
Temp	39 38 37 36 35			39 38 37 36 35
HEART RATE	170 160 150 140 130 120 110 100 90 80 70 60 50 40			170 160 150 140 130 120 110 100 90 80 70 60 50 40
Systolic blood pressure	200 190 180 170 160 150 140 130 120 110 100 90 80 70 60 50			200 190 180 170 160 150 140 130 120 110 100 90 80 70 60 50
Diastolic blood pressure	130 120 110 100 90 80 70 60 50 40			130 120 110 100 90 80 70 60 50 40
URINE	passed (Y/N)			passed (Y/N)
Proteinuria	protein ++			protein ++
	protein >++			protein >++
Amniotic fluid	Clear/Pink			Clear/Pink
	Green			Green
NEURO RESPONSE (√)	Alert			Alert
	Voice			Voice
	Pain			Pain
	Unresponsive			Unresponsive
Pain Score (no.)	0-1			0-1
	2-3			2-3
Lochia	Normal			Normal
	Heavy / Fresh Offensive			Heavy / Fresh Offensive
Looks unwell	NO (√)			YES (√)
	YES (√)			NO (√)
Total Yellow Scores				
Total Red Scores				

This Annex is available to download in PDF format from the CEMACH website – www.cemach.org.uk

20 Severe maternal morbidity - the Scottish experience 2003 to 2005

Gillian Penney, Dawn Kernaghan and Victoria Brace

For over 50 years, clinicians in the UK have used measures of maternal mortality as a means of monitoring the quality of maternity services. In addition, detailed study of the circumstances of individual cases has provided material for professional learning. Over the past decade, various groups internationally have investigated the rate of severe maternal morbidity, or 'near misses' as a complementary marker of standards of care.[1-7] The theory underlying this approach is described by Pattinson[5]: *'the sequence from good health to death in a pregnant woman is a clinical insult, followed by a systemic inflammatory response, organ failure and finally death. A near miss would be those women with organ dysfunction who survive'.* By viewing pregnancy and its potential outcomes as a continuum, beginning at normal pregnancy and concluding with maternal death, the number which can be studied meaningfully can be increased by examining the group of outcomes closest to death.

The Scottish Confidential Audit of Severe Maternal Morbidity began as a pilot study in 2001 and our growing experience has been reported in the last two Why Mothers Die Reports. Since 2003, data have been collected on a consistent national basis on 14 categories of severe maternal morbidity based on criteria originally described by Mantel et al.[8] We are now in a position to provide data for the triennium 2003-2005, to complement the maternal mortality data for the same period presented in the body of this Report.

Methods

As previously described[2,9], each month, every consultant-led maternity unit in Scotland reports the number of women meeting one or more of the 14 agreed definitions to the central office of the Scottish Programme for Clinical Effectiveness in Reproductive Health. The categories and definitions currently in use are summarised in Table 20.1. A minimal dataset on each case is collected, comprising: a unique identifier; age; date of event; and limited clinical information to verify that the case definitions are being met. These monthly returns are collated centrally and used to calculate national and unit-level rates of severe morbidity events.

In addition, case assessment proformas relating to the most common categories of severe morbidity events (major obstetric haemorrhage and eclampsia) have been developed. These proformas comprise both condition-specific (ie assessing adherence to national guidance) and general (ie root cause analysis) sections. These national proformas are used by local clinical risk management teams during assessment of cases of major obstetric haemorrhage (2003 to 2005) or eclampsia (from 2004). They serve to guide local teams through a systematic and structured assessment of each case. Risk management teams are required to make an overall assessment of quality of care using definitions of suboptimal care similar to those used by the Confidential Enquiries into Maternal Deaths. They are also required to formulate an action plan. The completed proformas are collated centrally in order to identify recurrent themes and draw generalisable lessons for Scotland as a whole. Thus, both case ascertainment (permitting the calculation of rates of events) and case assessment (permitting the learning of clinical lessons) take place.

Table 20.1
Inclusion criteria used in 2003-05

Code	Category	Definition
1	Major obstetric haemorrhage	Estimated blood loss ≥2,500ml, or transfused five or more units of blood, or received treatment for coagulopathy (fresh frozen plasma, cryoprecipitate, platelets). (Includes ectopic pregnancy meeting these criteria).
2	Eclampsia	Seizure associated with antepartum, intrapartum or postpartum symptoms and signs of pre-eclampsia.
3	Renal or Liver dysfunction	Acute onset of biochemical disturbance, urea > 15mmol/l, creatinine >400mmol/l, aspartate aminotransferase / alanine aminotransferase >200u/l.
4	Cardiac arrest	No detectable major pulse.
5	Pulmonary oedema	Clinically diagnosed pulmonary oedema associated with acute breathlessness and 0_2 saturation < 95%, requiring 0_2, diuretics or ventilation.
6	Acute respiratory dysfunction	Requiring intubation or ventilation for >60 minutes (not including duration of general anaesthetic).
7	Coma	Including diabetic coma. Unconscious >12 hours.
8	Cerebro-vascular event	Stroke, cerebral/cerebellar haemorrhage or infarction, subarachnoid haemorrhage, dural venous sinus thrombosis.
9	Status epilepticus	Unremitting seizures in a patient with known epilepsy.
10	Anaphylactic shock	An allergic reaction resulting in collapse with severe hypotension, difficulty breathing and swelling/rash.
11	Septicaemic shock	Shock (systolic blood pressure <80 mm/Hg) in association with infection. No other cause for decreased blood pressure. Pulse of 120 beats per minute or more.
12	Anaesthetic problem	Aspiration, failed intubation, high spinal or epidural anaesthetic.
13	Massive pulmonary embolism	Increased respiratory rate (>20 per minute), tachycardia, hypotension. Diagnosed as 'high' probability on V/Q scan or positive spiral chest CT scan. Treated by heparin, thrombolysis or embolectomy.
14	Intensive care or coronary care admission	Unit equipped to ventilate adults. Admission for one of the above problems or for any other reason. Include admissions to Coronary Care Units.

Results

During the 2003 to 2005 triennium, 845 women were reported as meeting one or more of our defined inclusion criteria. Using a denominator of 159,223 maternities, the rate of severe maternal morbidity during the triennium was 5.3 with a 95% confidence interval from 5.0 to 5.7 per 1000 maternities). During the triennium, 15 Direct or Indirect maternal deaths were reported to the Confidential Enquiry into Maternal Deaths in Scotland; giving a 'near-miss to death ratio' of 56:1, with a 95% CI from 34:1 to 100:1.

Many women met the definitions for more than one severe morbidity category. For example, some suffered major haemorrhage and were admitted to intensive care. Thus, during the triennium the 845 women who were reported to us experienced a total of 1,135 events meeting our inclusion criteria. Rates of the 14 individual categories of severe morbidity are summarised in Table 20.2. Major obstetric haemorrhage was the most numerous category occurring in 582 women during the triennium. Thus major haemorrhage occurred in 69% of all 845 women with severe maternal morbidity.

Table 20.2
Numbers and rates per 1,000 maternities of individual categories of severe maternal morbidity;
Scotland: 2003-05.

		Number of cases	Rate per 1,000 maternities	95 per cent CI	
1.	Major Obstetric Haemorrhage	582	3.66	3.37	3.96
2.	Eclampsia	55	0.35	0.26	0.45
3.	Renal or liver dysfunction	60	0.38	0.29	0.48
4.	Cardiac arrest	8	0.05	0.03	0.09
5.	Pulmonary oedema	42	0.26	0.20	0.36
6.	Acute respiratory dysfunction	58	0.36	0.28	0.47
7.	Coma	0	0.00	0.00	0.02
8.	Cerebro-vascular event	15	0.09	0.06	0.15
9.	Status epilepticus	2	0.01	0.00	0.04
10.	Anaphylactic shock	5	0.03	0.01	0.07
11.	Septicaemic shock	20	0.13	0.08	0.19
12.	Anaesthetic problem	26	0.16	0.11	0.24
13.	Massive pulmonary embolism	14	0.09	0.05	0.15
14.	Intensive care or coronary care admission	248	1.56	1.38	1.76
All women included		**845**	**5.31**	**4.96**	**5.68**

Overall Scottish rates of severe maternal morbidity in individual years from 2003 to 2005 are summarised in Table 20.3. The increase in rate from 4.6 per 1,000 in 2004 to 6.1 per 1,000 in 2005 is greater than would be expected by chance. The data in Table 20.3 suggest that this increase in severe maternal morbidity is almost entirely accounted for by an increase in major obstetric haemorrhage. The increase in rate of major haemorrhage from 3.2 per 1,000 in 2004 to 4.4 per 1,000 in 2005 was also statistically significant. In contrast, the increase in the rate of severe maternal morbidity if cases of haemorrhage are excluded is compatible with random variation. In commenting on these apparent increases between 2004 and 2005, it must be noted that there is no consistent upward trend over the three years studied to date.

Table 20.3
Numbers and rates of severe maternal morbidity (overall and from haemorrhage and non-haemorrhage causes) in individual years; Scotland: 2003 to 2005.

Year	Number of maternities	Number of women	Rate per 1000 maternities	95 per cent CI	
Women with severe maternal morbidity					
2003	51,902	270	5.2	*4.6*	*5.8*
2004	53,502	246	4.6	*4.0*	*5.2*
2005	53,819	329	6.1	*5.5*	*6.8*
Change 2004 to 2005			1.5	*0.6*	*2.4*
Major obstetric haemorrhage					
2003	51,902	176	3.4	*2.9*	*3.9*
2004	53,502	171	3.2	*2.8*	*3.7*
2005	53,819	235	4.4	*3.8*	*5.0*
Change 2004 to 2005			1.2	*0.4*	*1.9*
Non-haemorrhage severe morbidity					
2003	51,902	94	1.8	*1.5*	*2.2*
2004	53,502	75	1.4	*1.1*	*1.8*
2005	53,819	94	1.7	*1.4*	*2.1*
Change 2004 to 2005			0.3	*-0.1*	*0.8*

Detailed case assessments by hospital risk management teams, using the national proforma, have been conducted on cases of major obstetric haemorrhage throughout the triennium. Forms were returned for 517 of the 582 cases, but in 14 cases the space for the local assessment of sub-optimal care were left blank. Overall assessments of quality of care for the 503 cases for which information was returned are summarised in Table 20.4. The majority of cases (65%) were considered to be well-managed with only 3% of cases being judged as receiving major sub-optimal care. Similar detailed assessments of cases of eclampsia have been conducted since 2004. Again, only a small minority of cases were judged as receiving major sub-optimal care.

Table 20.4
Overall assessments of sub-optimal care in 503 cases of major obstetric haemorrhage.

Category	Number	Percentage
1 = Appropriate care, well managed.	327	65
2 = Incidental sub-optimal care – Lessons can be learnt although it did not affect the final outcome.	114	23
3 = Minor sub-optimal care – Different management may have resulted in a different outcome.	49	10
4 = Major sub-optimal care – Different management might have been expected to result in a more favourable outcome. The management of this case contributed significantly to the morbidity of this patient.	13	3

Discussion

The Scottish Confidential Audit of Severe Maternal Morbidity has collected data prospectively using 14 well-defined, consistent categories of morbidity for the triennium (2003-2005), contemporaneous with this maternal death enquiry. The audit is funded by NHS Quality Improvement Scotland. Continuous data collection under the auspices of a national agency, has two principal advantages. Firstly, aggregation of data over several years means that meaningful national rates of rare outcomes such as eclampsia can be calculated. Secondly, consistent methods mean that trends over time in overall rates of severe morbidity can be examined.

The causes of severe maternal morbidity found in our study differ from the causes of maternal death found in the Confidential Enquiries. Major haemorrhage accounted for 69% of our cases of severe morbidity but for only 11% of *Direct* maternal deaths in the UK in the 2003 to 2005 triennium. In contrast, venous thromboembolism was the principal cause of maternal death (28% of cases), but accounted for under 2% of our cases of severe morbidity. Thus, the pattern of morbidity and mortality appears to differ from the continuum described by Pattinson[5], with some clinical insults (e.g. major haemorrhage) being more amenable to alteration by prompt and appropriate treatment than others.

The approach used by the Scottish Confidential Audit relies on accurate and complete case identification at local hospital level. There have always been concerns that incident reporting systems under-estimate the true level of reportable events. In order to improve reproducibility, we have a designated member of staff within each unit with responsibility for reporting and we regularly update these participants. We would anticipate that with increasing familiarity with the study, case ascertainment would improve. Improved ascertainment may explain the apparent rise in the rate of severe morbidity.

Another explanation is that a rise in major obstetric haemorrhage has resulted from changes in the obstetric population: increasing numbers of mothers with complex medical conditions, increasing age at childbirth, increasing number of multiple pregnancies following assisted reproduction, and increasing number of caesarean sections with subsequent placenta praevia and accreta. Data from Information Services of NHS Scotland[10] show that the national rate of emergency caesarean section remained constant at 15.4% over the three years of this study but the rate of elective Caesarean section rose year on year, from 8.8% in 2003 to 9.5% in 2005 (Chi-squared test for trend, p<0.0001). The relationship between changes in the obstetric population and in obstetric practice and maternal morbidity requires continuing monitoring.

Although the number of women suffering major haemorrhage increased from 2004 to 2005, there was no concomitant rise in the number of women admitted to an intensive care unit. This suggests that high dependency facilities within labour wards are absorbing this rise. This pattern of care lends support to the continued use of definitions based on pathophysiological features, rather than aspects of clinical management such as admission to an intensive care unit, which may underestimate the burden of morbidity in our population.

In general, cases of major haemorrhage were considered to be well-managed, with only 3% judged to have major sub-optimal care. This is in marked contrast to assessments of cases of maternal death; in the 2003 to 2005 triennium, 10 of 17 cases (59%) of maternal deaths due to haemorrhage were judged by the Enquiry assessors to have major substandard care. These figures suggest that our cases of severe maternal morbidity should genuinely be thought of as 'great saves', rather than 'near misses': cases where appropriate care has prevented progression of morbidity to mortality.

Currently, the Scottish Confidential Audit of Severe Maternal Morbidity can only provide theories to explain any changes in morbidity in maternity units across Scotland. Although we cannot make broad assumptions based on a rising rate in a single year, it does highlight the need for continuing monitoring. Changes in the obstetric population and in obstetric practice result in changes to the risks of childbirth for both mother and baby; continuous monitoring of mortality and morbidity represents an essential element of reflective clinical practice.

References

1 Baskett TF,.O'Connell CM. *Severe obstetric maternal morbidity: a 15-year population-based study.* J.Obstet.Gynec. 2005;25:7-9.

2 Brace V, Penney G, Hall M. *Quantifying severe maternal morbidity: a Scottish population study.* BJOG 2004;111:481-4.

3 *Severe acute maternal morbidity and maternal death audit - a rapid diagnostic tool for evaluating maternal care.* S.Afr.Med.J. 2003;93:700-2.

4 *'Near-miss' obstetric events and maternal deaths in Sagamu, Nigeria: a retrospective study.* Reprod. Health. 2005;2:9.

5 Pattinson RC, Buchmann E, Mantel GD, Schoon M, Rees H. *Can enquiries into severe acute maternal morbidity act as a surrogate for maternal death enquiries?* BJOG 2003;110:889-93.

6 Waterstone M, Bewley S, Wolfe C. *Incidence and predictors of severe obstetric morbidity: case-control study.* BMJ 2001;322:1089-93.

7 Wen SW, Huang L, Liston R, Heaman M, Baskett TF, Rusen ID et al. *Severe maternal morbidity in Canada, 1991-2001.* CMAJ 2006;173:759-64.

8 Mantel GD, Buchmann E, Rees H, Pattinson RC. *Severe acute maternal morbidity: a pilot study of a definition for a near-miss.* Brit.J.Obstet.Gynaec. 1998;105:985-90.

9 Penney G, Brace V. *'Near misses' and severe maternal morbidity; the Scottish experience.* In Lewis G, ed. Why Mothers Die 2000-2002, pp 267-71. London: RCOG Press, 2004.

10 ISD *Scotland Live births by mode of delivery and induced.* http://www.isdscotland.org/isd/files/mat_bb_table5.xls

APPENDIX 1: Method of Enquiry

Naufil Alam

The Confidential Enquiry into Maternal and Child Health (CEMACH) has five regional offices in England and works with partner offices in Wales, Northern Ireland and Scotland. The work is co-ordinated by a Central Office in London. Each of the regional offices has contacts within every Trust that provides maternity care, at the Maternity-Unit level.

The Enquiry has its own Board with representation from the Royal College of Obstetricians and Gynaecologists (which hosts the Enquiry), Royal College of Midwives, Royal College of Pathologists, Faculty of Public Health, Royal College of Paediatrics and Child Health, and the Royal College of Anaesthetists. Recent additions to the Board include the Royal College of General Practitioners and the Royal College of Psychiatrists.

From 2003 to 2005, CEMACH was commissioned by the National Institute for Clinical Excellence (NICE) to conduct the Maternal Death Enquiry (MDE) in England and Wales. Since 2005, this commissioning role has been carried out by the National Patient Safety Agency (NPSA). In Northern Ireland CEMACH is commissioned by the Northern Ireland Department of Health, which contributes funds for their participation in the Enquiry. In Scotland, the Scottish Programme for Clinical Effectiveness in Reproductive Health (SPCERH), acting on behalf of NHS Quality Improvement Scotland (NHSQIS) conducts its own Enquiry programme, but cases are forwarded to the Enquiry's central assessors and included in the triennial Report.

England and Wales

It is a government requirement that all maternal deaths should be subject to this Confidential Enquiry, and all health professionals have a duty to provide the information required. In participating in the Confidential Enquiry, the professionals concerned are asked for three things:

(i)   to provide a full and accurate account of the circumstances leading to the woman's death, with supporting records

(ii)   to reflect on any clinical or other lessons that have been learned, either personally or as part of the wider context.

The responsibility for initiating an enquiry into maternal death lies with the CEMACH Regional Manager (RM). Following a pregnancy-associated-maternal-death, a notification is usually made by one of the health professionals involved in the care of the woman to the relevant CEMACH RM. Cases are also reported by the coroners, Local Supervising Authority Midwifery Officers (LSAMO), and others. Data are also cross validated with data received from the Office for National Statistics (ONS). The data received from ONS are discussed more fully below (see "Verification of ascertainment").

The enquiry is initiated using a standard data collection form (Maternal Enquiry pro forma; MDR-1) which is completed by obstetricians, anaesthetists, pathologists, general practitioners, midwives and any other professionals that were involved in the care of the woman. Copies of case notes are obtained, where relevant, and in some cases additional written statements are supplied. Each case is then prepared for a two stage review and assessment process, the first occurring at a regional level, and the second occurring at a central level. Following collection of all the relevant information, the records are anonymised and circulated by the CEMACH Regional Manager to Regional Assessors (RA). The obstetric and midwifery assessors review all cases. Anaesthetic assessors review all cases where there was involvement of an anaesthetic or intensive care. Every possible attempt is made to obtain full details of any autopsy and pathological investigations, and these are reviewed by the pathology assessor. The assessors add their comments and opinions regarding the cause or causes of death, before returning the completed form to the relevant Regional Office where core notification data are entered onto a database.

The Director of the Maternal Death Enquiry then reviews all cases and allocates the cases for further assessment as necessary. There are a number of central assessors in different specialities, e.g. cardiac disease, psychiatric illness etc. or clinical practice, e.g. midwifery, general practice etc. The Director will make a decision as to which is the most appropriate central assessor to review each case, although a case may be sent to more than one assessor. The Director then works in collaboration with the central assessors to review all available recorded facts about each case, and assess the factors that may have led to death. All details regarding the death, including the agreed clinical cause of death are recorded in a database.

All data and databases are held in accordance with CEMACH's information security procedures. This ensures anonymity at different stages of the Enquiry process, guarantees confidentiality, and safeguards any identifiable information for the duration it is held.

After preparation of the Report, and before its publication, all maternal death report forms, related documents and files relating to the period of the Report are destroyed, and all electronic data are irreversibly anonymised.

These processes are summarised in figure 1.

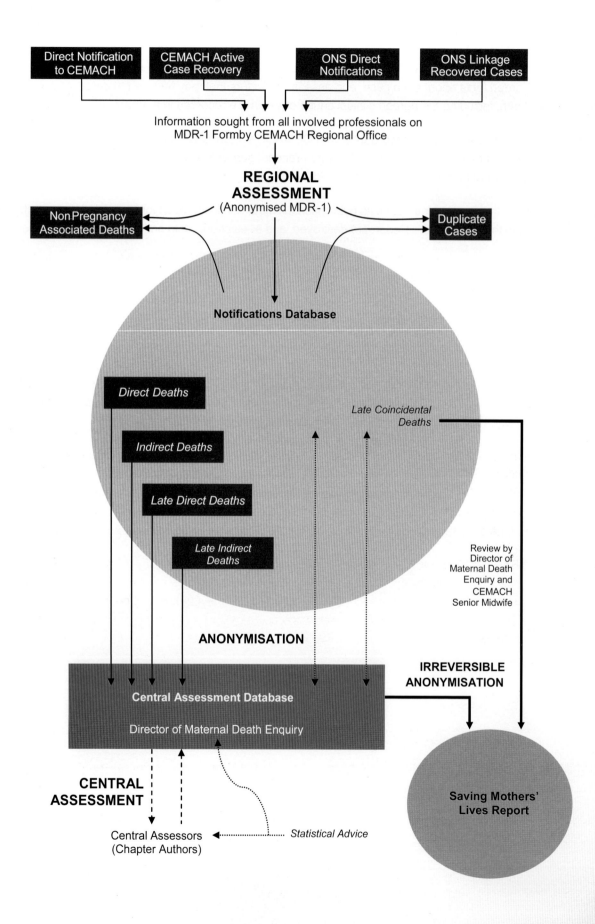

Verification of ascertainment

Ascertainment is checked with reference to data supplied by ONS. This data are supplied in two forms:

(i) Direct Notifications; these are deaths of women where "pregnancy" is mentioned anywhere on the ONS death registration. These cases are coded as a maternal death according to the International Classification of Diseases, Injuries and Causes of Death tenth revision (ICD10). This would identify all women where pregnancy may have been a contributing factor to their death.

(ii) Linkage Notifications; these are deaths of women where the name of the woman appeared on the registration of a birth in the current or preceding calendar year. This would allow for the identification of women who had died up to 364 days following delivery.

This data is cross-matched with the data that has been directly acquired by CEMACH. Any cases that have been identified by one organisation but not the other would then be established. These outstanding cases are then further investigated to ensure that they are pregnancy-associated-deaths, and that they warrant inclusion in the Enquiry and then an enquiry initiated using the standard data collection form.

Regional assessment

Each CEMACH region has one or more sets of Regional Assessors (RA) depending on requirements. Each set includes an obstetric assessor, midwifery assessor, pathology assessor, an anaesthetic assessor and a perinatal psychiatric assessor. Assessors are appointed for the term of the triennium (about 4 years, allowing for completion of assessment). Nominations for medical assessors are sought from the presidents of the Royal Colleges, and nominations for midwives are sought from the LSAMO.

An RA must be an active clinical practitioner in the National Health Service (NHS), in the relevant speciality. If medical, the Regional Assessor should be at consultant level, or, if a midwife, must be at supervisory level. The Regional Assessor should have knowledge and experience of organisation of care, as well as the respect of his/her peers. It is important that the Regional Assessor is able to realistically commit enough time to assess and return enquiry forms in a timely manner. The position is honorary.

The role of the Regional Assessor is to review the information reported in the MDR-1 form, and any other documents that have been assembled by the CEMACH Regional Manager. The Regional Assessor will then make a short report in the relevant section of the enquiry form. All the information provided to the Regional Assessor is anonymised. This report includes a comment on the case, an evaluation of the clinical management and the resources of the organisation responsible for the care of the woman. The assessor is also asked to make a judgement as to whether the care was substandard and, if so, if this was a contributing factor in the death of the mother.

Central assessment

The Central Assessors review each case thoroughly, taking into account the case history, the results of pathological investigations, and findings of autopsy that may have been conducted. Following this detailed investigation, each case is allotted to a specific chapter in the final report.

This assessment occasionally varies with the underlying cause of death as given on the death certificate, and classified by the Registrars General using the ICD10. This is because a death may be coded for a specific cause-of-death, but the pathogenesis of this condition may have been precipitated by an obstetric event. For example, although a given death may be coded as multiple-organ failure as the terminal event, it could have been precipitated by an obstetric event such as septicaemia from an infected caesarean section. Although each pregnancy-associated-maternal-death reported to this Enquiry is only counted once and assigned to one chapter, it may be referred to in additional chapters. For example, a death assigned to "hypertensive disorder of pregnancy", in which haemorrhage and anaesthesia also played a part, may be discussed in all three chapters.

Authors

Chapters are initially drafted by individual Central Assessors, and then discussed in detail by the whole panel before the Report is finalised. Other acknowledged professionals who have a particular and expert interest in specific diseases or areas of practice may be asked to review and comment on the recommendations prior to publication.

Statistical analysis and data presentation advice to each author is provided by both an independent statistical advisor, and data analysts at CEMACH.

Confidentiality

After preparation of the Report, and before its publication, all maternal death report forms, related documents and files relating to the period of the Report are destroyed, and all electronic data are irreversibly anonymised.

Denominator data

Denominator data and other relevant statistical data are supplied by organisations such as ONS, the Scotland General Registrar Office (GRO), Northern Ireland Statistical Research Agency (NISRA) and Hospital Episode Statistics (HES).

Northern Ireland

In Northern Ireland the same government requirement applies, in that all maternal deaths should be subject to Confidential Enquiry. During this triennium the responsibility for initiating an enquiry remained with the Director of Public Health (DPH) of the health and social services board in which the woman was resident. Maternal deaths were reported to the relevant DPH, who was responsible for organising completion of the MDR-1 by those involved in the care of the dead woman, and obtaining the autopsy report, where one had been conducted. On completion, the forms were sent to the Medical Coordinator at the Department of Health, Social Sciences, and Public Safety. The Medical Coordinator, acting on behalf of the Chief Medical Officer, anonymised the forms, and then coordinated the input of the pathology, anaesthetic, midwifery and obstetric assessors. A single panel of assessors dealt with all cases. Assessed MDR-1 forms, and other collected documentation, were forwarded to the CEMACH Central Office and submitted to the MDE Director for central assessment, as outlined for England and Wales, and illustrated in figure 1. All data and databases are held in accordance with CEMACH's information security procedures as for England and Wales.

Ascertainment is checked with reference to data supplied by the General Registrar's Office in Northern Ireland.

From 2006 the notification is made directly to the CEMACH Regional Manager, who initiates the enquiry on behalf of the DPH and, in conjunction with CEMACH Unit Co-ordinators and professional staff, arranges for completion of the MDR-1 form. The same process of anonymisation and regional assessment is followed as before.

Scotland

A single panel of assessors covers the whole of Scotland. A single assessor representing each of anaesthetics, pathology, psychiatry and midwifery comments on all cases, and each of three obstetric assessors comments on cases from a defined geographical area. The panel of assessors meets twice a year to assess and classify each case. SPCERH administers the Enquiry on behalf of NHSQIS. SPCERH receives copies of all relevant death certificates from the Scotland General Register Office (GRO), and then the SPCERH Administrator notifies the DPH of the health board of the residence of the woman concerned. The SPCERH Administrator takes responsibility for organising completion of the MDR(UK)-1 by all the professional staff involved in caring for the woman. The completed form, with any additional relevant documents, is passed to the appropriate obstetric assessor. He/she determines whether any further documentation is required before the information is submitted for discussion and classification by the full panel of assessors. In cases where an anaesthetic has been given, an autopsy or a pathological investigation undertaken, or where there were significant psychiatric or midwifery issues, the obstetric assessor passes the form to the assessors from relevant disciplines for their further comments. The form is then returned to the SPCERH medical director, who retains it from that time until it has been fully considered, classified and used for preparation of the report. The completed MDR(UK)-1, and addition documentation, is held under conditions of strict confidentiality and is anonymised before being forwarded to the UK Central Office. The cases are then passed to Chapter authors for inclusion in the triennial report.

APPENDIX 2: Assessors for the Maternal Deaths Enquiry for the triennium 2003-2005 and CEMACH personnel

Director of Enquiry

Dr G Lewis *MSc MRCGP FFPH FRCOG*

Central Assessors and authors

Obstetrics	**Professor J Drife** *MD FRCIG FRCP(Ed) FRCS(Ed) FCOG(SA)* **Professor J Neilson** *MD FRCOG*
Anaesthetics	**Dr G Cooper** *OBE FRCA FRCOG* **Dr JH McClure** *RCA*
Intensive Care	**Dr T Clutton-Brock** *MRCP FRCA*
Pathology	**Dr GH Millward-Sadler** *FRCPath MHSH*
Medicine	**Professor M de Swiet** *MD FRCP FRCOG* **Dr C Nelson-Piercy** *FRCP FRCOG*
Midwifery	**Dr G Edwards** *RN RM ADM Cert Ed Med PhD* **Dr J Rogers** *BA PhD DPSM SRN RM* **Mrs V Beale** *RN RM Dip Man MSc*
Psychiatry	**Dr M Oates** *DPM FRCPsych*
General Practice	**Dr J Shakespeare** *MRCP FRCGP*
Emergency Medicine	**Dr D Hulbert** *FRCS FFAEM*

CEMACH personnel involved in Enquiry work

Central Office

Chief Executive	**Mr R Congdon**
Director of Research and Development	**Ms S Golightly**
Programme Director	**Mrs A Miller**
Administrative Officer	**Mrs M Wilson**

CEMACH Regional Managers

East of England	**Mrs C Hay**
East Midlands	**Mrs S Wood**
London	**Mrs S Roberts** **Mrs V Clements** **Mrs R Thomas**
South East	**Miss M Gompels**
South West	**Mrs R Thompson**
North East	**Mrs M Renwick**
Northern Ireland	**Dr M Scott** **Dr A Bell**
North West	**Mrs J Maddocks**
Wales	**Mrs J Stewart** **Mrs J Hopkins** **Mrs D Roberts**
West Midlands	**Mrs P McGeown** **Mrs J Maddocks**
Yorkshire and Humber	**Mrs L Anson** **Mrs S Wood**

Regional Assessors in Obstetrics

East of England	**Mr B Lim** *FRCOG FRANZCOG*
East Midlands	**Miss HJ Mellows** *FRCOG*
London	**Miss G Henson** *FRCOG* **Mr ME Setchell** *FRCS FRCOG* **Mr GHW Ward** *FRCOG FRANZCOG*
North East	**Professor JM Davison** *MD FRCOG*
North West	**Miss P Buck** *FRCOG* **Mr SJ Duthie** *FRCOG* **Mr S Walkinshaw** *FRCOG*
South East	**Miss P Hurley** *FRCOG* **Miss C Iffland** *FRCOG* **Dr K Morton** *FRCOG*

South West	**Miss I Montague** MRCOG DOM
	Miss S Sellers MD FRCOG
	Professor P Soothill MD FRCOG
West Midlands	**Mrs G Masson** FRCOG
	Mr DHA Redford FRCOG
Yorkshire/Humber	**Mr SF Spooner** FRCOG
Mr D Tuffnell FRCOG	**Professor J Walker MD** FRCP FRCOG

Regional Assessors in Anaesthetics

East of England	**Dr Nicholl** FRCA
	Dr J Bamber FRCA
East Midlands	**Dr D Bogod** FRCA
London	**Dr W Aveling** DRCOG FRCA
	Dr I Findley DRCOG FRCA
	Dr S Yentis MD FRCA
North East	**Dr D Hughes** FRCA
North West	**Dr K Grady** FRCA
	Dr EL Horsman FRCA
	Dr S Wheatly FRCA
	Dr R G Wilkes FRCA
South East	**Dr H Adams** FRCA
	Dr MB Dobson MRCP FRCA
South West	**Dr L Shutt** FRCA
	Dr M Wee FRC
West Midlands	**Dr M Lewis** FRCA
Yorkshire/Humber	**Dr G Kesseler** FFARCS
	Dr IF Russell FRCA

Regional Assessors in Pathology

East of England	**Dr A Cluroe** *FRCPA Dip Forens Path* **Dr C Womack** *FRCPath*
East Midlands	**Dr LJR Brown** *FRCPath*
London	**Dr A Bates** *MD PhD MRCPath* **Dr C Corbishley** *FRCPath* **Dr M Jarmulowicz** *FRCPath*
North West	**Dr R Hale** *FRCPath* **Dr G Wilson** *FRCPath*
North East	**Dr JN Bulmer** *PhD FRCPath*
South East	**Dr M Hall** *FRCPath* **Dr N Kirkham** *MD FRCPath* **Dr H Millward-Sadler** *FRCPath MHSH*
South West	**Dr L Hirschowitz** *FRCPath* **Dr C Keen** *FRCPath*
West Midlands	**Dr T Rollason** *FRCPath*
Yorkshire/Humber	**Dr A Andrew** *FRCPath* **Dr DR Morgan** *FRCPath*

Regional Assessors in Midwifery

East of England	**Miss J Fraser** *MSc DPSM RM RN*
East Midlands	**Miss JM Savage** *RN RM*
London	**Ms P Cooke** *RM ADM MSc PGCEA* **Ms A Cuthbertson** *MSc RM RGN* **Ms S Truttero** *MBA LLB ADM RN RM* **Mrs M Wheeler** *RN RM ADM BSc(Hons)*
North East	**Ms K Mannion** *RM RN ADM MSc* **Miss L Robson** *MA RN RM ADM PGCE*
North West	**Ms D Birchall** *RGN RM LLB MSc* **Ms N Parry** *RGN RM BSc* **Ms A Pedder** *RN RM BSc MA* **Ms M Sidebotham** *RGN RM DPSM/ADM MA*

South East	**Ms C Drummond** *RGN RM*
	Ms S Sauter *RM DNLS ADM Dip Ethics*
	Ms A Weavers *RM*
South West	**Mrs V Beale** *RN RM Dip Man MSc*
	Mrs J Drury *RM RN MSc DpSM SEN*
	Ms D Morrall *RN RM*
	Mrs A Remmers *RGN RM MSc*
West Midlands	**Mrs C McCalmont** *RN RM DPSM*
	Mrs E Newell *RGN RM DPSM BSc(Hons)*
	Mrs S Smithson *BSc(Hons) RN ADM ONC*
Yorkshire/Humber	**Mrs JM Jackson** *RN RM*
	Ms J Lovett *RGN RM*
	Ms D Watkins *RN RM ADM MSc*

SCOTLAND

Chairman of Enquiry	**Professor MH Hall** *FRCOG*
	Dr W Liston *FRCOG*
Medical Coordinator:	
Scottish Programme for Clinical	
Effectiveness in Reproductive Health	**Dr G Penney** *FRCOG*
CMO's Representative:	
Scottish Executive Health Department	**Dr I Bashford** *MRCOG*
Obstetric Assessors	**Professor MH Hall** *FRCOG*
	Dr D A Lees *FRCOG*
	Dr WA Liston *FRCOG*
	Dr CB Lunan *FRCOG*
	Professor D Murphy *MRCOG*
	Dr H MacPherson *FRCOG*
	Professor J Norman *MD FRCOG*
Anaesthetic Assessor	**Dr JH McClure** *FRCA*
Pathology Assessor	**Dr R Nairn** *FRCPath*
Midwifery Assessor	**Mrs J Reekie** *RGN RM*

NORTHERN IRELAND

Department of Health and Social Services: Northern Ireland	**Dr C Willis** *MB ChB BAO MFPH*
Obstetric Assessor	**Miss A Harper** *OBE FRCOG*
Anaesthetic Assessor	**Dr IM Bali** *MD PhD FFARCS* **Dr D Hill** *FCARCSI*
Pathology Assessor	**Dr G McCusker** *FRCPath*
Midwifery Assessor	**Mrs E Bannon** *RN RM BSc(Hons) MSc* **Mrs E Millar** *RN RM NDNC MHSCert*

WALES

Welsh Assembly Government	**Dr J Ludlow** *FFPHM*
Obstetric Assessor	**Mr R Vlies** *FRCS(Ed) FRCOG*
Anaesthetic Assessor	**Dr P Clyburn** *FRCA*
Pathology Assessor	**Dr Lesley Murray** *FRCPath*
Midwifery Assessor	**Ms J Keats** *RN RM* **Mrs K McGrath** *SRN RM Dip Mid MSc (Health Management)*

CEMACH Board

Professor M Weindling	*Chair*
Dr J Chapple	*Faculty of Public Health*
Mr R Congdon	*Chief Executive CEMACH*
Dr G Cooper	*Royal College of Anaesthetists*
Dame Karlene Davis	*Royal College of Midwives*
Ms S Golightly	*Director of Research and Development CEMACH*
Dr S Gould	*Royal College of Pathologists*
Dr S Hollins	*Royal College of Psychiatrists*
Dr Mary Macintosh	*Medical Director CEMACH (until April 2006)*
Dr J McAughey	*Royal College of General Practitioners*
Professor N McIntosh	*Royal College of Paediatrics and Child Health*
Mrs A Miller	*Programme Director CEMACH*
Professor A Templeton	*Royal College of Obstetrics and Gynaecology*